Oxford Textbook of

Cardiac Anatomy

OXFORD TEXTBOOKS IN CARDIOLOGY SERIES

Oxford Textbook of Heart Failure 2e
Edited by Andrew L. Clark, Roy S. Gardner, and Theresa A. McDonagh

Oxford Textbook of Interventional Cardiology 2e
Edited by Simon Redwood, Nick Curzen, and Adrian Banning

Oxford Textbook of Advanced Heart Failure and Cardiac Transplantation
Edited by Michael J. Domanski, Mandeep R. Mehra, and Marc A. Pfeffer

Oxford Textbook of

Cardiac Anatomy

Demosthenes G. Katritsis

Department of Cardiology, Hygeia Hospital, Athens, Greece and Cardiology, Johns Hopkins Medicine, Baltimore, MD, USA

Robert H. Anderson

Biosciences Division, Newcastle University, UK and University College London, UK

Diane E. Spicer

Heart Insitute, Johns Hopkins All Children's Hospital, St Petersburg, FL, USA

Damián Sánchez-Quintana

Department of Human Anatomy and Cell Biology, Faculty of Medicine and Health Sciences, University of Extremadura, Badajoz, Spain

Justin T. Tretter

Department of Pediatric Cardiology, Cleveland Clinic Children's, and The Heart, Vascular, and Thoracic Institute, Cleveland Clinic, Cleveland, OH, USA

OXFORD
UNIVERSITY PRESS

OXFORD
UNIVERSITY PRESS

Great Clarendon Street, Oxford, OX2 6DP,
United Kingdom

Oxford University Press is a department of the University of Oxford.
It furthers the University's objective of excellence in research, scholarship,
and education by publishing worldwide. Oxford is a registered trade mark of
Oxford University Press in the UK and in certain other countries.

Published in the United States of America by Oxford University Press
198 Madison Avenue, New York, NY 10016, United States of America.

British Library Cataloguing in Publication Data
Data available

Library of Congress Control Number: 2026930056

ISBN 978–0–19–790472–5

DOI: 10.1093/med/9780197904725.001.0001

Printed in the UK by
Bell & Bain Ltd., Glasgow

Foreword

In recent years, the field of cardiac anatomy has undergone an explosive transformation. New evidence, and recognition of the value of this information in the clinical context, have reshaped our perception of the heart as an anatomic and functional entity. Cardiac surgeons have long acknowledged the importance of such knowledge. Recent advances in transcatheter approaches for both electrophysiological and structural interventions have now similarly underlined the importance of a precise and updated description of all cardiac structures. A quantitative assessment of the atrioventricular and ventriculo-arterial anatomy, for example, is critical for transcatheter valvar implantation, which is now becoming feasible for all four valves. Variations in the anatomy such as the "mitral disjunction" have acquired clinical significance. Tachycardias may originate from, and be ablated in, the atrioventricular and ventriculo-arterial junctions. Epicardial or endocardial arrhythmic focuses may be detected in the left ventricular summit and the area of the cardiac crux. All these regions, previously of only limited anatomical interest, have now acquired a clinical significance. They need to be clearly described and presented to the practising cardiologist. Since a textbook already exists that emphasizes the importance of cardiac anatomy for the surgeon, this textbook was initially aimed at serving as a manual providing aid for interventionists and electrophysiologists. During the writing, and with the encouragement of our publishers, we realized that the scope of the book should be broadened by means of revisiting the anatomy of the heart in detail and summarizing new evidence in the context of evolving concepts. We have, therefore, attempted to write a comprehensive, but still user-friendly, manual using photographs of our own anatomical preparations. Our intention is to provide the "gold standard" of cardiac anatomy, but at the same time to discuss the clinical dimensions of each described cardiac structure as they stand today in the contemporary literature.

We are indebted to Jose Angel Cabrera and Shumpei Mori, who permitted us to relabel images prepared by themselves and to use them specifically for this textbook. We also thank Gemma Morgan, who prepared the originals for many of the drawings we have used. We are also indebted to Rachel Goldsworthy, from Oxford University Press. Without her help, and constant encouragement, we would have been unable to navigate the troubled waters that still exist between the submission of an idea and its appearance in print.

Demosthenes G. Katritsis
Robert H. Anderson
Damian Sanchez-Quintana
Diane E. Spicer
Justin T. Tretter

Contents

1

The Need for the Attitudinally Appropriate Approach

One of the most important principles of anatomy is that all structures should be described in reference to the coordinates of the body as seen with the subject standing in the anatomical position and facing the observer.[1] When assessed in this fashion, it is conventional to account for the relationships of the bodily structures by describing their locations as observed in the three orthogonal planes (Figure 1.1). Of these planes, two are in the long axis of the body and cut it in frontal and sagittal fashion. When assessed in the frontal plane, components can be judged to be right- or left-sided. Interrogation in the sagittal plane shows whether the same structures are positioned anteriorly as opposed to posteriorly, with biologists frequently describing such coordinates as being ventral and dorsal. The third orthogonal plane is transverse and cuts the body in its short axis. Depending on the location of this plane relative to the long axis planes, structures can be described as being superior or cranial, as opposed to being inferior or caudal (Figure 1.1).

Throughout the ages, however, when describing the components of the heart, the organ has been considered as if removed from the body and positioned with its apex pointing down, an arrangement truly reminiscent of the heart as illustrated for the purposes of St Valentine's Day. It is only in this "Valentine" position, when the planes are created in the long axis of the heart itself, that the chambers are seen in right-sided and left-sided locations and with the atrial chambers on top of their respective ventricles (Figure 1.2). The Valentine arrangement, whilst showing the cardiac chambers in locations that match their names, does not represent the fashion in which the heart is positioned within the chest during life.

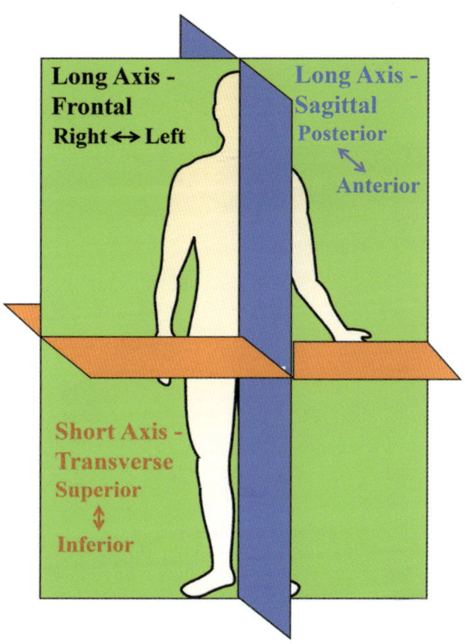

Figure 1.1. The drawing shows the adjectives used to describe the bodily structures when assessed with the subject standing in the so-called anatomical position, which is facing the observer. One of the first rules of human anatomy is that the relationships of all bodily components should be described in the setting of the organs as seen in the anatomical position.

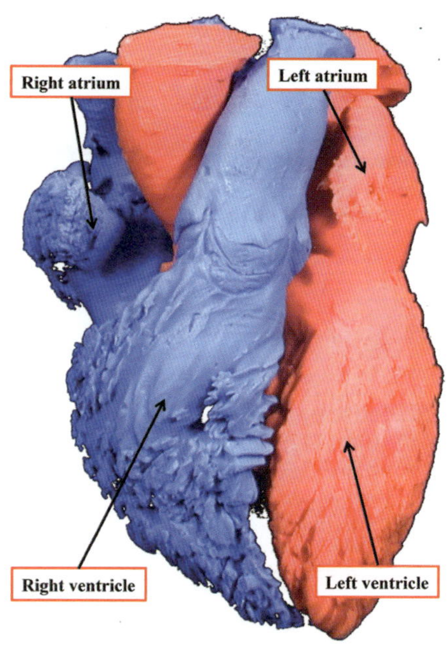

Figure 1.2. The chambers of the heart have been filled with blue resin to show the morphologically right components and red resin to show their morphologically left counterparts. The heart is photographed as if positioned on its apex. It is only in this "Valentine" arrangement that the morphologically right structures are seen directly to the right of their counterparts, and with the atrial chambers on top of the ventricles.

In order to understand the arrangement as found in the living patient, the heart, and its component parts, should be described relative to the bodily planes, rather than its own long and short axis planes (Figure 1.3).[2] Unfortunately, it has been the incorrect Valentine approach that has been used conventionally by clinicians, in particular by interventional cardiologists and electrophysiologists, to describe the cardiac components. Even those who had listed the arguments supporting the attitudinally appropriate approach continued to use the inappropriate terms when producing textbooks of cardiac anatomy.[3,4] Thus, when electrophysiologists described the atrioventricular junctions, which are best seen in the left anterior oblique projection favoured by angiographers (Figure 1.4), it had become accepted that the superior components of the heart should be described as being anterior, with the true anterior and posterior quadrants being described incorrectly as right and left lateral (Figure 1.5).

In reality, it is these two "lateral" quadrants that are positioned closest to the sternum and vertebral column, respectively. It is these quadrants that should properly have been described as being anterior and posterior also by those using electroanatomical mapping (Figure 1.6). Most of the seminal advances in cardiac electrophysiology published in the 20th century and in the first two decades of the 21st century had been based on the incorrect terminology, despite the fact that its imperfections had already been identified by the end of the 20th century.[5]

Fortunately, it is now becoming generally acknowledged that the Valentine approach is inappropriate for those working in the clinical setting.[6,7] The imperfections of the Valentine approach have always been evident to the cardiac surgeon. Thus, when entering the chest through a sternotomy, it is obvious that the most anterior cardiac chamber is the right ventricle. This fact is also evident when the chest itself is sectioned in its short axis. The right ventricle is closest to the sternum, and anterior. The left atrium is closest to the vertebral column, and hence posterior (Figure 1.7). The correct location of the cardiac chambers, as viewed in attitudinal fashion, can now readily be demonstrated by segmenting three-dimensional computed tomographic datasets (Figure 1.8).[2]

Computed tomographic images confirm that the left atrium is the most posterior of the cardiac chambers, while the pulmonary venous component of the chamber forms its roof (Figure 1.8 panel A). It is the body and vestibule of the atrium, rather than the pulmonary venous components, which lie directly adjacent to the vertebral column,[8] with the oesophagus and descending aorta also passing posterior to the left atrial chamber as they extend to perforate the diaphragm and enter the abdomen (Figure 1.9). When the right atrial chamber is segmented and added to the images prepared from the three-dimensional computed tomographic dataset (Figure 1.8 panel B), it forms the right border of the cardiac silhouette, matching the images as shown when the cardiac casts are viewed in attitudinal fashion (Figure 1.3). The addition of the left ventricle (Figure 1.8 panel C) then confirms that, rather than being beneath the atrial chambers, as suggested by the Valentine approach (Figure 1.2), the ventricular chambers are orientated with their long axis in posterior to anterior fashion. The images produced from the computed tomographic dataset also show well how the aortic root fills the indentation seen on the anterior wall of the left atrium (compare Figure 1.8 panels A and C). It is the addition of the right ventricle and the pulmonary trunk that completes the cardiac silhouette (Figure 1.8 panel D). The right ventricle occupies the inferior border of the silhouette, rather than the inferior part of the right border, as is suggested when the heart is viewed in Valentine fashion (Figure 1.2).

For most of the time that has elapsed since structural intervention and electrophysiology became specialties in their own right, practitioners have used the inaccurate Valentine nomenclature to account for interventions on the cardiac valves, and when describing the locations of accessory pathways and the arrangement of the atrioventricular conduction axis relative to the atrioventricular junctions.

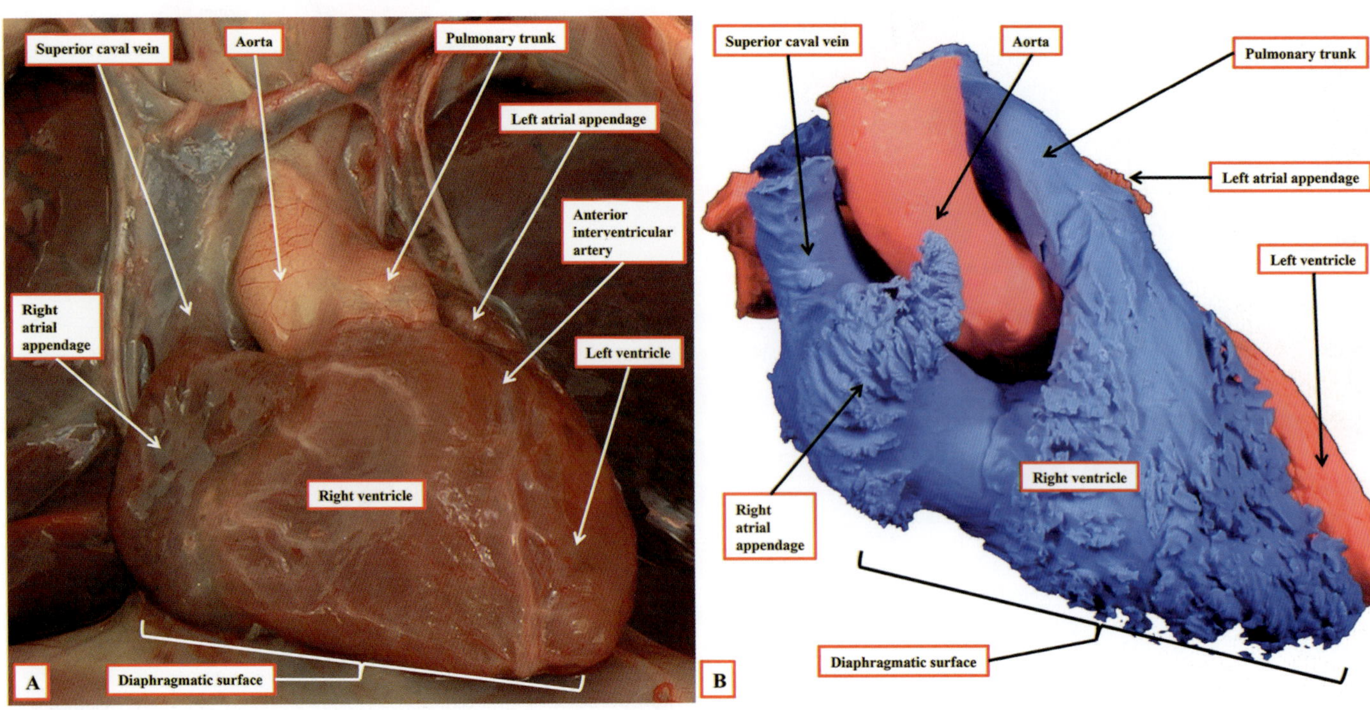

Figure 1.3. Panel A shows the heart as it lies within the chest during life. Panel B shows the same heart as illustrated in Figure 1.2, but with the cast rotated so as to demonstrate the cardiac components in attitudinally appropriate location.

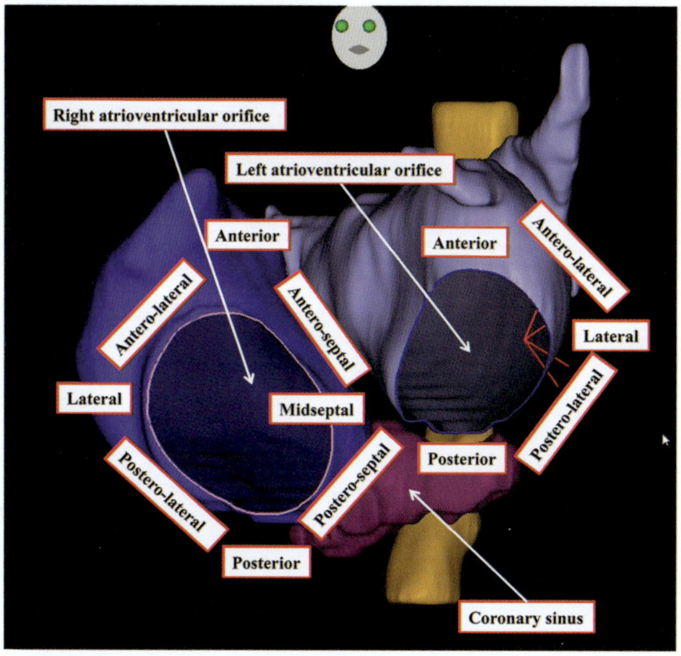

Figure 1.4. The electroanatomical map of the atrioventricular junctions shows the junctions as viewed in left anterior oblique projection. The icon showing the head provides the appropriate information for describing the quadrants in attitudinally appropriate fashion. The image is labelled using the incorrect Valentine approach. Until very recently, electrophysiologists have described the quadrants that are superior (see Figure 1.5) as being "anterior", with the opposite quadrants, which are supported by the diaphragm, said to be "posterior". Courtesy of Dr Jose Angel Cabrera.

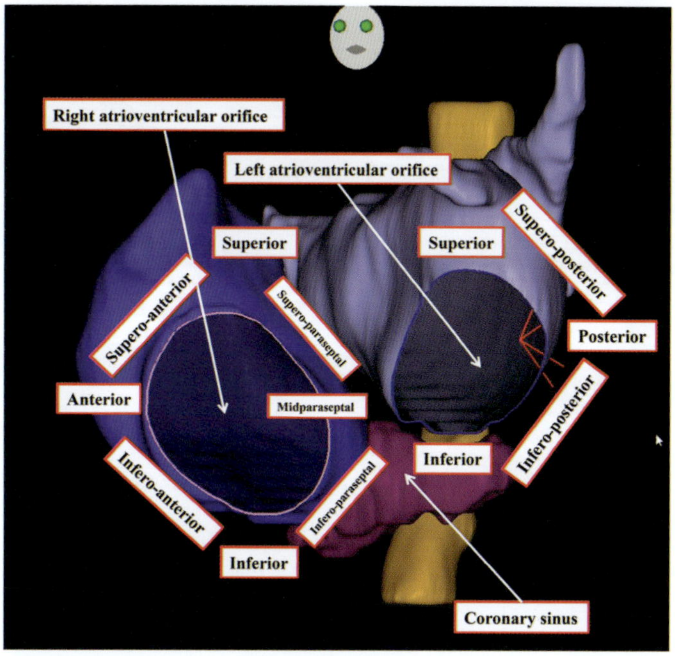

Figure 1.6. The electroanatomical map, as labelled incorrectly in Figure 1.4, has been labelled in the correct attitudinally appropriate fashion in this image. It is these adjectives that show the appropriate relationships of the quadrants of the atrioventricular junctions to the body when the heart is assessed during life, and as is now confirmed by attention to computed tomograms as shown in Figure 1.5. The labels also show that, when assessed accurately, the so-called septal components are paraseptal. Courtesy of Dr Jose Angel Cabrera. The white arrows pointing to the AV orifices and CS are not on this illustrations as they are in Fig. 1.4.

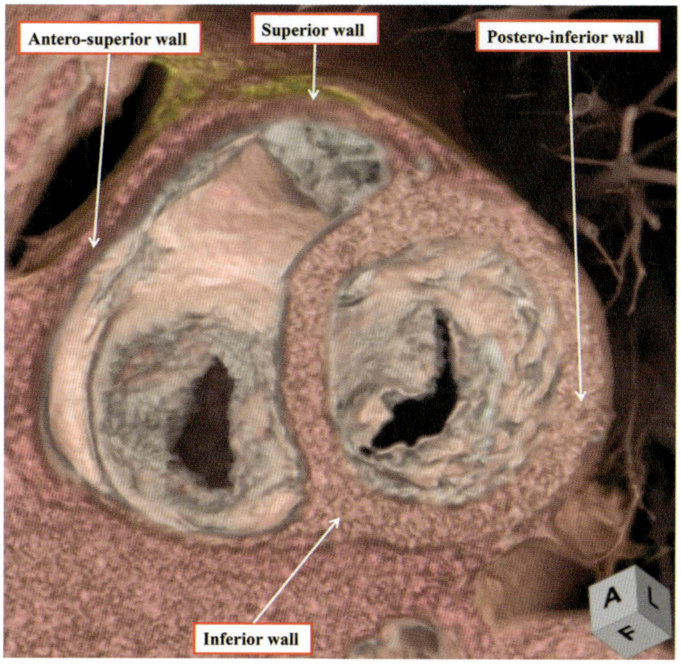

Figure 1.5. Supplementing the information provided by the icon to which reference was made in the legend for Figure 1.4, the "compass block" shown in the lower right-hand corner of this computed tomographic image confirms that when assessed within the body, the part of the ventricular cone supported by the diaphragm is positioned inferiorly, rather than "posteriorly" as it would incorrectly be described when using the Valentine approach. The borders can correctly be identified by following the "compass".

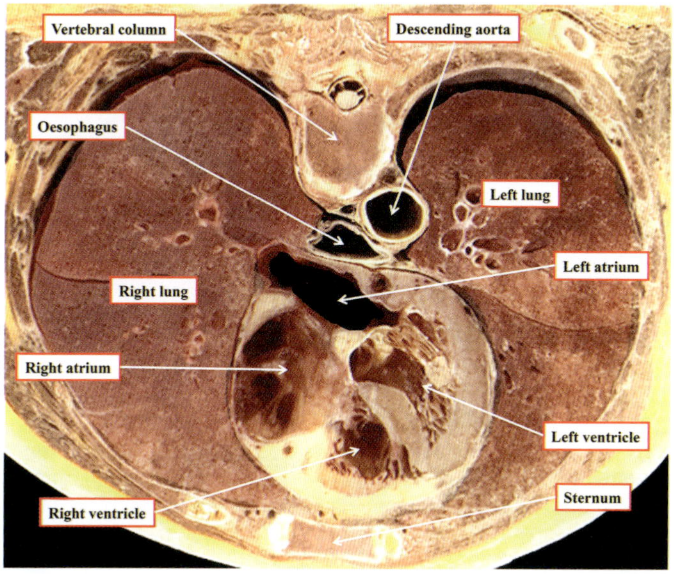

Figure 1.7. The thorax has been sectioned in its short axis and the section viewed from above. By taking note of the locations of the sternum and vertebral column, it can be seen that the right ventricle is the most anterior of the cardiac chambers, with the left atrium being the most posterior. The wall of the right atrial appendage forms the right border of the cardiac silhouette, with the wall of the left ventricle forming the left border.

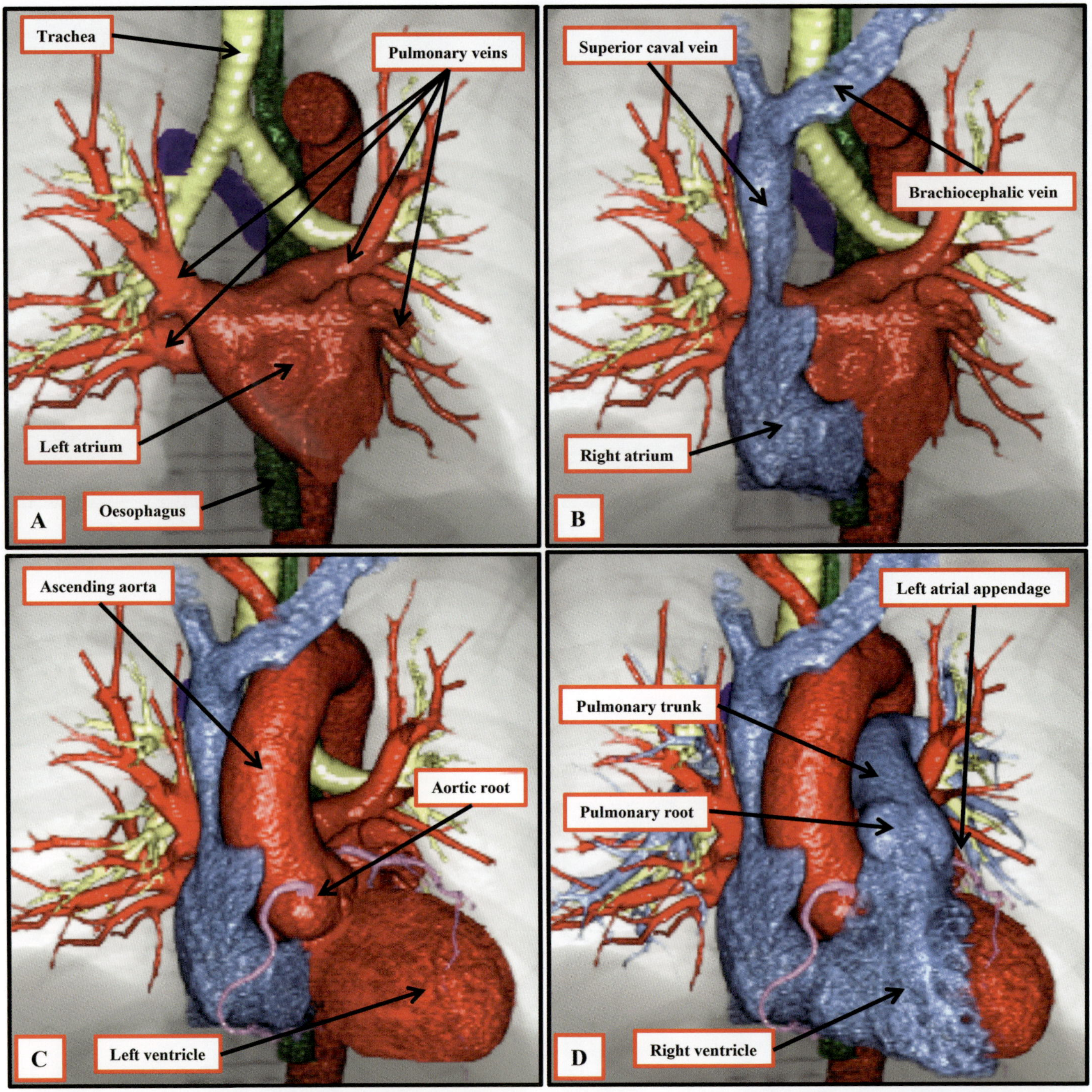

Figure 1.8. The images have been prepared by segmenting a three-dimensional computed tomographic dataset. Panel A shows that the left atrium is the most posterior of the cardiac chambers, with the pulmonary veins forming the roof of the chamber, and the appendage protruding from its anterior wall. In panel B, the right atrium has been added to the image, showing that this chamber forms the right margin of the cardiac silhouette. In panel C, the left ventricle and aorta have been added. It can be seen that the aortic root fills the depression on the anterior wall of the left atrium, while the left ventricle extends anteriorly from its atrioventricular junction. The cardiac silhouette is completed in panel D by the addition of the right ventricle and the pulmonary trunk. The inferior border of the silhouette is formed by the right ventricle, with only the tip of its appendage now remaining visible as regards the left atrium. Courtesy of Dr Shumpei Mori.

Three-dimensional echocardiography and electroanatomic mapping now permit projections to be chosen and displayed in a three-dimensional environment that is attitudinally appropriate, matching the images that can be produced using computed tomography and magnetic resonance imaging (Figure 1.10).[6]

During structural and electrophysiological procedures, the cardiac components remain relatively stable, with any movement influenced only by respiration and the heart's contractile function. It is an accurate knowledge of the true anatomic relationships of the heart within the chest that permits the operator properly to orientate

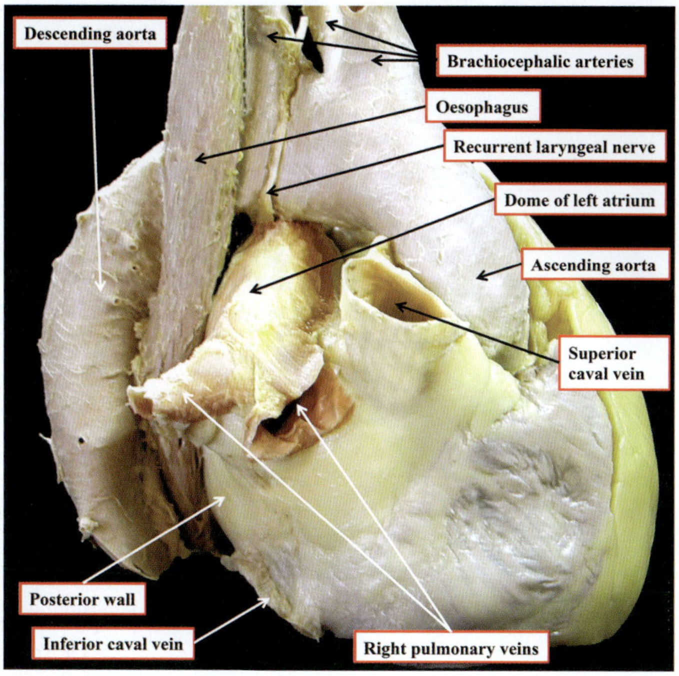

Figure 1.9. The heart, along with the aortic arch, the descending aorta, and the oesophagus, has been removed from the body but retained in its appropriate attitudinal position. It is photographed from the right side and slightly from behind. The pulmonary veins join the roof of the left atrium, with the wall between the origins of the right and left veins forming its dome. The descending aorta and the oesophagus pass behind the posterior wall of the atrium which is formed by the body and the vestibule of the chamber.

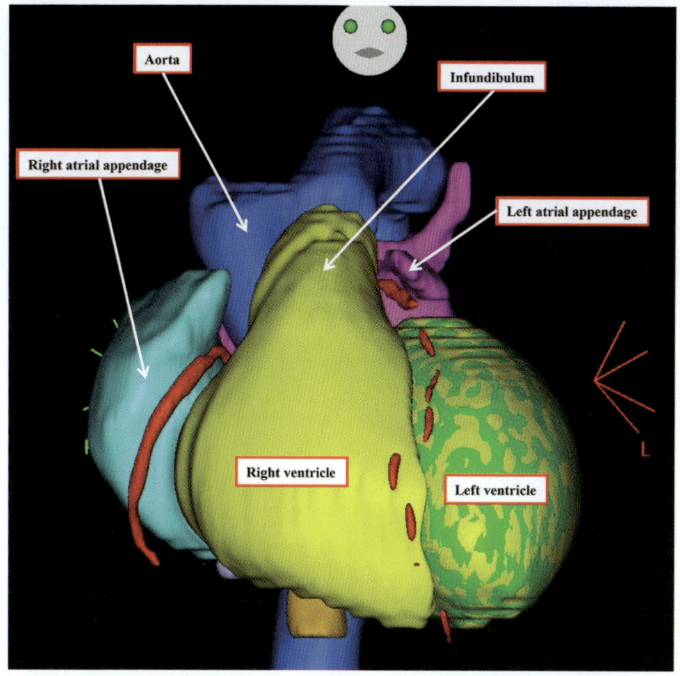

Figure 1.10. The electoanatomical map, which was used to prepare Figures 1.4 and 1.6, is shown here as seen in the frontal projection. The icon showing the face confirms that the image is being viewed from the front. The reconstruction shows how the cardiac chambers can now be reconstructed by the electrophysiologist in attitudinally appropriate fashion, mimicking the arrangement that can now be obtained using computed tomography (see Figure 1.8 panel D). Courtesy of Dr Jose Angel Cabrera.

his or her mapping and to correctly place catheters and devices used for intervention. The components of the atrioventricular junctions, furthermore, must be described not only in attitudinally appropriate fashion, but also by recognizing those components that are paraseptal as opposed to being truly septal. It is knowledge of the correct location of the heart within the thorax that also permits interventionists to be aware of the relationships of the chambers they are invading with their catheters to adjacent structures outside the pericardial cavity, such as the oesophagus, the phrenic nerves, and the aortic root (Figure 1.9).[9] The attitudinally appropriate terms will be used for the description of significant anatomical features of the cardiac components throughout the subsequent chapters of this book.

REFERENCES

1. Cook AC, Anderson RH. Attitudinally correct nomenclature. *Heart*. 2002;**87**:503–506. doi: 10.1136/heart.87.6.503
2. Mori S, Tretter JT, Spicer DE, Bolender DL, Anderson RH. What is the real cardiac anatomy? *Clin Anat*. 2019;**32**:288–309. doi: 10.1002/ca.23340
3. Anderson RH, Becker AE. *Cardiac Anatomy: An Integrated Text and Colour Atlas*. Edinburgh: Churchill Livingstone; 1980.
4. McAlpine WA. *Heart and Coronary Arteries: An Anatomical Atlas for Clinical Diagnosis, Radiological Investigation, and Surgical Treatment*. Berlin: Springer; 1975.
5. Cosio FG, Anderson RH, Kuck KH, Becker A, Benditt DG, Bharati S, Borggrefe M, Campbell RW, Gaita F, Guiraudon GM, et al. ESCWGA/NASPE/P experts consensus statement: living anatomy of the atrioventricular junctions. A guide to electrophysiologic mapping. Working Group of Arrhythmias of the European Society of Cardiology. North American Society of Pacing and Electrophysiology. *J Cardiovasc Electrophysiol*. 1999;**10**:1162–1170. doi: 10.1111/j.1540-8167.1999.tb00291.x
6. Anderson RH, Back Sternick E, Mahmud R, Cabrera JA, Katritsis D, Farre J, Tretter JT, Spicer DE, Cook AC, Sanchez-Quintana D. How best to describe the location of the substrates for abnormal cardiac rhythms. *Heart Rhythm*. 2024;**21**:2377–2385. doi: 10.1016/j.hrthm.2024.05.066
7. Richardson TD, Attia ZI, Chorin E, Delmar M, Di Biase L, Ellenbogen KA, Ernst S, Gollob MH, Indik JH, Kannankeril PJ, et al. Describing cardiac anatomy: the truth is staring us in the face. *Heart Rhythm*. 2024;**21**:2386–2387. doi: 10.1016/j.hrthm.2024.07.125
8. Elbatran AI, Anderson RH, Mori S, Saba MM. The rationale for isolation of the left atrial pulmonary venous component to control atrial fibrillation: a review article. *Heart Rhythm*. 2019;**16**:1392–1398. doi: 10.1016/j.hrthm.2019.03.012
9. Ernst S, Sanchez-Quintana D, Ho SY. Anatomy of the pericardial space and mediastinum: relevance to epicardial mapping and ablation. *Card Electrophysiol Clin*. 2010;**2**:1–8. doi: 10.1016/j.ccep.2009.11.003

2

Cardiac Development

Not all components of the definitive heart are present at the stage when the developing organ is first seen in the form of a straight tube. The major part of the straight tube forms little more than the left ventricle, with ongoing contributions from the heart-forming areas of the embryonic disc subsequently entering the arterial and venous poles of the primary tube so as to provide the primordiums of the remaining cardiac components.[1] When it exists as a straight tube, the heart is recognized at the end of the fourth week of human development. The different parts of the heart, in the human, then develop in concert throughout the next 4 weeks of embryonic life to produce the four-chambered organ. Further subtle changes continue during the early weeks of fetal development. The changes are taking place at more or less the same time in different parts of the developing organ. It helps, nonetheless, to account for the changing morphology in regional fashion. The timings can be described in terms of the stages identified by those working at the Carnegie Institute in the USA.[2] Each Carnegie stage accounts for around 2 days of development, with the arrangement when the tube is straight (Figure 2.1) recognized as stage number 10.

The Straight Tube Stage

By the end of the fourth week of development in the human, initially paired endothelial tubes have joined together and have been enveloped in a myocardial covering. Cardiac jelly fills the space

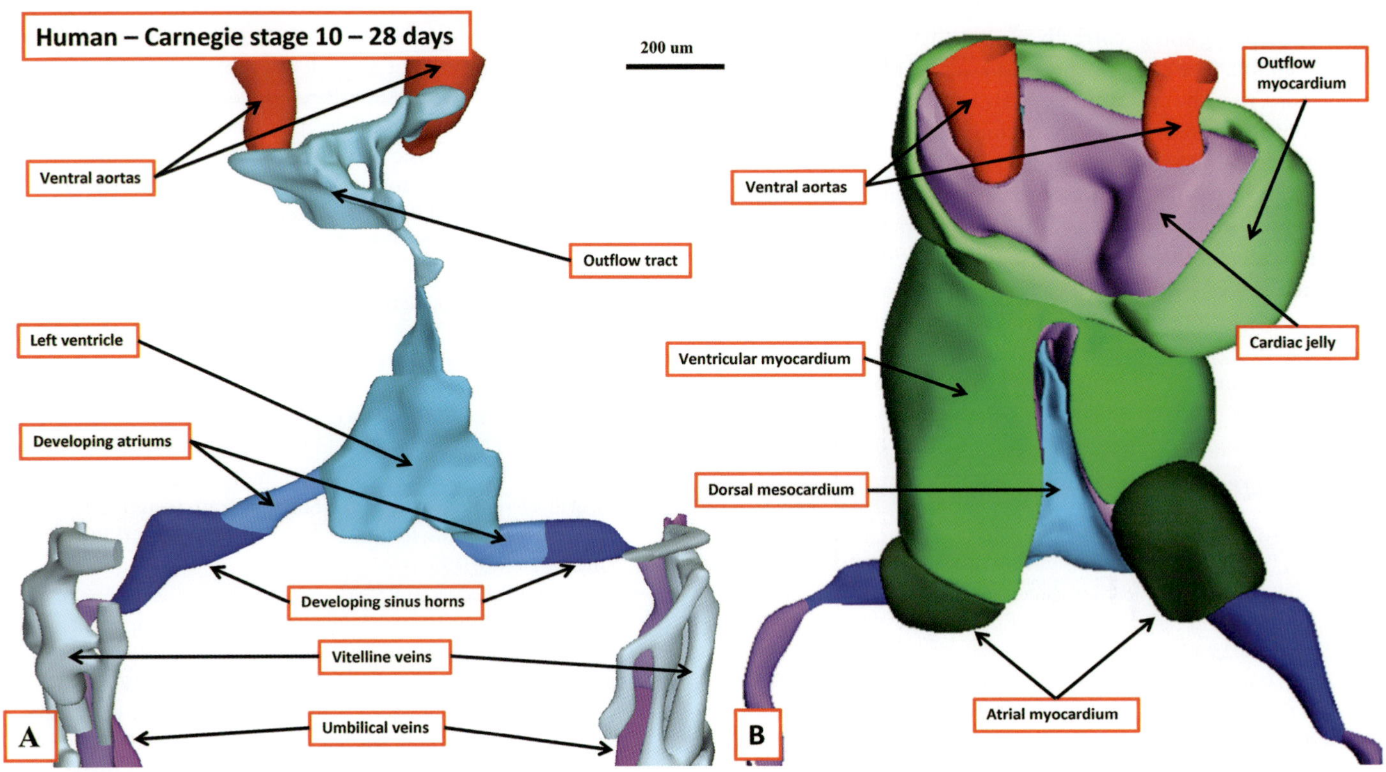

Figure 2.1. Reconstructions made from an interactive pdf of a segmented human heart at Carnegie stage 10, when around 28 days have elapsed subsequent to conception. Panel A shows a reconstruction of the cavities as seen from the front. Panel B shows the view from the back, with inclusion of the developing myocardial walls. Note the location of the dorsal mesocardium, where the myocardial walls at the venous pole are contiguous with the pharyngeal mesenchyme.

throughout the tube between the endocardial and myocardial layers. The myocardial tube itself is already encased in a pericardial sac. Venous tributaries entering the tube caudally bring back the venous returns from the yolk sac and placenta, with ventral aortas emerging from the cranial end (Figure 2.1 panel A).[2] During the stages that led to formation of the straight tube, its developing layers had initially been in continuity throughout its length with the supporting pharyngeal mesenchyme through the dorsal mesocardium. By Carnegie stage 10, the mesocardium has broken down through its larger part, although the connections with the pharyngeal mesenchyme are still recognizable at the caudal end of the tube (Figure 2.1 panel B). This dorsal mesocardial connection, having grown in absolute terms, is now much shorter when assessed relative to the size of the venous pole. It will eventually provide the portal for the developing pulmonary vein to enter the left atrium. At the end of the fourth week, there is no venous return to the heart tube from either the systemic or the pulmonary circuits. Indeed, at this initial stage there is scant formation of the lungs or trachea. The cavity of the tube itself shows a marked constriction between the part destined to become the left ventricle and the part that will provide the basis for formation of the right ventricle and both ventricular outflow tracts (Figure 2.1 panel A). The myocardium that envelops the developing left ventricle is derived from the so-called first heart field, with the myocardium at the arterial pole of the tube formed from the second field.[3,4] Ongoing migrations from the heart-forming areas will eventually provide the myocardial and non-myocardial components of the atrial chambers and the intrapericardial outflow tracts.[5]

The Process of Ventricular Looping

The precise mechanisms underscoring the key process of looping of the heart tube remain uncertain.[6] The morphological changes in shape of the tube, nonetheless, take place concomitant with the addition of new material to the heart at both its venous and arterial poles. The addition of the new material at the venous pole makes it possible to recognize the primordium of the atrial chambers. The atrial component itself initially connects only with the cavity of the developing left ventricle, which forms the inlet of the ventricular loop (Figure 2.2 panel A). The ventricular loop, as viewed from the front of the developing embryo, extends to the right. The outflow tract, which exits from the outlet of the loop, then turns cranially. By this stage, which is stage 11 in the Carnegie sequence, changes have taken place at the arterial pole such that the outflow tract merges beyond the margins of the pericardial cavity with the manifold in the pharyngeal mesenchyme known as the aortic sac, from which arteries extend through the first two pharyngeal arches. The arteries then join at the back of the embryo to form the dorsal aortas.[5] A further significant change in the outer curvature of the ventricular loop becomes visible at the next stage in the Carnegie sequence. This is the process of so-called ballooning of the apical components of the developing ventricles (Figure 2.2 panel B).[7]

The apical part of the developing left ventricle balloons from the inlet part of the loop, with the apical part of the developing right ventricle emerging from its outlet component. With the ballooning of the two apical components, it becomes possible to recognize, for the first time,

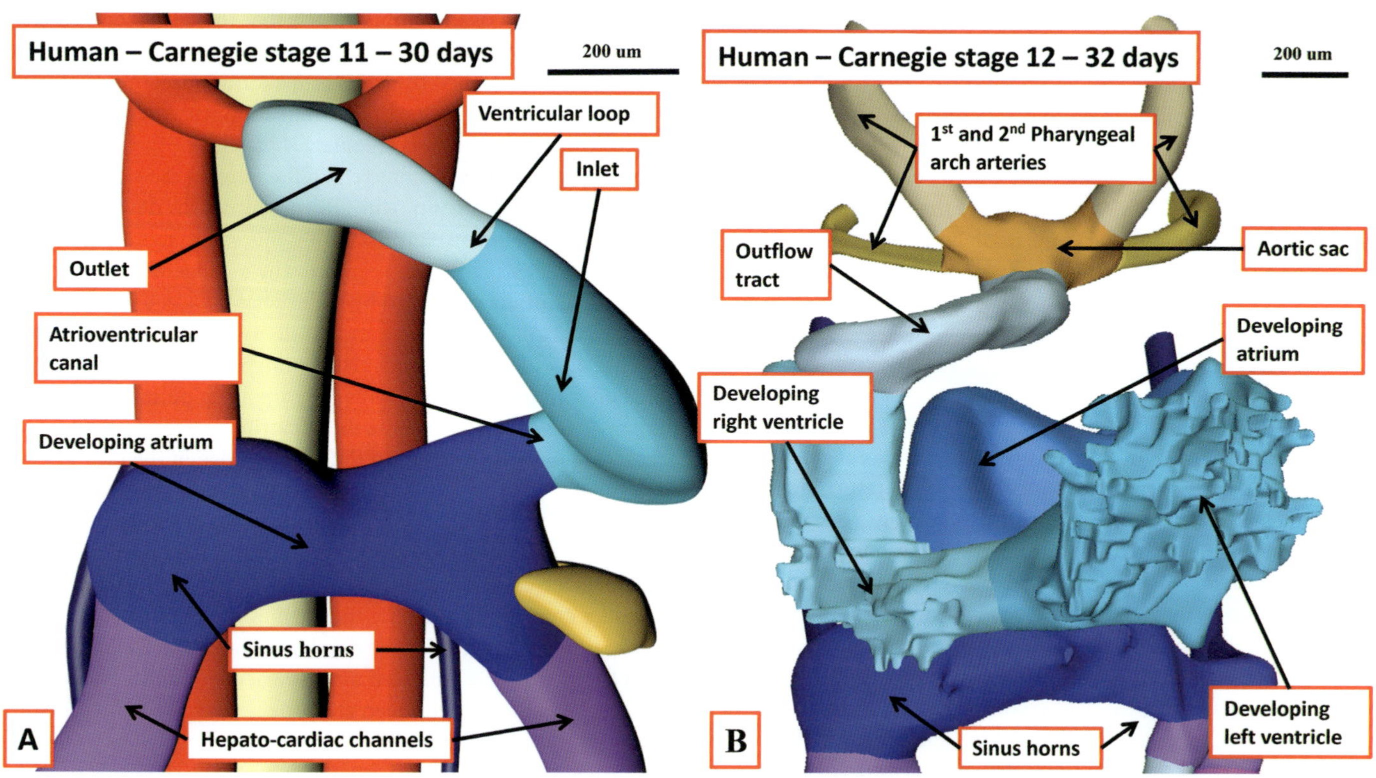

Figure 2.2. The images show comparable reconstructions of the developing cardiac cavities as were prepared to produce Figure 2.1A. They reveal the formation of the ventricular loop at Carnegie stage 11 and the beginning of formation of the apical ventricular components by the process of ballooning at Carnegie stage 12. Both reconstructions are viewed from the front.

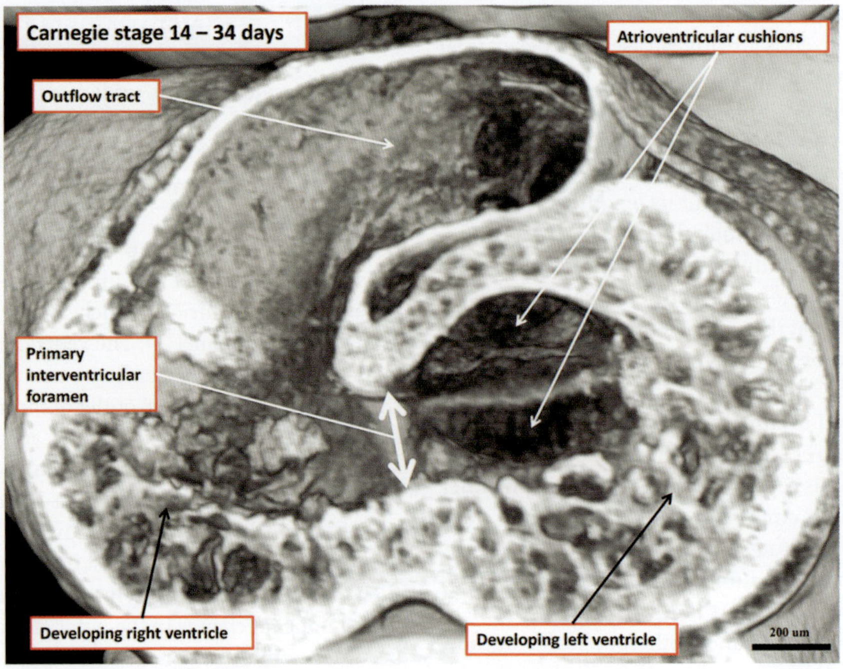

Figure 2.3. The image shows a section from a human embryo at Carnegie stage 14, which is nearly at the end of the fifth week of development, prepared using the technique of episcopic microscopy. The section shows the base of the developing ventricular mass as viewed from the apex. At this stage, the atrioventricular canal opens exclusively into the developing left ventricle, with the developing right ventricle supporting the entirety of the outflow tract. The space between the developing ventricles is the primary interventricular foramen.

the interventricular foramen. This key area is bounded caudally by the developing muscular ventricular septum and cranially by the inner heart curvature. Remodelling of this primary foramen will initially provide the developing right ventricle with its inlet component. Subsequent additional remodelling will permit the subaortic component of the outflow tract to be transferred to the left ventricle.[8] By Carnegie stage 14, it is possible to recognize the apical part of the right ventricle, which at this early stage supports the entirety of the developing outflow tract. The atrioventricular canal at the same stage empties exclusively into the developing left ventricle (Figure 2.3). When considered in the context of congenital malformations, therefore, it can be said that the developing heart shows a double inlet left and double outlet right ventricle.

Formation of the Atrial Chambers

Prior to ventricular looping, the venous tributaries bring blood back to the inlet component of the heart tube only from the vitelline and umbilical circulations, with the veins themselves returning in symmetrical fashion.[2] By Carnegie stage 11, the venous return from the embryo itself has obtained a connection to the venous pole through the cardinal veins, which are again bilaterally symmetrical. The venous tributaries then enter the developing atrial chamber through each side via the sinus horns, with each horn itself also connecting in symmetrical fashion (Figure 2.4 panel A). With the passage of time, the dorsal mesocardium has reduced significantly in size when considered relative to the overall developing heart, but still provides a direct connection between the heart and the pharyngeal mesenchyme. A midline strand can be recognized within the pharyngeal mesenchyme supporting the mesocardium at this early stage, but it does not yet possess a cavity.[9] With ongoing development, the strand will canalize to become the pulmonary vein.[10] Before the strand canalizes, a major change takes place in the arrangement of the systemic venous tributaries. This occurs as anastomotic channels develop within the body of the embryo such that the left-sided venous returns from both the body and the placenta are channelled to the right-sided tributaries. This results in a diminution in size of the left sinus horn, which loses its direct connection with the developing left side of the atrial chambers (Figure 2.4 panel B).

All of the systemic venous return then enters the right side of the initially common atrium, with prominent valves developing at the venoatrial junctions (Figure 2.5). By this stage, significant changes have also taken place with regard to the arrangement of the dorsal mesocardium. Its rightward boundary has enlarged markedly, with new tissues growing into the atrial walls as a spine directed ventrally.

First observed in the mid-19th century, the spine serves two important functions. First, it walls the canalizing pulmonary vein into the cavity of what will become the left atrium. Second, along with the mesenchymal cap formed on the leading edge of the primary atrial septum, or "septum primum", it will myocardialize to become part of the true second atrial septum.[10] The ingrowth of the vestibular spine coincides with the canalization of the mid-pharyngeal strand as it becomes the common pulmonary vein. When first observed as providing a connection between the cavities of the left atrium and the intraparenchymal veins of the developing lungs, the vein opens adjacent to the vestibule of the left atrioventricular junction (Figure 2.6). This arrangement can be seen at Carnegie stage 15, which is subsequent to the commitment of the systemic venous sinus to the right atrium. It is the shift of the systemic veins to the right side of the initially common atrial chamber that sets the scene for atrial septation.

The first sign of septation is the appearance of a bulge in the roof of the atrial component of the primary heart tube (Figure 2.7 panel A).

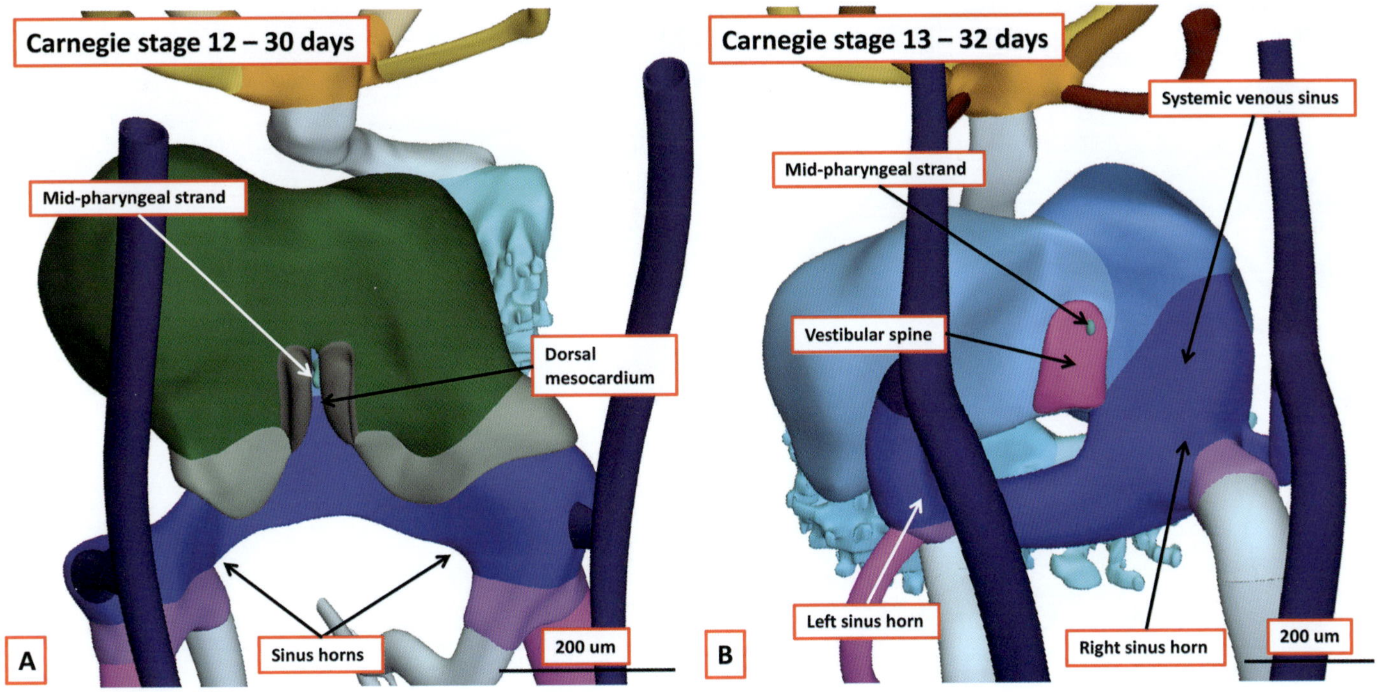

Figure 2.4. The images show further reconstructions made from interactive pdf files from human embryos. Each reconstruction is viewed from the back. In panel A, the reconstruction includes the myocardium enclosing the cavity of the primary atrial chamber and the proximal parts of the sinus horns. Note the continuing attachment of the venous pole to the pharyngeal mesenchyme through the dorsal mesocardium. At Carnegie stage 12, each sinus horn drains into the primary atrial chamber. By Carnegie stage 13, as shown in panel B, the systemic venous sinus has remodelled so as to open to the right side of the primary atrium. The right margin of the dorsal mesocardium has begun to expand to form the vestibular spine. At this stage, it is possible to recognize a midline strand that will eventually canalize to form the pulmonary vein.

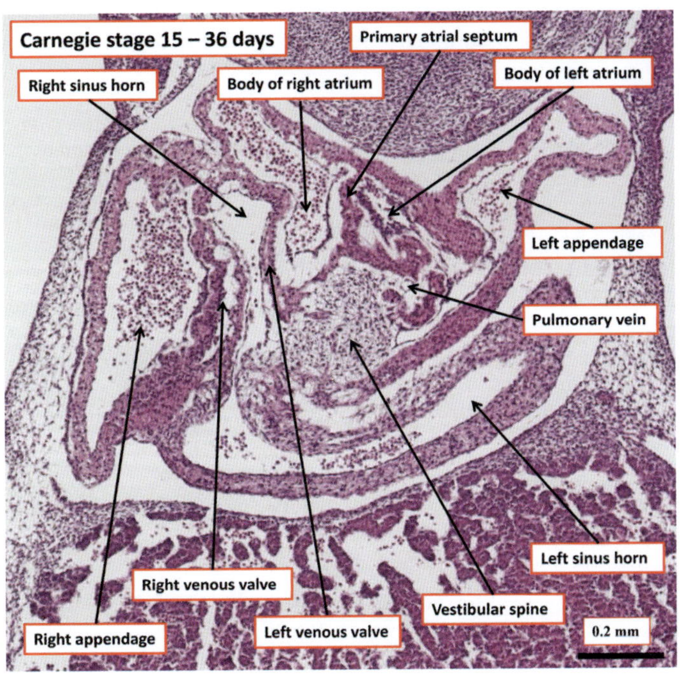

Figure 2.5. The image shows a frontal section through the developing atrial chambers at Carnegie stage 15, which is the beginning of the sixth week of development. The section is stained with hematoxylin and eosin. It shows how the junction between the systemic venous tributaries and the developing right atrium is formed by the venous valves. Note the mesenchymal mass that has grown into the heart to produce the vestibular spine, and the location of the canalized pulmonary vein.

From the outset, the bulge carries on its atrial margin a cap of mesenchyme. With time, the bulge becomes the primary atrial septum, or "septum primum", which grows towards the atrioventricular canal. The canal itself is separated into right- and left- sided components by the formation of superior and inferior mesenchymal masses. These are the atrioventricular cushions. As the primary septum, along with its cap, grows towards the cushions, so the space between its leading edge and the atrial surface of the cushions diminishes in size.[11] This space is the primary atrial foramen, or foramen primum (Figure 2.7 panel B). When patent, it permits the richly oxygenated blood being delivered to the developing embryo to reach the left side of the heart and the atrioventricular canal. Continued flow to the developing left-sided structures is integral to ongoing development. With reduction in size of the primary foramen, it is necessary for the embryo to provide an alternative route for the left-sided flow. This is achieved by the breakdown of the cranial attachment of the septum, thus producing the secondary atrial foramen (Figure 2.7 panel B).

By Carnegie stage 16, the cushions have approximated each other within the atrioventricular canal, and the mesenchymal cap has grown sufficiently to begin to close the primary atrial foramen (Figure 2.8 panel A). The area of fusion between the cap and the cushions is then reinforced caudally by the additional contribution made by the vestibular spine, which merges with the inferior atrioventricular cushion to become part of the true second atrial septum (Figure 2.8 panel B). This process also serves to commit the newly formed pulmonary vein to the cavity of the left atrium (Figure 2.8 panel C).

The pulmonary vein, which is a common vessel draining the blood from both lungs, initially opens into the developing left atrium

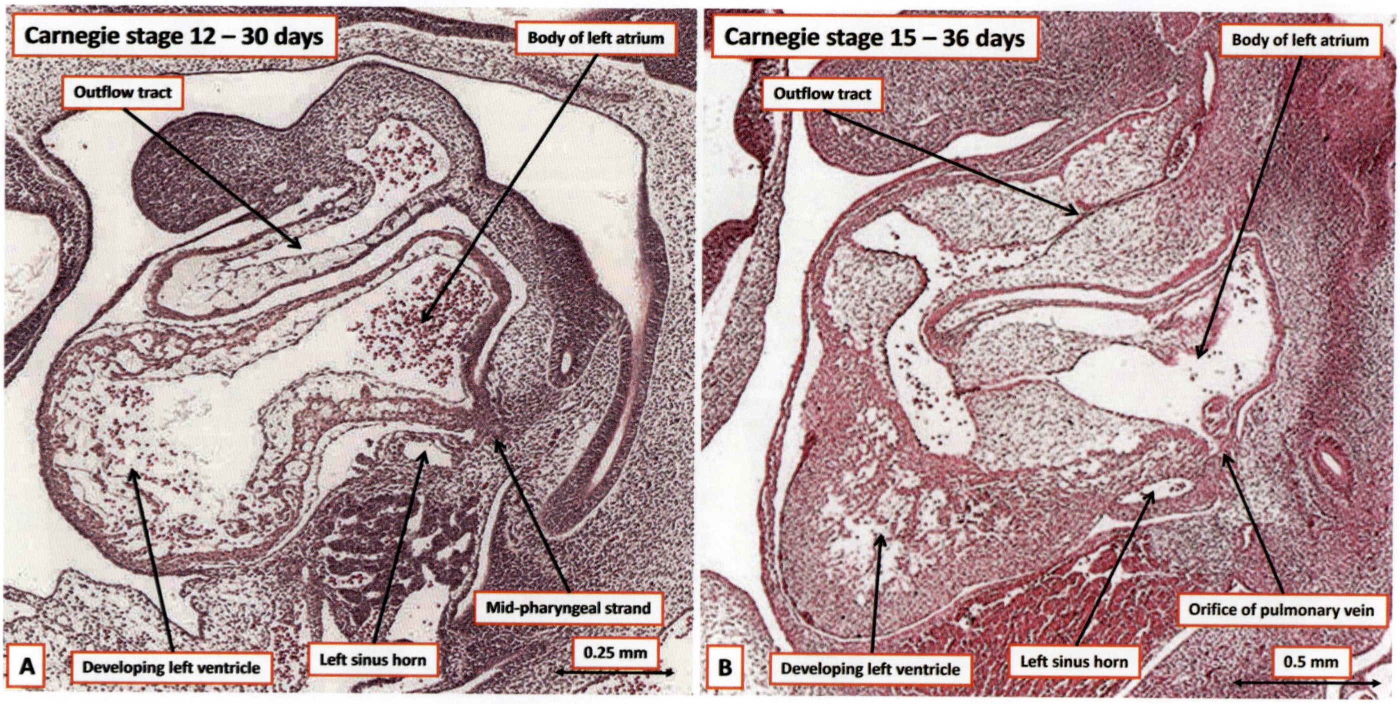

Figure 2.6. The images show sagittal sections through the hearts of embryos at Carnegie stages 12 (panel A) and 15 (panel B). They show how the mid-pharyngeal strand has canalized to become the common pulmonary vein. Note that, when first formed, the vein is adjacent to the developing left atrioventricular junction. Note also the presence of the left sinus horn in the left junction.

adjacent to the atrioventricular canal. Only towards the end of the embryonic period, concomitant with integration of the proximal parts of the pulmonary veins into the developing left atrial chamber, do the pulmonary veins begin to attain separate origins to the atrial wall.[12] And not until the fetal period of development is the arrangement produced in which two pulmonary veins open from each side so as to form the atrial roof (Figure 2.9). This process, which has become known as cannibalization, involves the incorporation of the

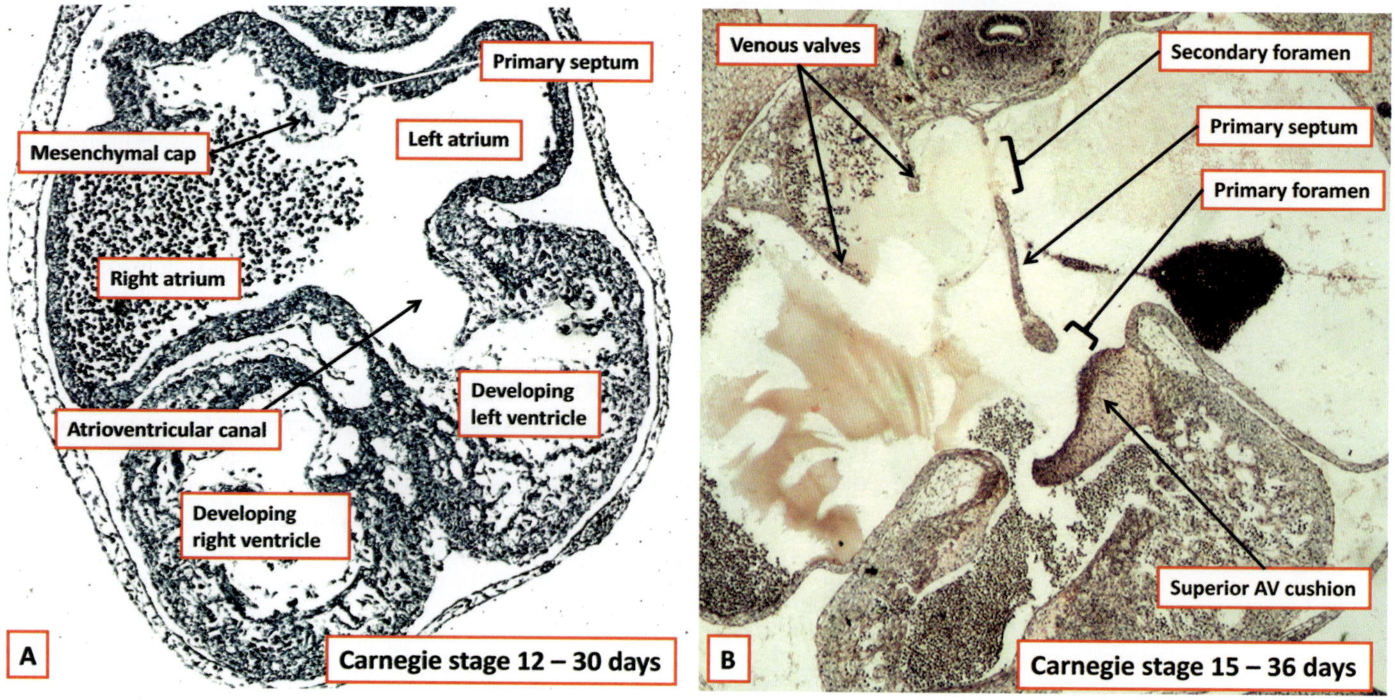

Figure 2.7. The images illustrate the growth of the primary septum. At Carnegie stage 12 (panel A), the septum originates as a bulge in the roof of the primary atrium and grows towards the atrioventricular cushions that have developed in the atrioventricular canal, carrying on its leading edge a cap of mesenchyme. As shown in panel B, by the beginning of the sixth week, at Carnegie stage 15, the cranial margin of the septum has broken down to produce the second atrial foramen, also known as "ostium secundum", with the primary foramen itself representing the "ostium primum".

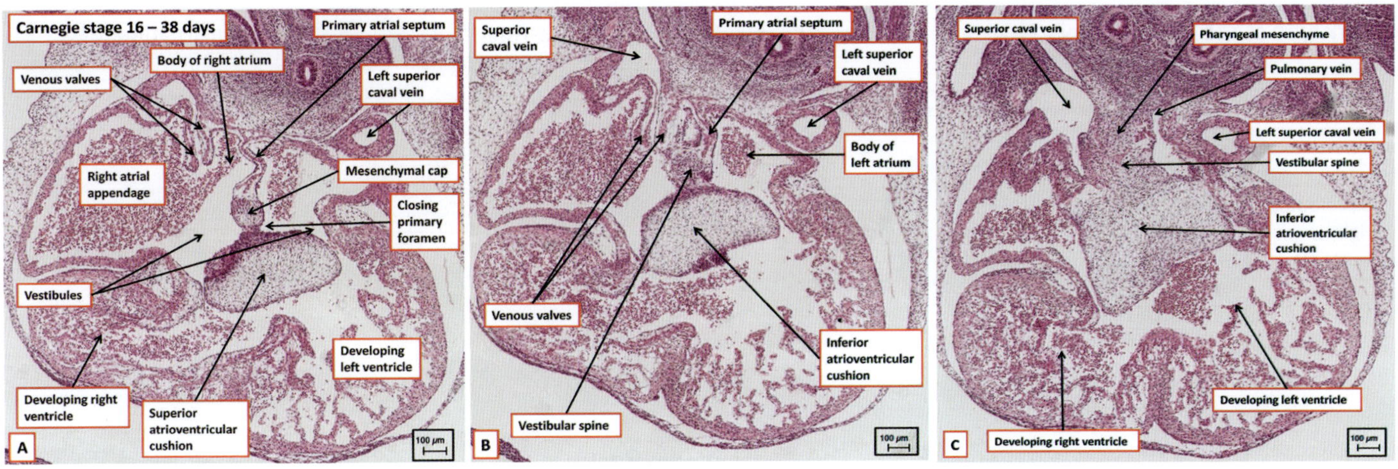

Figure 2.8. The images, in the frontal plane, are all from the same embryo, which was obtained at Carnegie stage 16. They show, in panel A, how the mesenchymal cap is fusing with the superior atrioventricular cushion to close the primary atrial foramen, with panel B showing how the vestibular spine fuses with the inferior cushion to reinforce the area of closure. Panel C then shows how this process commits the common pulmonary vein to the cavity of the left atrium.

walls of the individual veins to form the left- and right-sided carinas. The process of cannibalization on the right side also produces a deep cranial fold between the adjacent walls of the right and left atrial chambers. It is this fold that produces the structure against which the cranial margin of the primary atrial septum abuts in postnatal life to close the secondary atrial foramen.[11] It used to be thought that the fold, which produces the cranial rim of the oval foramen, grew into the heart as a second septum. This is not true. As long ago as the end of the 19th century, it had been pointed out that the structure in question, known as the "septum secundum", was a fold. The true second atrial septum is formed by muscularization of the mesenchymal cap and vestibular spine that helps to obliterate the primary atrial foramen. These myocardialized components form the antero-inferior buttress of the atrial septum, with the newly formed cardiomyocytes also providing the fast pathway into the atrioventricular node.

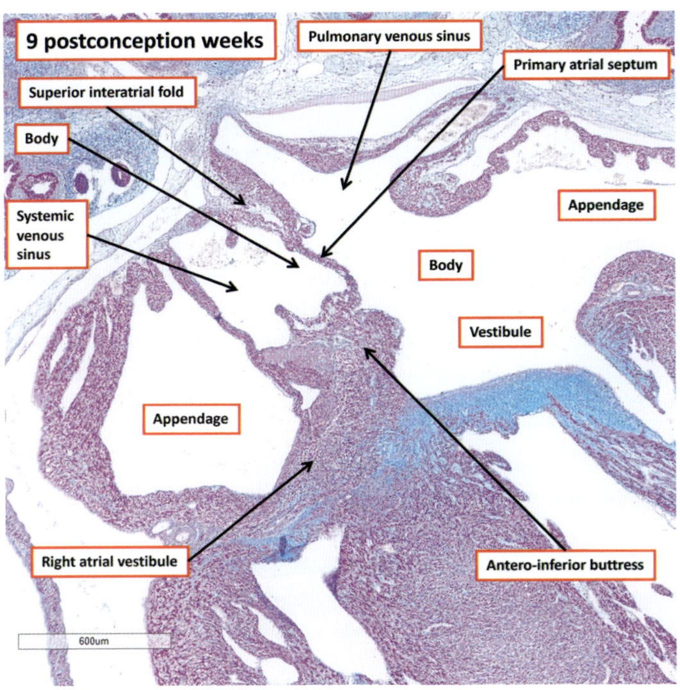

Figure 2.9. A frontal section through the atrial chambers is shown from a heart obtained at the first week of fetal life. The section shows how, with the pulmonary veins now beginning to open into the roof of the left atrium, there is an extensive superior fold against which the primary atrial septum is able to abut to close the secondary atrial foramen. The section shows how each atrium retains part of the primary atrium as its body, but also possesses an appendage, a vestibule, and a venous component. Note how the vestibular spine and mesenchymal cap have muscularized to form the antero-inferior buttress of the atrial septum. This is the true second atrial septum.

The atrial chambers, therefore, are formed by contributions from multiple embryonic primordiums. The initial atrial component of the primary heart tube produces the bodies of both the chambers, with the larger part committed to the definitive left atrium. The myocardium of the atrioventricular canal is committed to both chambers as the atrial vestibules. The atrial appendages balloon on each side from the initial body of the atrium. The venous components are initially formed extrapericardially, with the systemic venous tributaries committed to the developing right atrium as the systemic venous sinus. The pulmonary vein canalizes from the mid-pharyngeal strand, with its branches then being cannibalized to produce the pulmonary venous sinus. The primary atrial septum becomes the floor of the oval fossa, with the myocardialized cap and vestibular spine producing the true second atrial septum. The remaining rims of the oval fossa are infoldings of the atrial walls.

Formation of the Ventricles

Atrial development involves contributions being made from multiple developmental primordiums. The arrangement is much simpler for the ventricles, which arise exclusively from the part of the primary heart tube known as the ventricular loop.[6] The proximal part of the ventricular part of the tube is derived from the first heart field. Material derived from the second heart field then produces the outlet part of the loop.[3,4] The ingrowth of the new material from the second heart field provides the site for 'ballooning' of the apical component of the right ventricle, with the apical component of

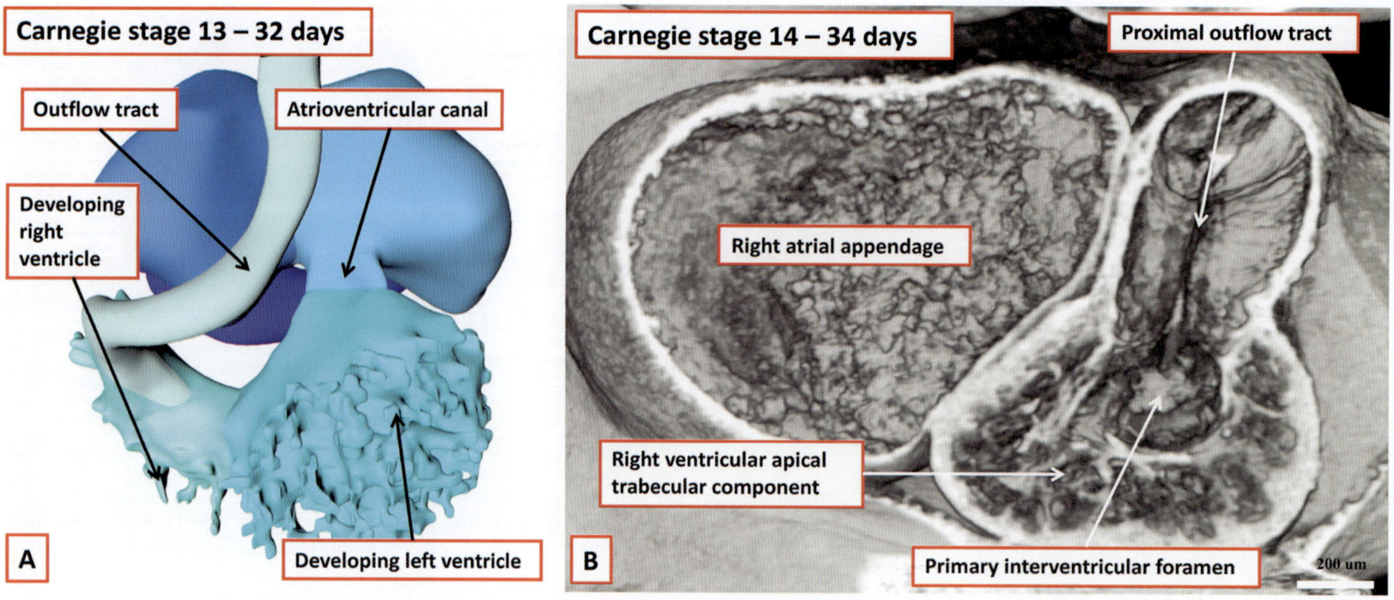

Figure 2.10. Panel A is a reconstruction of the cavities of the developing ventricles at Carnegie stage 32, which is midway through the fifth week of development. The apical components of the ventricles are beginning to balloon from the ventricular component of the primary heart tube. Panel B shows an oblique cut taken from a dataset prepared using the technique of episcopic microscopy. The developing right ventricle supports the entirety of the outflow tract, but has no direct connection with the atrial chambers. It receives the blood from the developing left ventricle through the primary interventricular foramen.

the left ventricle ballooning from the inlet part of the loop (Figure 2.2).[7] When first formed, the right ventricle lacks a direct inlet from the atrial chambers, but supports the entirety of the outflow tract (Figure 2.10 panel B).

Although having no direct inlet from the atrial chambers, the wall of the developing ventricle, from the outset, is in continuity with the wall of the developing right atrium through the rightward margin of the atrioventricular canal (Figure 2.11 panel B). All that is required, therefore, to provide the right ventricle with its inlet is expansion of the atrioventricular canal.[8] This is achieved by Carnegie stage 16, which is at the end of the fifth week of development (Figure 2.11 panel B). By then, the myocardium of the atrioventricular canal has been committed to the atrial chambers as their vestibules (Figure 2.11 panel B), although atrioventricular myocardial continuity persists throughout the newly formed atrioventricular junctions.

Having obtained its inlet by expansion of the canal, the developing right ventricle continues to support the entirety of the developing outflow tract. The outflow tract itself, by this stage, is becoming separated into aortic and pulmonary channels by the formation of additional cushions, which spiral throughout its length. As will be described, subsequent to ingrowth of additional non-myocardial tissues from the heart-forming areas, and straightening of the outflow tract, the distal parts of the cushions will excavate to form the adjacent leaflets of the arterial valves. The proximal parts of the cushions, in contrast, fuse so as to commit the subaortic component of the proximal outflow tract to the left ventricle (Figure 2.12). This is achieved because, as they fuse, the cushions block off the larger part of the space beneath the developing aortic root from the supporting cavity of the right ventricle.

This space beneath the aortic root, however, although now separated in larger part from the cavity of the supporting right ventricle, remains in continuity with the cavity of the left ventricle through the secondary interventricular foramen, but also with the right ventricle through a space which can be considered to represent a tertiary interventricular foramen (Figure 2.13 panel A). The area providing continuity with the right ventricle is closed by the formation of tubercles from the rightward margins of the atrioventricular cushions (Figure 2.13 panel B). By means of these changes, the subaortic area, which initially was part of the cavity of the right ventricle, becomes the outflow tract of the left ventricle. The secondary interventricular foramen, which is an integral part of the new pathway, is never closed (Figure 2.13 panel B). As the aortic root is eventually remodelled during the fetal period so as to be wedged between the developing atrioventricular junctions, the fused tubercles of the cushions remodel to become the membranous part of the septum. Eventual delamination of the septal leaflet of the tricuspid valve then produces the interventricular as opposed to the atrioventricular parts of the septum.[13] The fused proximal components of the outflow cushions then myocardialize, separating from the aortic root to become the free-standing infundibulum of the right ventricle.[14]

Formation of the Arterial Roots and the Intrapericardial Arterial Trunks

Subsequent to the formation of the ventricular loop, and at the beginning of the ballooning of the ventricular apical components (Figure 2.2 panel B), the outflow tract is supported exclusively above the cavity of the right ventricle (Figure 2.3). At this stage of development, which is in the fifth week subsequent to conception, and stage 12 in the Carnegie sequence, the entirety of the walls of the outflow tract, extending to the margins of the pericardial cavity, are myocardial (Figure 2.14 panel A).[15] At the margins of the pericardial cavity, the cavity of the outflow tract is continuous with that

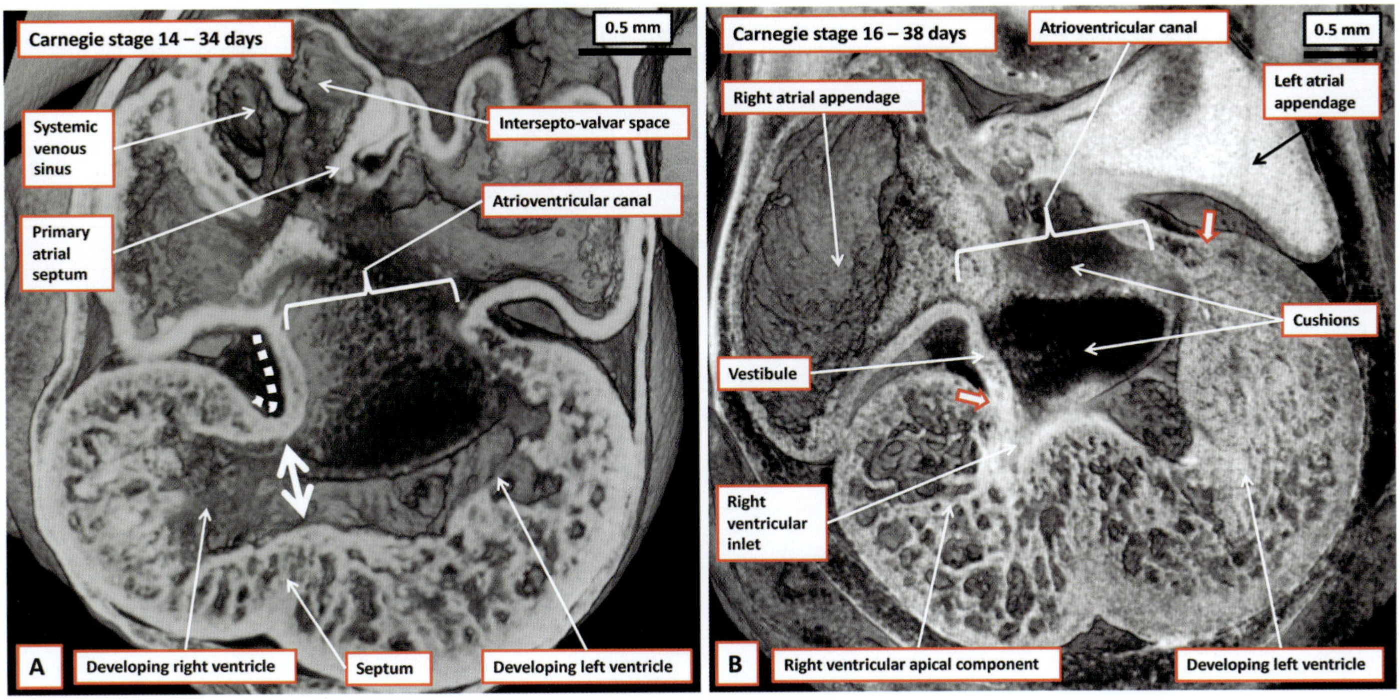

Figure 2.11. Panel A shows a different cut through the episcopic dataset used to prepare Figure 2.10B. The "four-chamber" section shows that, although the atrioventricular is supported exclusively by the developing left ventricle, the walls of the right atrium and ventricles are already continuous (dashed white line) at the right margin of the primary interventricular foramen (double-headed white arrow). All that is required to provide the right ventricle with its direct inlet is expansion of the atrioventricular canal, which has taken place by Carnegie stage 16, as can be seen in panel B. The formation of the plane of insulation then sequestrates the atrioventricular canal myocardium as the atrial vestibules (white arrows with red borders).

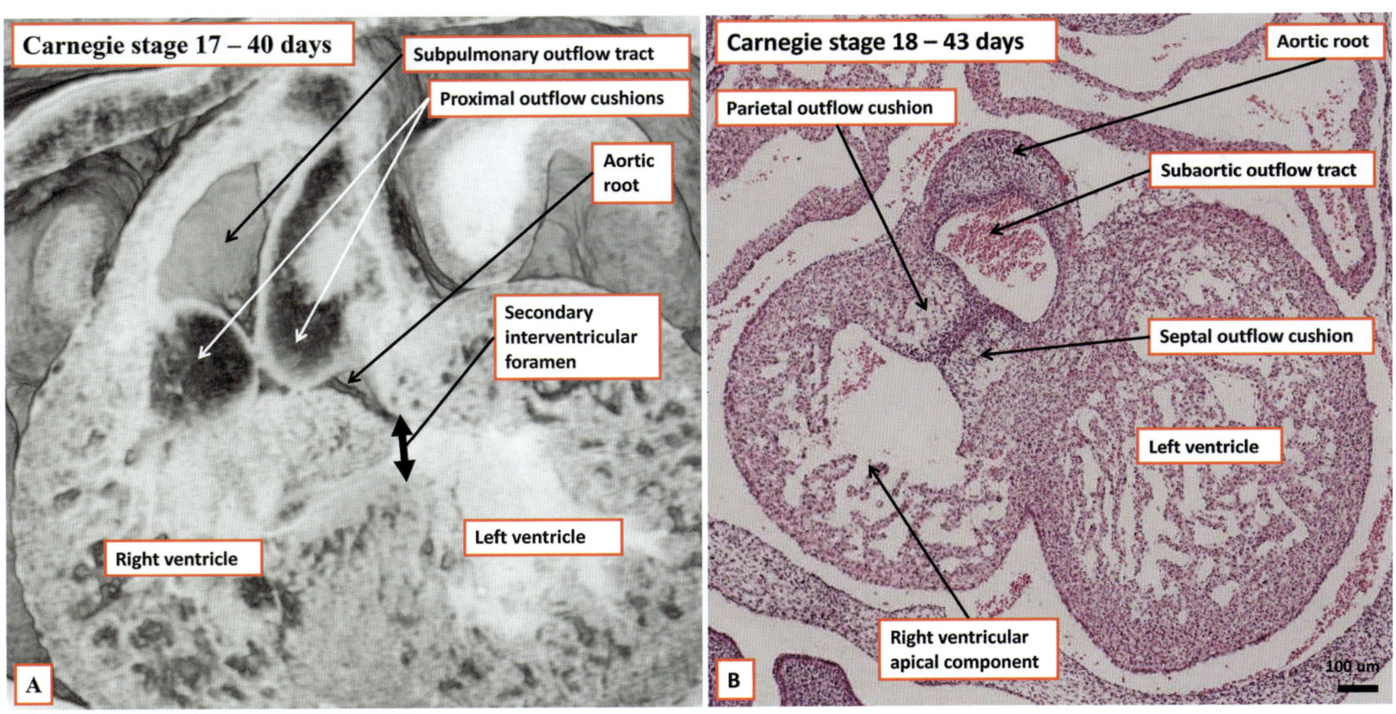

Figure 2.12. The panels show how the subaortic component of the outflow tract becomes separated from the right ventricle by fusion of the proximal parts of the outflow cushions. Panel A is an episcopic image from a heart at Carnegie stage 17, which shows the proximal cushions prior to their fusion. The blood from the left ventricle reaches the outflow tract through the secondary interventricular foramen. Panel B is a histological section one stage later, when the proximal cushions have fused with each other. This process places the subaortic part of the outflow tract in communication with the left ventricle through the secondary interventricular foramen.

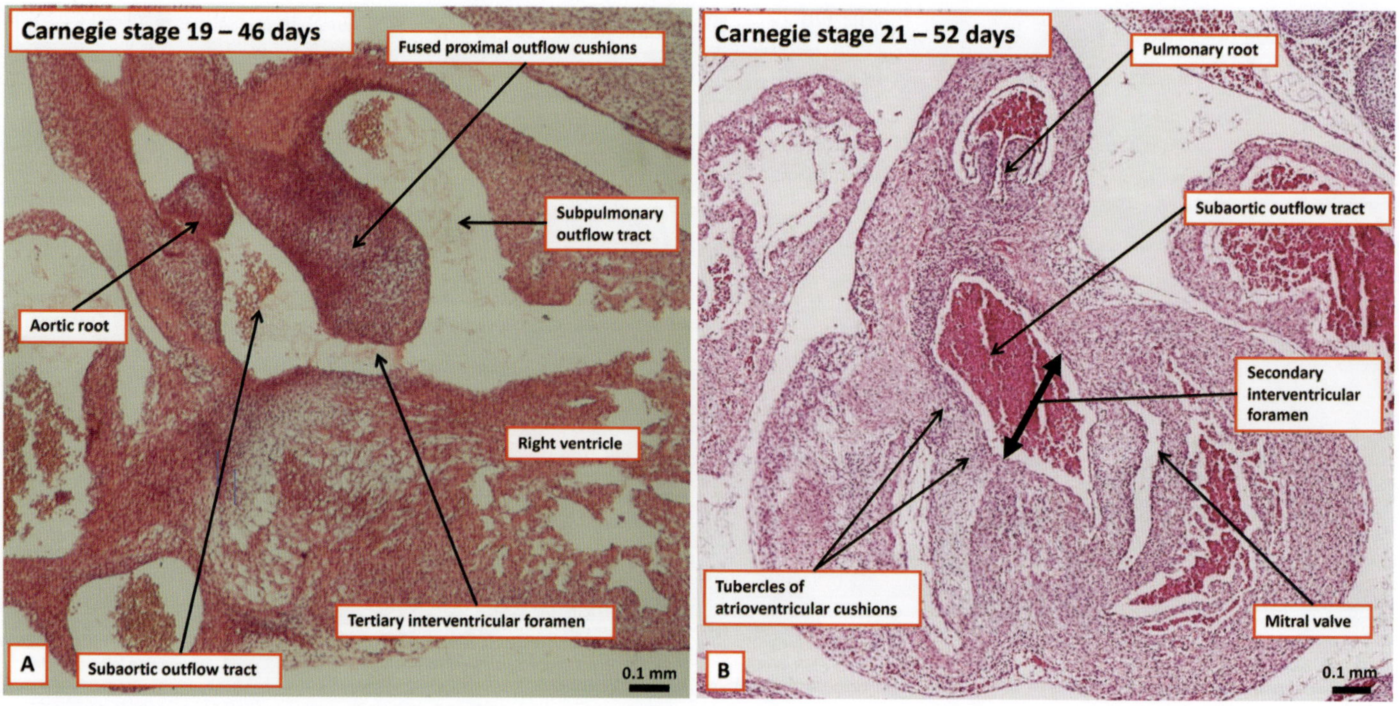

Figure 2.13. The histological sections, from embryos at Carnegie stages 19 and 21, show how the subaortic component of the right ventricle becomes committed as the outlet of the left ventricle by the fusion of tubercles from the atrioventricular cushions, which close the space between the subaortic space and the cavity of the right ventricle that represents a tertiary interventricular foramen. Panel A is an oblique section, whereas panel B is in the "four-chamber" plane. The fused tubercles of the atrioventricular cushions will become the membranous part of the ventricular septum, with part eventually becoming atrioventricular subsequent to the delamination of the septal leaflet of the tricuspid valve. The secondary interventricular foramen is never closed. It becomes the outflow tract for the definitive left ventricle.

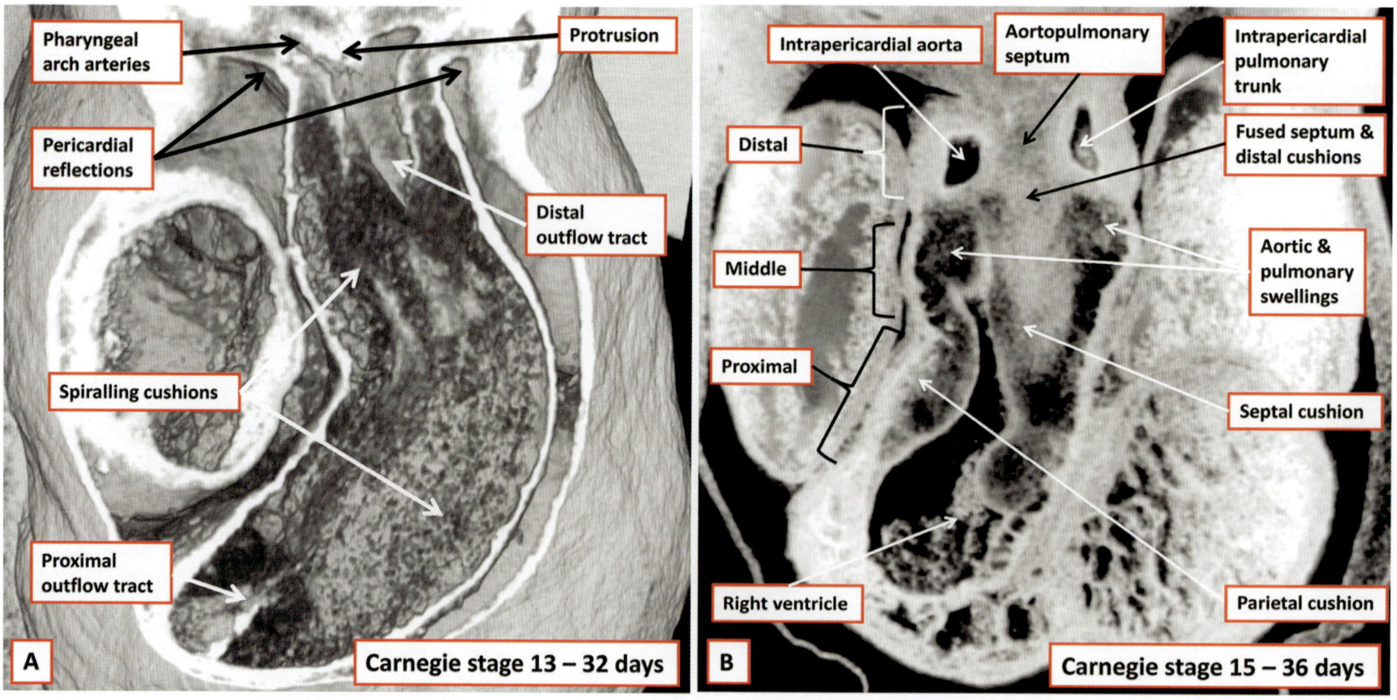

Figure 2.14. These sections across the developing outflow tract in the frontal plane are taken from episcopic datasets prepared from embryos at Carnegie stage 13 (panel A) and late stage 15 (panel B). At stage 13, the walls of the outflow tract are myocardial to the level of the pericardial reflections, with the cavity separated by spiralling cushions into pulmonary and aortic channels. By stage 15, the outflow tract has straightened, and non-myocardial tissues have entered the arterial pole such that the myocardial walls now surround only the proximal and middle parts of the outflow tract. The cushions have fused with each other in the middle part of the tract and also with the protrusion that has grown as the aortopulmonary septum from the dorsal wall of the aortic sac. The cushions remain unfused in the proximal part of the tract.

of the aortic sac. Arising from the aortic sac are the paired arteries that percolate through the mesenchyme of the pharyngeal arches, joining dorsally to form the descending aorta. New migrations of non-myocardial tissues from the heart-forming areas then enter the arterial pole of the heart tube during the end of the fifth week of development. These tissues form the walls of the intrapericardial arterial trunks.[15] Entering the cavity of the distal outflow tract at the same time is a protrusion from the dorsal wall of the aortic sac. This separates the cranial pharyngeal arteries, which will form the systemic arterial channels, from the caudal arteries, which eventually feed the lungs. By the beginning of the sixth week of development, the non-myocardial tissues have formed the distal part of the outflow tract, which has straightened concomitant with the addition of the new material.

The part that has retained its myocardial walls can now be distinguished as forming the middle and proximal components of the developing outflow tract. Within the middle part, the cushions separating the tract into the aortic and pulmonary channels have fused with each other. They have also fused with the protrusion from the dorsal wall of the aortic sac, which formed an aortopulmonary septum, separating the distal part of the outflow tract into its aortic and pulmonary components.[14] The cushions have fused in the middle part, but they have still to fuse in the proximal part (Figure 2.14 panel B). In the middle part of the outflow tract, however, there has been formation of additional mesenchymal swellings. These new intercalated swellings interdigitate with the unfused parietal ends of the major cushions. In this way, they form the primordiums of the arterial roots, which are still encased within the myocardium of the outflow tract (Figure 2.15 panel A).[14] With further development, the distal ends of the major cushions, along with the swellings, excavate to become the leaflets of the arterial valves. Still further ingrowth of non-myocardial tissues from the heart-forming areas then produces the walls of the arterial valvar sinuses (Figure 2.15 panel B).[16]

By the end of the embryonic period, at Carnegie stage 23, when 8 weeks have elapsed subsequent to conception, the myocardial wall of the outflow tract has effectively regressed proximally such that it continues to support all three developing leaflets of the pulmonary valve (Figure 2.16). In the developing aortic root, however, the outflow tract myocardium attenuates still further during the initial weeks of fetal development such that the parts supporting the non-adjacent sinus are completely effaced, thus producing the area of fibrous continuity between the leaflets of the aortic and mitral valves. During the same period, the proximal outflow cushions themselves myocardialize, separating from the aortic root to become the free-standing infundibular sleeve (Figure 2.15 panel B).[14] As already described, it was fusion of the proximal cushions with the tubercles of the atrioventricular cushions that served to close the tertiary interventricular foramen, thus committing the area beneath the aortic root to the left ventricle as its definitive outflow tract (Figure 2.13 panel B).[17]

Remodelling of the Arteries of the Pharyngeal Arches

At the stage of the straight heart tube, the ventral aortas exit from its cranial end, turning to become the paired dorsal aortas (Figure 2.1).[2] Within the fifth week of development, the arrangement

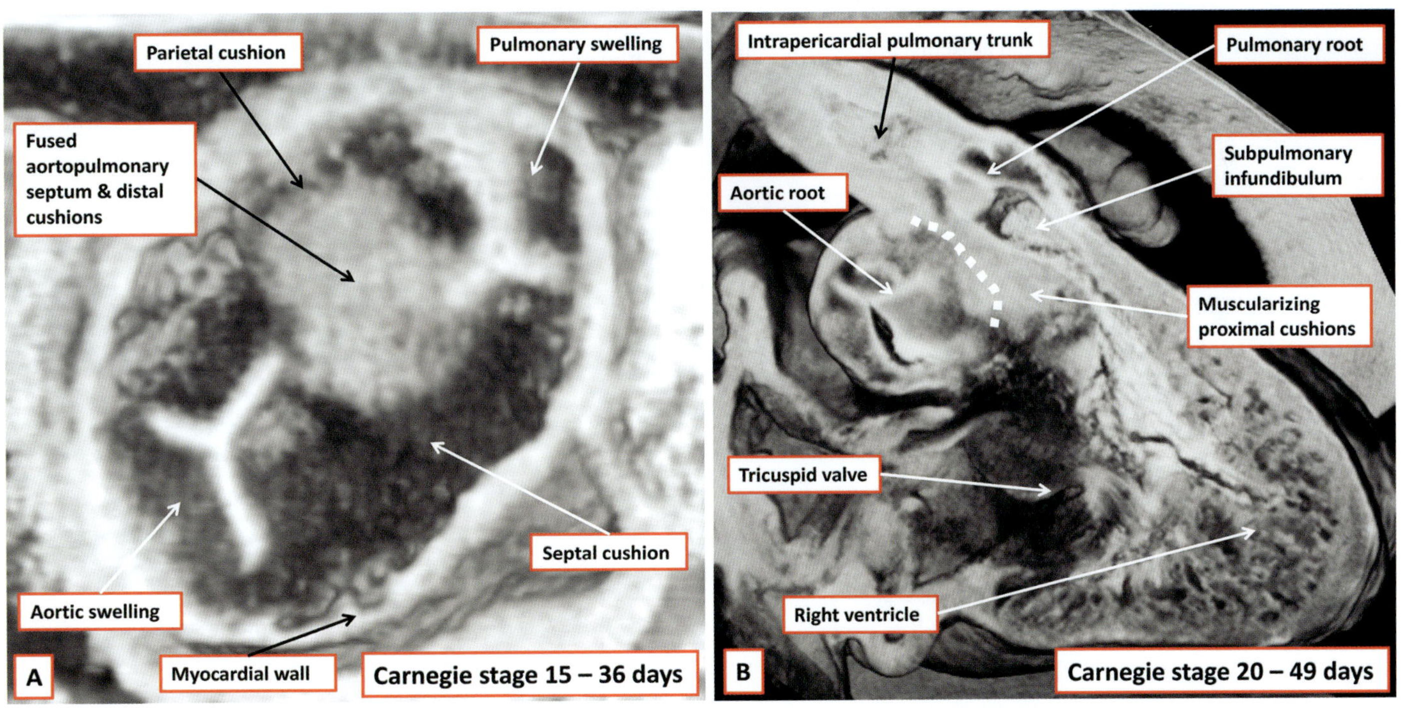

Figure 2.15. Panel A is a short axis section taken through the middle part of the outflow tract from the same episcopic dataset as shown in Figure 2.14B. It shows how the interdigitations between the fused major outflow cushions and the swellings that have appeared in the middle part of the outflow tract provide the primordiums for development of the arterial roots. Panel B is an oblique long axis section through a dataset at Carnegie stage 20, showing how excavation of the distal cushions produces the leaflets of the arterial valves. The section also shows the muscularizing proximal cushions which separate from the aortic root (white dashed line) to form the free-standing subpulmonary infundibulum.

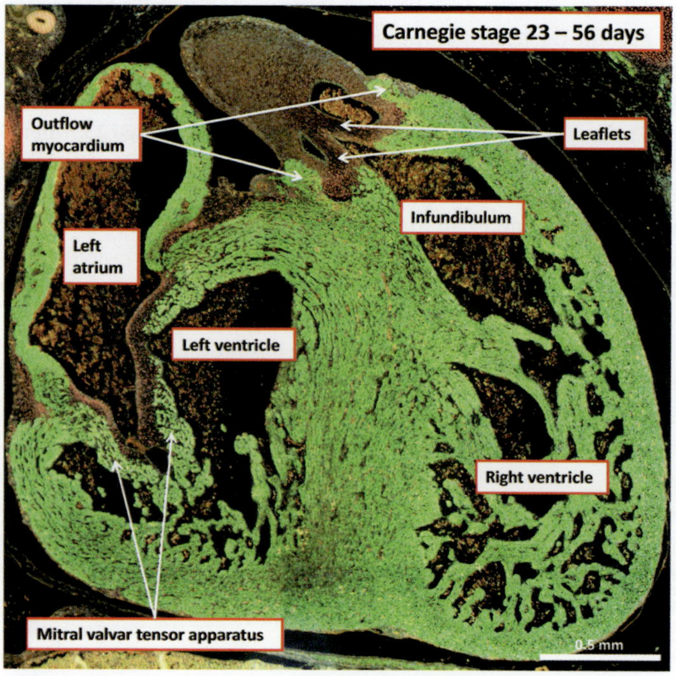

Figure 2.16. This histological section, in the same plane as the section shown in Figure 2.15, has been stained to show the extent of the myocardium (in green) and the non-myocardial components of the pulmonary root (shown in brown). The outflow tract myocardium is supporting the excavating leaflets of the pulmonary valve. Note the coalescing trabeculations in the left ventricle that are supporting the developing leaflets of the mitral valve.

changes markedly, coinciding with the development of the pharyngeal arches.[18] As they are formed, each of the paired arches contains an artery, along with a cranial nerve, and muscular and skeletal components. At Carnegie stage 12, at the beginning of the fifth week, there is evidence of formation of the first two pharyngeal arches, with each block of pharyngeal mesenchyme bordered caudally by a pharyngeal pouch (**Figure 2.17** panel A). During the fifth week, there is rapid growth of the third and fourth arches, along with their arteries, which are bilaterally symmetrical (**Figure 2.17** panel B). By the end of the fifth week, there has been formation of one additional set of arches with contained arteries, but no formation of additional pouches (**Figure 2.17** panel C). During normal development in the human, therefore, there is formation of five bilaterally symmetrical pharyngeal pouches, with each pouch containing an artery on each side. Contrary to traditional belief, there is never formation of six arches, with the fifth arch being transient.[19] It is the arteries of the ultimate arches that give rise to the right and left pulmonary arteries. It would be accurate, therefore, to label these ultimate arches as being fifth in number. There is so much literature, however, addressing presumed 'persistent arteries of the fifth pharyngeal arches' that it would now be confusing to seek to distinguish the arteries correctly in numerical fashion. It is better, therefore, simply to describe the ultimate set of arteries as belonging to the pulmonary arches.[20]

By the middle of the fifth week of development, the arteries percolating through the pharyngeal arches had remained essentially bilaterally symmetrical, although already the right-sided pulmonary arch artery and the right dorsal aorta are beginning to attenuate (**Figure 2.18** panel A). It is the ongoing attenuation of these right-sided components that underscores the remodelling to produce the definitive arrangement of the extrapericardial systemic and pulmonary arterial pathways. It is the artery of the left pulmonary arch that persists as the arterial duct, or ductus arteriosus, with the artery of the right pulmonary arch disappearing (**Figure 2.18** panel B). The seventh cervical intersegmental arteries become the subclavian arteries, with the arteries of the third pharyngeal arches becoming the common carotid arteries. The right horn of the cranial component of the aortic sac remodels to become the brachiocephalic artery, with the artery of the right fourth arch feeding the seventh cervical intersegmental artery as it becomes the right subclavian artery. The artery of the left fourth arch becomes part of the transverse aortic arch,

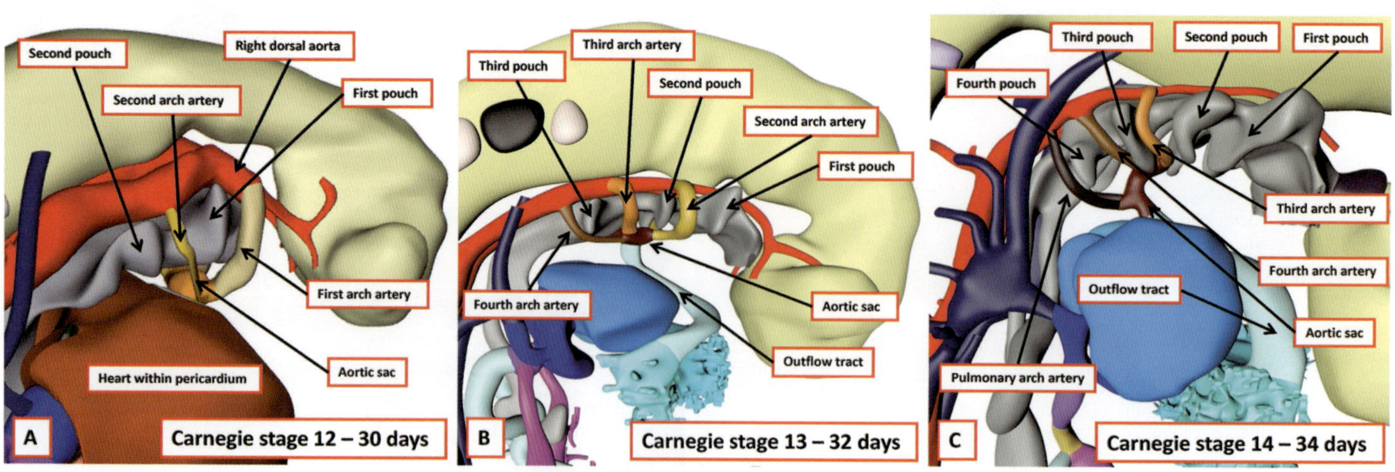

Figure 2.17. The reconstructions show the right side of the developing embryo during the fifth week of development, illustrating the formation of the pharyngeal arches. Each arch is a block of pharyngeal mesenchyme bordered caudally by the cavity of a pharyngeal pouch, with the arches being bilaterally symmetrical. At Carnegie stage 12, as seen in panel A, there are two arches formed, each with its contained artery. By Carnegie stage 13, as shown in panel B, the third and fourth arch arteries have formed, but the arteries of the first arch have regressed. At Carnegie stage 14, shown in panel C, there has been formation of arteries caudal to the fourth pouch, with the arteries of the second arches having also regressed. There is never any evidence of formation of a sixth pharyngeal arch. Because of the frequent incorrect use of "fifth arch artery", it is better to describe the arteries of the ultimate arches as the pulmonary arch arteries.

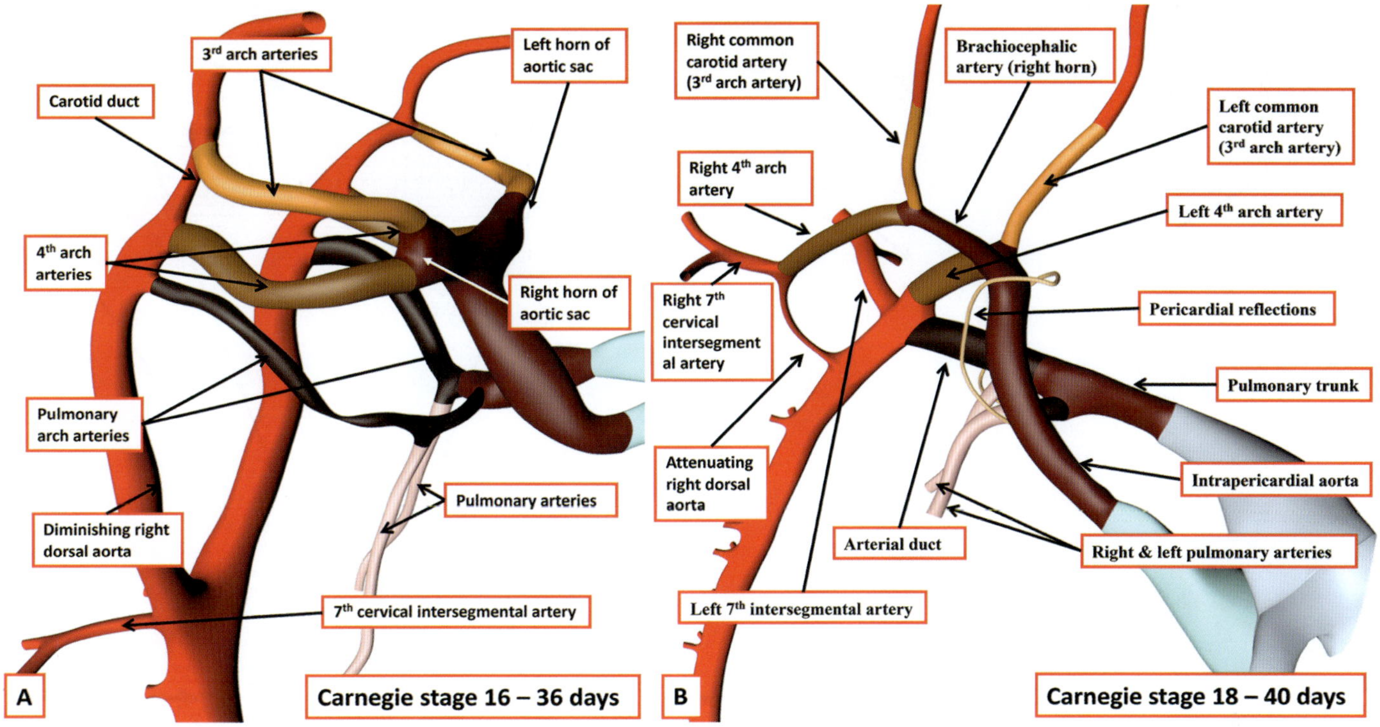

Figure 2.18. These reconstructions illustrate the remodelling of the aortic sac and the arteries of the third, fourth, and pulmonary arches, along with the seventh cervical intersegmental artery. As shown in panel A, the arrangement is initially bilaterally symmetrical, with the third and fourth arch arteries arising from the cranial component of the aortic sac and the pulmonary arteries from the caudal component. With ongoing development, as shown in panel B, there is regression of the artery of the right pulmonary arch artery and the right dorsal aorta. The left pulmonary arch artery persists as the arterial duct. Further cranial migration of the left seventh cervical intersegmental artery is required as it becomes the left subclavian artery. The right horn of the aortic sac becomes the brachiocephalic artery.

with the left seventh cervical intersegmental artery having to cross the insertion of the left pulmonary arch artery to the descending aorta as it remodels to become the left subclavian artery (Figure 2.18 panel B).

Formation of the Cardiac Valves

As was discussed when describing the formation of the arterial roots, it is excavation of the distal margins of the major outflow cushions and the intercalated valvar swellings that produces the leaflets of the arterial valves.[14] As also discussed, during this process of excavation the cushions and swellings are initially supported within the distal parts of the myocardial walls that initially clothed the entirety of the outflow tract (Figure 2.14 panel A). It is the addition of new non-myocardial tissues from the heart-forming areas that produces the fibrous walls of the arterial valvar sinuses.[15] With the addition of the non-myocardial components, there is effective regression of the distal myocardial border towards the ventricular base. The precise mechanics of this process, along with the formation of the walls of the valvar sinuses, have still to be determined. The myocardial support of the adjacent leaflets and sinuses of the aortic and pulmonary roots, nonetheless, is provided by muscularization of the proximal parts of the outflow cushions, with the large part of the newly myocardialized area becoming the free-standing infundibular sleeve of the right ventricle.[14] The myocardium supporting the non-coronary leaflet and part of the left coronary leaflet of the aortic root disappears during development. This is why, in the definitive heart, myocardium is almost always found at the bases of all the sinuses of the pulmonary root, but only at the bases of the sinuses of the aortic root that give rise to the coronary arteries.

The development of the atrioventricular valves is equally as complex, with the finer details just as poorly understood as for the arterial valves. Early in development, the atrioventricular canal is separated by the formation within its orifice of superior and inferior cushions. By the end of the sixth week of development, the major cushions have fused with each other and also fused with the crest of the muscular ventricular septum. The manner of fusion with the ventricular septum is such that rightward margins drape themselves across the septal crest, leaving the bulk of the fused cushion mass positioned above the cavity of the left ventricle (Figure 2.19 panel A). Earlier in development, the atrioventricular canal had expanded to provide the right ventricle with its own inlet. Part of this remodelling resulted in the entirety of the atrioventricular canal myocardium becoming sequestrated on the atrial aspect of the atrioventricular junctions, forming the vestibules of the developing atrial chambers (Figure 2.11 panel B). During the period of expansion of the canal, additional cushions had been formed in the lateral margins of the newly separated ventricular inlets. It is these lateral cushions, along with the fused major cushions, that then provide the primordiums for development of the leaflets of the atrioventricular valves (Figure 2.19 panel A). The lateral cushion in the left atrioventricular junction will provide the primordium for the mural leaflet of the mitral valve. The lateral cushion in the right atrioventricular

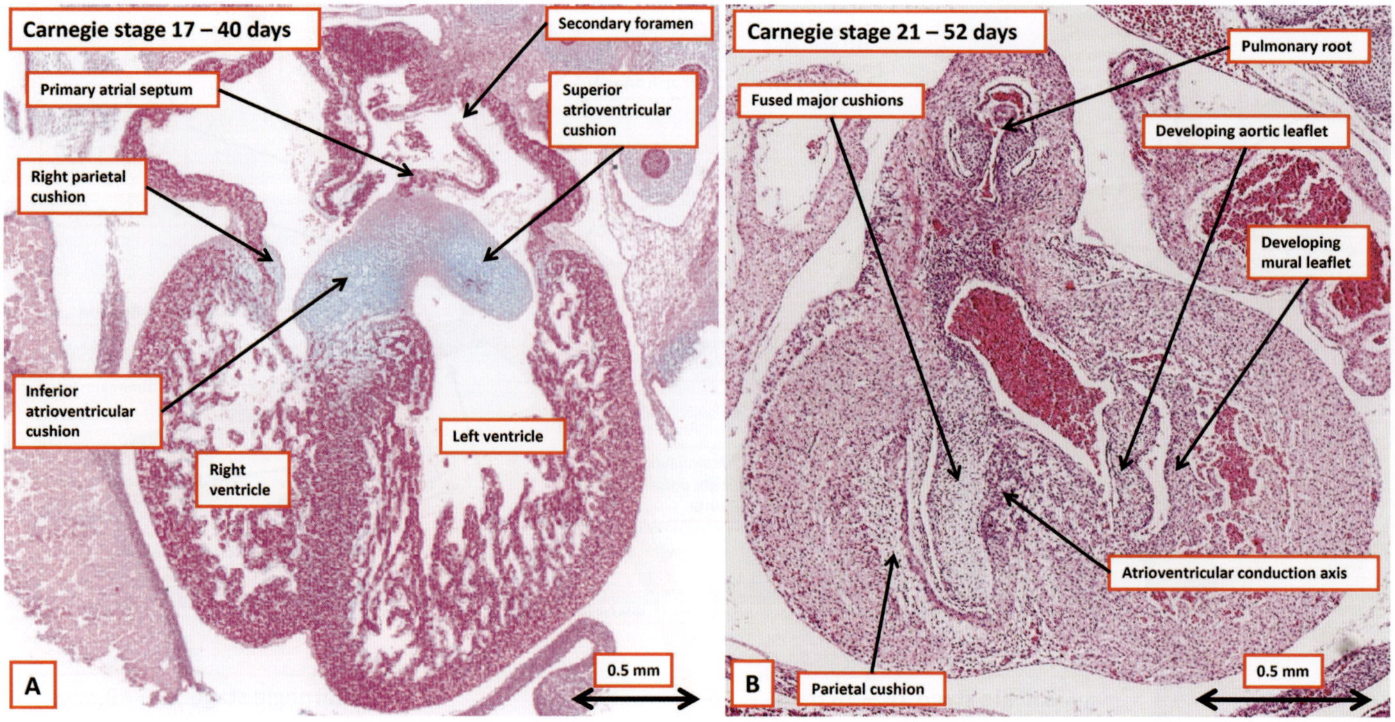

Figure 2.19. The histological sections reveal the locations of the cushions that provide the primordiums for development of the leaflets of the atrioventricular valves. Panel A shows a four-chamber section at Carnegie stage 17. The major cushions have fused to separate the atrioventricular canal into the tricuspid and mitral valvar orifices, with new cushions formed parietally in both junctions, although little is seen of the parietal cushion in the left junction in this section. Note that the large part of the major junctions remains above the cavity of the developing left ventricle. Panel B shows the situation at Carnegie stage 21, as seen in a short axis section viewed from the apex looking towards the base. There is still no evidence of formation of the inferior leaflet of the tricuspid valve, and as yet the developing mural leaflet of the mitral valve is comparable in size to the aortic leaflet, which still shows evidence of the fusion of the superior and inferior cushions.

canal will eventually remodel to produce both the antero-superior and inferior, or mural, leaflets of the tricuspid valve. The rightward margins of the conjoined atrioventricular cushions, subsequent to draping themselves across the crest of the muscular ventricular septum, provide the substance for formation of the septal leaflet of the tricuspid valve.

Delamination of this leaflet, however, does not take place until the fetal period of development. As has already been described, tubercles from these rightward margins of the cushions will already have closed the space between the developing aortic root and the right ventricle that can be described as the tertiary interventricular foramen (Figure 2.13 panel B).[17] On the left side, the developing mitral valve initially has a trifoliate configuration, reflecting the contributions made by both major atrioventricular cushions and the parietal cushion. At the end of the embryonic period, the developing mural leaflet of the valve retains similar dimensions to the aortic leaflet, which is formed by fusion of the major cushions (Figure 2.20 panel A). Only later, during the fetal period, does the left atrioventricular junction expand inferiorly to provide the full extent of the mural leaflet. A significant part of the fused major cushions then persists as the fibrous roof of the infero-septal recess of the left ventricular outflow tract (Figure 2.19 panel A). In both ventricles, it is coalescence of the initial trabecular layers of the ventricular walls that forms the papillary muscles, which initially support the overall length of the developing leaflets (Figure 2.20 panel B). It is delamination of the cushions from the parietal wall of the right ventricle, and from the muscular septum, which serves to produce the inferior and septal leaflets of the tricuspid valve. Comparable delamination from the parietal wall of the left ventricle produces the mural leaflet of the mitral valve. The junctions between the cushions and the extensive support provided by the trabecular myocardium then remodel to produce the tendinous cords, with leaflets and cords both having an endocardial rather than a myocardial lineage.[21] The transformation into tendinous cords does not take place until the tenth and eleventh weeks of development.

Development of the Conduction System

It is relatively late in development that areas of myocardium can be recognized as satisfying the histological criterions of the so-called conducting tissues.[22] It is possible to record an electrocardiogram from the developing embryo long before the tissues become recognizable histologically. This is because all myocardial cells within the heart have the ability to conduct the cardiac impulse. The electrocardiogram is seen as soon as the heart tube has developed, creating areas permitting fast as opposed to slow conduction. This is seen concomitant with the ballooning of chamber myocardium from the primary heart tube. The chamber myocardium conducts faster than the slowly conducting primary myocardium. The walls of the atrioventricular canal, and those of the outflow tract, are made of primary myocardium, as is a floor extending from the atrioventricular canal to incorporate the orifices of the systemic venous tributaries. Most of this primary myocardium becomes isolated from the ventricular

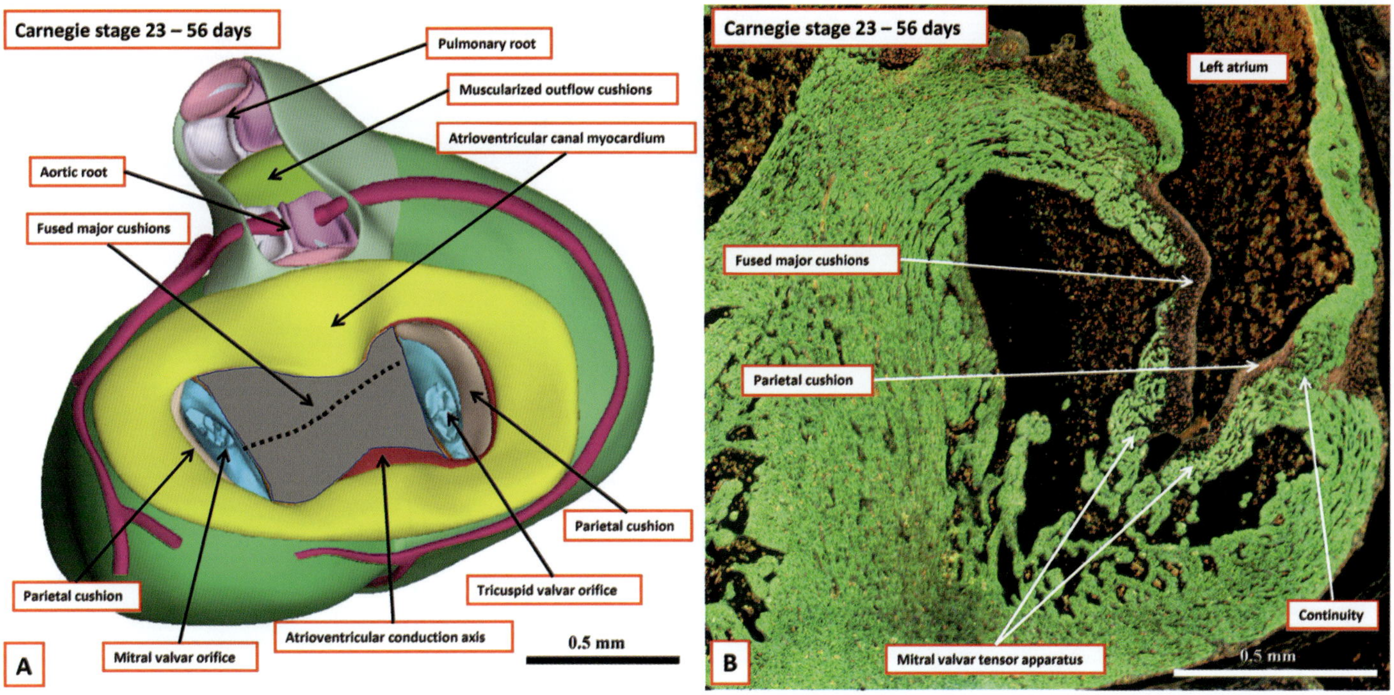

Figure 2.20. The images reveal the stage of development of the atrioventricular valves at the end of the embryonic period. Panel A shows a reconstruction viewed from the atrial aspect looking towards the apex. As yet, there has been limited inferior expansion of the junctions, so that the dimensions of the developing mural leaflet of the mitral valve still match that of the developing aortic leaflet, with the aortic root yet to be translocated to its definitive wedged position. There is still no evidence of formation of the inferior leaflet of the tricuspid valve. Panel B shows a long axis section of the developing mitral valve. The tension apparatus still remains exclusively myocardial, with the myocardium supporting the entirety of the ventricular surfaces of the developing leaflets. Note that, as yet, myocardial continuity persists across the parietal atrioventricular junction.

component subsequent to the formation of the insulating tissues of the atrioventricular grooves. It is of limited importance to the development of the substrates for atrioventricular conduction. The location of primary myocardium within the atrial vestibules, around the mouth of the coronary sinus, and along the terminal crest, nonetheless, offers some explanation for the origins of abnormal activity in patients with atrial arrhythmias. The sinus node itself, which is the pacemaker, can be recognized at the junction of the superior caval vein with the developing right atrium at Carnegie stage 15, when the embryo is just beginning its sixth week of development. By Carnegie stage 19, the node has established its definitive position within the terminal groove, with an obvious body and a well-formed tail (Figure 2.21). While the pulmonary venous myocardial sleeves are very frequently a substrate for atrial fibrillation, they have never been exposed to the same morphogenetic processes that underscore the formation of the definitive components of the conduction system. Their contained cardiomyocytes are exclusively of the working type.

The basis for formation of the atrioventricular conduction axis is the ring of cardiomyocytes that initially surrounds the primary interventricular communication. In the human heart, this ring is marked by an antibody to the nodose ganglion of the chick.[8] Subsequent to expansion of the atrioventricular canal, the part of the ring carried on the crest of the muscular ventricular septum becomes the ventricular component of the axis.[23] With expansion of the canal, the dorsal part of the ring becomes incorporated within the right atrioventricular junction as part of the vestibule of the right atrium (Figure 2.22). With the formation of the insulating tissues of

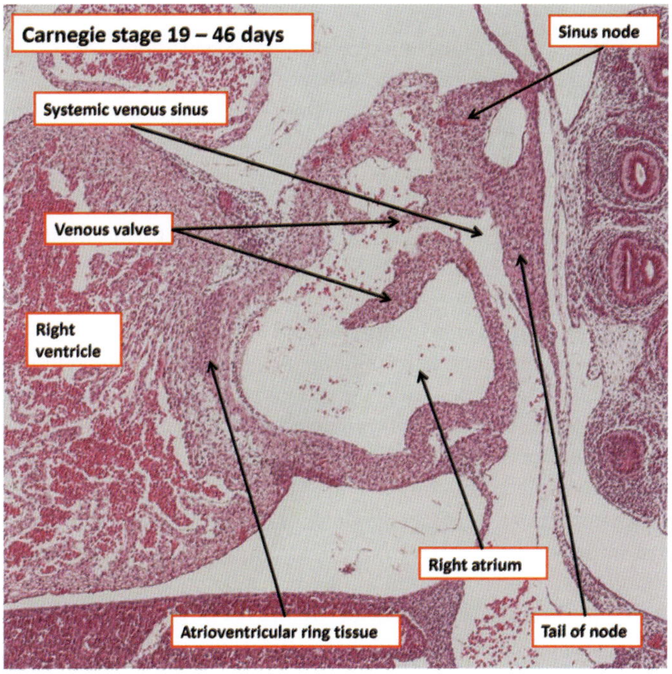

Figure 2.21. The histological section, showing the long axis of the developing right atrium in a human embryo almost at the end of the seventh week of development, shows the sinus node to be well formed and histologically discrete. It occupies the larger part of the terminal groove, with an extensive tail reaching towards the orifice of the inferior caval vein.

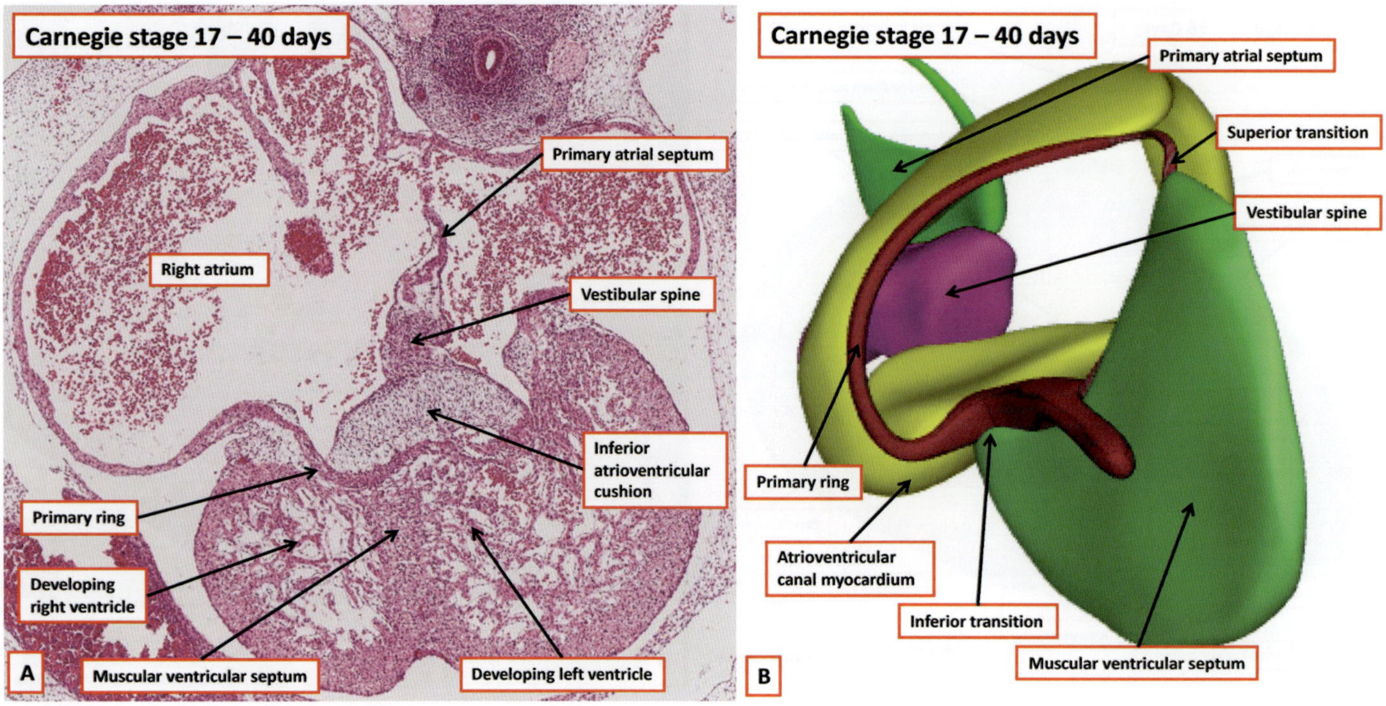

Figure 2.22. The histological section as shown in panel A and the reconstruction shown in panel B are both from human embryos at Carnegie stage 17, which is towards the end of the sixth week of development. At this stage it is still possible to recognize the extent of the primary ring, which initially encircled the primary interventricular foramen. At this stage, subsequent to expansion of the atrioventricular canal to provide the right ventricle with its own inlet, part of the ring now encircles the right atrioventricular junction, being sequestrated at the distal end of the right half of the atrioventricular canal myocardium, which now forms the vestibule of the right atrium. As shown in the reconstruction (panel B), the initial ring transitions from the ventricular to the atrial components superiorly and inferiorly. The inferior transition will eventually become the atrioventricular node, whereas the superior transition will provide the primordium of the retroaortic node.

the atrioventricular junctions, two potential transitions are created between the primary ring and the atrial myocardium. The inferior transition, as it crosses the plane of developing insulation, will become the junction between the atrioventricular node and the non-branching bundle. The tissues that will become the atrioventricular node are then in continuity with the vestibules of both the right and left atrioventricular junctions. Part of the primary ring itself is a component of the right junction. It will become the right inferior extension of the atrioventricular node.

The node also develops an inferior and leftward extension. This left extension is part of the atrioventricular canal myocardium, but does not contain any component of the primary ring. The nodal inputs are then completed concomitant with myocardialisation of the vestibular spine. This process provides the inputs from the atrial septum, which merge with the atrial component of the primary ring to form the compact part of the node. Components of the trabecular meshwork that initially filled the larger part of both ventricular apical components then remodel to produce the ventricular bundle branches and their apical ramifications. Further remnants of the initial primary ring also persist in the vestibule of the tricuspid valve as the so-called atrioventricular ring tissues. When first formed, the ring encircled the primary interventricular foramen, part of which remodelled to become the entrance to the aortic root (Figure 2.13 panel B). The ring initially ascended the crest of the muscular ventricular septum in this area to reach its second superior transition with the atrioventricular canal myocardium. The larger parts of the ring on the septal crest cranial to the non-branching bundle attenuate and disappear, although some remnants can extend into the aortic root as the so-called dead-end tract.[24] The superior transition can still be identified in many postnatal hearts as the retro-aortic node (Figure 2.22).[23]

Development of the Coronary Circulation

The coronary arteries are derived from the epicardium, which in turn is derived from the pro-epicardial organ. Cells derived from this organ subsequently expand over the epicardial surface of the heart, reaching as far as the distal outflow tract. The cells then penetrate the developing myocardial walls, providing not only the fibrous matrix of the compact myocardium, but also the muscular walls of the coronary arteries and veins.[25] It had long been suggested that stems budded out from the aortic root to connect with the developing epicardial coronary arteries, with additional stems said to bud from the pulmonary root. More recently, it has been argued that the proximal epicardial coronary arteries grow into the aortic root.[26] The evidence now shows that stems do, indeed, grow out from the proximal margins of the distal non-myocardial outflow tract as the walls become converted into the arterial valvar sinuses (Figure 2.23).[25]

The establishment of direct flow from the aortic root to the epicardial coronary arteries is directly linked to the maturation of ventricular mural architecture. Prior to the establishment of direct nourishment, for example at Carnegie stage 18 (Figure 2.24 panel A), the trabecular layer of the ventricular walls is appreciably thicker than the compact layer. With ongoing development, the growth of

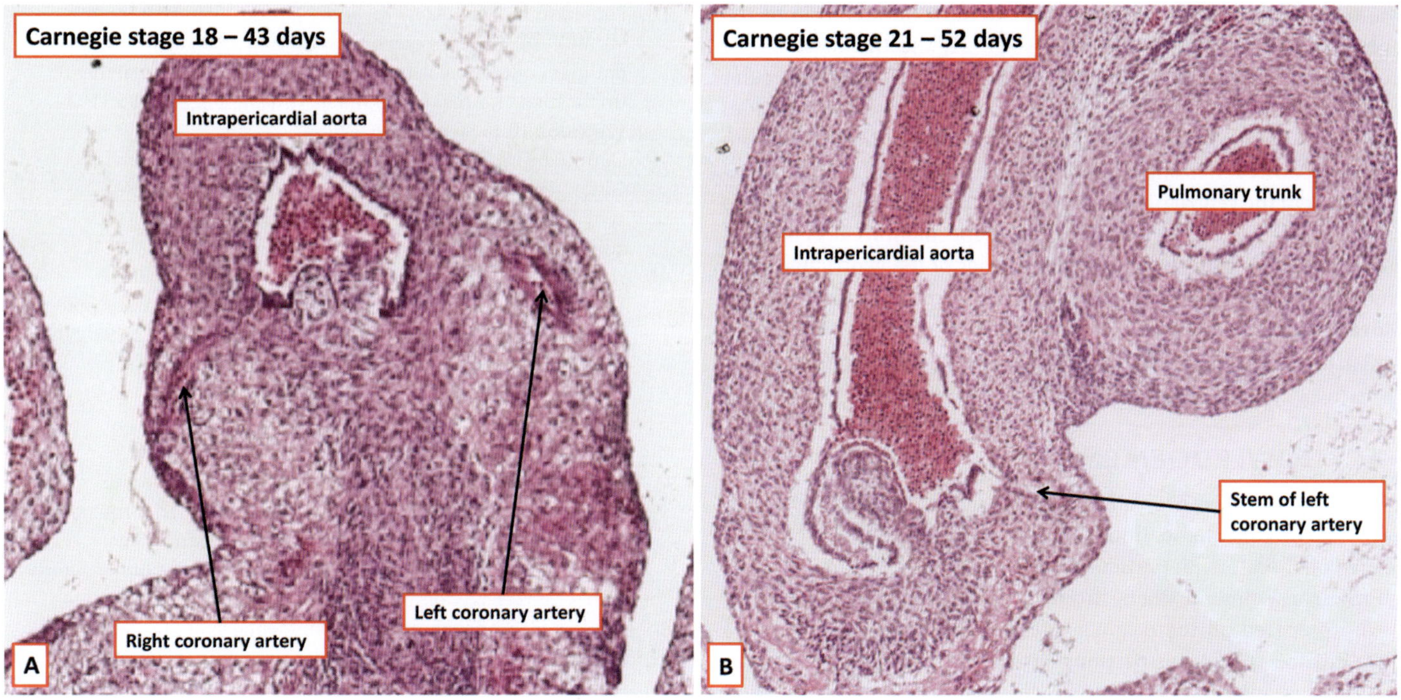

Figure 2.23. The histological sections, both in the long axis of the developing aortic root, show the steps involved in commitment of the developing coronary arteries to the sinuses of the aortic root. The major coronary arteries develop with the epicardial coverings of the heart. At Carnegie stage 18, as shown in panel A, they are contained within the myocardial turret that supports the developing aortic root. At this stage, the arteries are not in direct communication with the lumens of the valvar sinuses. It is later in development, concomitant with formation of the valvar sinuses, as shown in panel B, that stems grow out from the sinuses to contact the epicardial arteries.

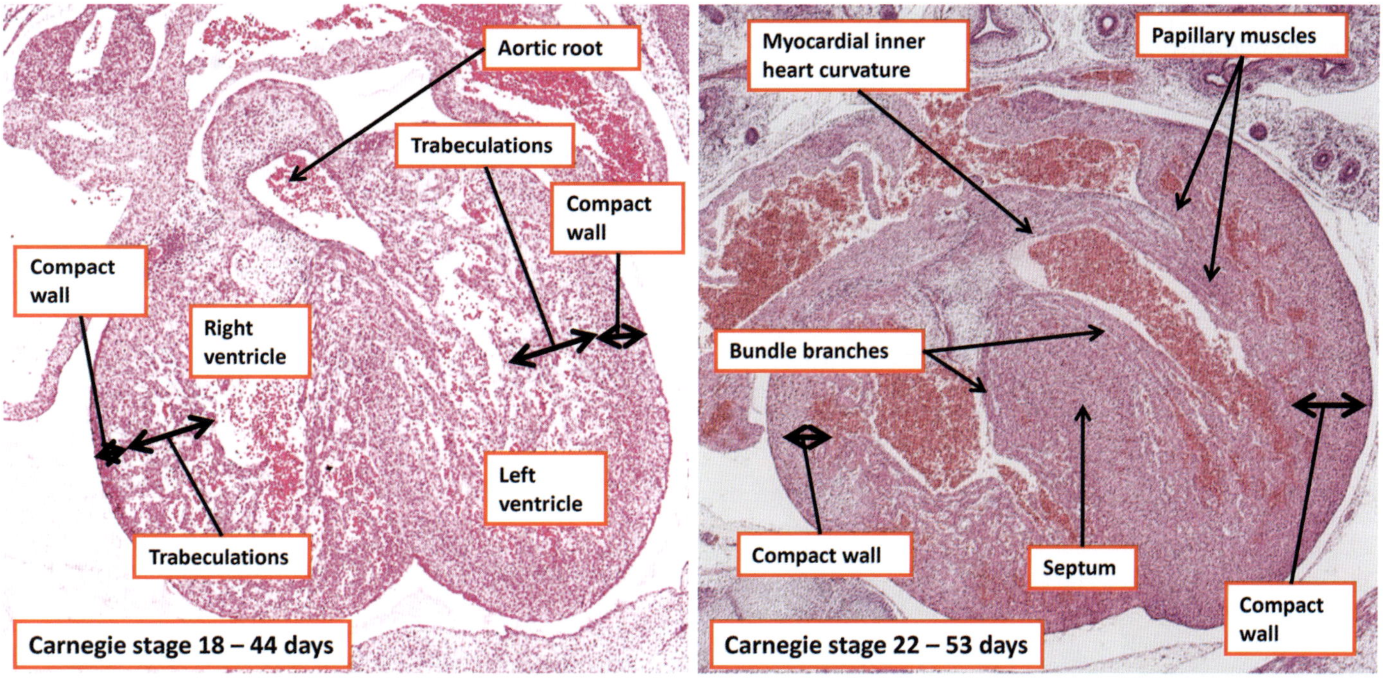

Figure 2.24. The histological sections, both shown in four-chamber fashion, show the steps involved in formation of the walls of the ventricular chambers. At Carnegie stage 18, as shown in panel A, at the beginning of the seventh week of development, even though the ventricular septum is complete in this specimen, there has been minimal formation of the compact components of the ventricular walls. It is the trabecular myocardium that makes up the greater part of the mural thickness. Only towards the end of the embryonic period, as shown in panel B, is there proliferation of the compact myocardium. The trabecular myocardium coalesces to form the ventricular conduction and the papillary muscles of the atrioventricular valves. It does not make any significant contribution by "compacting" to form the compact layer of the ventricular wall.

the trabeculations fails to match the extent of proliferation of the compact component. By Carnegie stage 22, the thickness of the compact wall has exceeded the thickness of the remaining trabecular layer (**Figure 2.24** panel B). Much has been written in recent decades regarding the significance of so-called non-compaction. There is no evidence, however, to suggest that a substantial fraction of the compact layer of the ventricular myocardium is produced by coalescence of pre-existing trabeculations.[27,28] The trabeculations do coalesce, nonetheless, to form the insulated branches of the ventricular conduction system and also the papillary muscles of the atrioventricular valves. They also persist as the characteristic apical trabeculations, which are much coarser in the right than in the left ventricle.

ACKNOWLEDGEMENT

We would not have been able to produce all the figures used to illustrate this chapter without the help of several of our colleagues and collaborators. In particular, we thank Dr Jill Hikspoors, and Professor Wouter Lamers, from the University of Maastricht, who prepared all the original interactive pdf files from which we created the reconstructions shown in many of the figures. We also thank Dr Tim Mohun, who prepared all the episcopic datasets. The hsitological images could not have been prepared without the help ofg the staff of the Human Biology Development Resource at Newcastle University. Most of the sections, along with the interactive pdf files, can now be interrogated within the website of the Developmental Resource.

REFERENCES

1. Moorman A, Webb S, Brown NA, Lamers W, Anderson RH. Development of the heart: (1) formation of the cardiac chambers and arterial trunks. *Heart*. 2003;**89**:806–814. doi: 10.1136/heart.89.7.806
2. Hikspoors J, Kruepunga N, Mommen GMC, Kohler SE, Anderson RH, Lamers WH. A pictorial account of the human embryonic heart between 3.5 and 8 weeks of development. *Commun Biol*. 2022;**5**:226. doi: 10.1038/s42003-022-03153-x
3. Kelly RG, Brown NA, Buckingham ME. The arterial pole of the mouse heart forms from Fgf10-expressing cells in pharyngeal mesoderm. *Dev Cell*. 2001;**1**:435–440. doi: 10.1016/s1534-5807(01)00040-5
4. Mjaatvedt CH, Nakaoka T, Moreno-Rodriguez R, Norris RA, Kern MJ, Eisenberg CA, Turner D, Markwald RR. The outflow tract of the heart is recruited from a novel heart-forming field. *Dev Biol*. 2001;**238**:97–109. doi: 10.1006/dbio.2001.0409
5. Moorman AF, Christoffels VM, Anderson RH, van den Hoff MJ. The heart-forming fields: one or multiple? *Philos Trans R Soc Lond B Biol Sci*. 2007;**362**:1257–1265. doi: 10.1098/rstb.2007.2113
6. Manner J. The anatomy of cardiac looping: a step towards the understanding of the morphogenesis of several forms of congenital cardiac malformations. *Clin Anat*. 2009;**22**:21–35. doi: 10.1002/ca.20652
7. Christoffels VM, Habets PE, Franco D, Campione M, de Jong F, Lamers WH, Bao ZZ, Palmer S, Biben C, Harvey RP, et al. Chamber formation and morphogenesis in the developing mammalian heart. *Dev Biol*. 2000;**223**:266–278. doi: 10.1006/dbio.2000.9753
8. Lamers WH, Wessels A, Verbeek FJ, Moorman AF, Viragh S, Wenink AC, Gittenberger-De Groot AC, Anderson RH. New findings concerning ventricular septation in the human heart. Implications for maldevelopment. *Circulation*. 1992;**86**:1194–1205. doi: 10.1161/01.cir.86.4.1194
9. DeRuiter MC, Poelmann RE, Mentink MM, Vaniperen L, Gittenberger-De Groot AC. Early formation of the vascular system in quail embryos. *Anat Rec*. 1993;**235**:261–274. doi: 10.1002/ar.1092350210
10. Sizarov A, Anderson RH, Christoffels VM, Moorman AF. Three-dimensional and molecular analysis of the venous pole of the developing human heart. *Circulation*. 2010;**122**:798–807. doi: 10.1161/CIRCULATIONAHA.110.953844
11. Jensen B, Spicer DE, Sheppard MN, Anderson RH. Development of the atrial septum in relation to postnatal anatomy and interatrial communications. *Heart*. 2017;**103**:456–462. doi: 10.1136/heartjnl-2016-310660
12. Webb S, Kanani M, Anderson RH, Richardson MK, Brown NA. Development of the human pulmonary vein and its incorporation in the morphologically left atrium. *Cardiol Young*. 2001;**11**:632–642. doi: 10.1017/s1047951101000993
13. Allwork SP, Anderson RH. Developmental anatomy of the membranous part of the ventricular septum in the human heart. *Br Heart J*. 1979;**41**:275–280. doi: 10.1136/hrt.41.3.275
14. Anderson RH, Lamers WH, Hikspoors J, Mohun TJ, Bamforth SD, Chaudhry B, Eley L, Kerwin J, Crosier M, Henderson DJ. Development of the arterial roots and ventricular outflow tracts. *J Anat*. 2024;**244**:497–513. doi: 10.1111/joa.13973
15. Anderson RH, Chaudhry B, Mohun TJ, Bamforth SD, Hoyland D, Phillips HM, Webb S, Moorman AF, Brown NA, Henderson DJ. Normal and abnormal development of the intrapericardial arterial trunks in humans and mice. *Cardiovasc Res*. 2012;**95**:108–115. doi: 10.1093/cvr/cvs147
16. Henderson DJ, Eley L, Chaudhry B. New concepts in the development and malformation of the arterial valves. *J Cardiovasc Dev Dis*. 2020;**7**:38. doi: 10.3390/jcdd7040038
17. Anderson RH, Spicer DE, Mohun TJ, Hikspoors J, Lamers WH. Remodeling of the embryonic interventricular communication in regard to the description and classification of ventricular septal defects. *Anat Rec*. 2019;**302**:19–31. doi: 10.1002/ar.24020
18. Graham A. Development of the pharyngeal arches. *Am J Med Genet A*. 2003;**119A**:251–256. doi: 10.1002/ajmg.a.10980
19. Graham A, Poopalasundaram S, Shone V, Kiecker C. A reappraisal and revision of the numbering of the pharyngeal arches. *J Anat*. 2019;**235**:1019–1023. doi: 10.1111/joa.13067
20. Anderson RH, Bamforth SD, Gupta SK. How best to describe the pharyngeal arch arteries when the fifth arch does not exist? *Cardiol Young*. 2020;**30**:1708–1710. doi: 10.1017/S1047951120003807
21. de Lange FJ, Moorman AF, Anderson RH, Manner J, Soufan AT, de Gier-de Vries C, Schneider MD, Webb S, van den Hoff MJ, Christoffels VM. Lineage and morphogenetic analysis of the cardiac valves. *Circ Res*. 2004;**95**:645–654. doi: 10.1161/01.RES.0000141429.13560.cb
22. Moorman AF, Christoffels VM, Anderson RH. Anatomic substrates for cardiac conduction. *Heart Rhythm*. 2005;**2**:875–886. doi: 10.1016/j.hrthm.2005.04.025
23. Hikspoors J, Macias Y, Tretter JT, Anderson RH, Lamers WH, Mohun TJ, Sanchez-Quintana D, Farre J, Back Sternick E. Miniseries 1—Part I: The development of the atrioventricular conduction axis. *Europace*. 2022;**24**:432–442. doi: 10.1093/europace/euab287

24. Anderson RH, Spicer DE, Mori S. Of tracts, rings, nodes, cusps, sinuses, and arrhythmias—a comment on Szili-Torok et al.'s paper entitled "The 'dead-end tract' and its role in arrhythmogenesis". *J Cardiovasc Dev Dis*. 2016;**3**:11. doi: 10.3390/jcdd3020017
25. Anderson RH, Turner JE, Henderson DJ. The morphogenesis of abnormal coronary arteries in the congenitally malformed heart. *J Thorac Cardiovasc Surg*. 2022;**164**:344–349. doi: 10.1016/j.jtcvs.2021.08.084
26. Bogers AJ, Gittenberger-de Groot AC, Poelmann RE, Peault BM, Huysmans HA. Development of the origin of the coronary arteries, a matter of ingrowth or outgrowth? *Anat Embryol (Berl)*. 1989;**180**:437–441. doi: 10.1007/BF00305118
27. Anderson RH, Jensen B, Mohun TJ, Petersen SE, Aung N, Zemrak F, Planken RN, MacIver DH. Key questions relating to left ventricular noncompaction cardiomyopathy: is the emperor still wearing any clothes? *Can J Cardiol*. 2017;**33**:747–757. doi: 10.1016/j.cjca.2017.01.017
28. Petersen SE, Jensen B, Aung N, Friedrich MG, McMahon CJ, Mohiddin SA, Pignatelli RH, Ricci F, Anderson RH, Bluemke DA. Excessive trabeculation of the left ventricle: JACC: Cardiovascular Imaging Expert Panel paper. *JACC Cardiovasc Imaging*. 2023;**16**:408–425. doi: 10.1016/j.jcmg.2022.12.026

3

The Pericardium

The pericardium is the dense fibrous sac that envelops the heart and the origins and terminations of the great arteries and veins. When observed externally, it makes up the larger part of the mediastinum (**Figure 3.1** panel A). The fibrous sac is continuous inferiorly with the central parts of the diaphragm. It is attached to the posterior surface of the sternum by the anterior sterno-pericardial ligaments (**Figure 3.1** panel B) and posteriorly to the vertebral column by comparable ligaments.[1,2]

Opening the ***fibrous pericardium*** reveals the pericardial space (**Figure 3.2**). The space is bounded by two layers of a serous sac, the ***serous pericardium***. The ***visceral*** component is the epicardium, which forms the external surface of all the cardiac components within the fibrous sac, including the intrapericardial arterial trunks. The ***parietal*** layer provides the internal surface of the fibrous sac itself. The thickness of the combined serous and fibrous layers of the parietal pericardium varies from 0.8 to 2.5 mm.[3] The two layers of the serous pericardium are reflected back on one another at the exits of the arterial trunks into the superior mediastinum and the entrances of the systemic and pulmonary veins at the cardiac base. The reflections enclose two areas that have been described as the cardiac hilums.[4] The names are appropriate, since it is through these areas that the cardiac nerves enter the heart. The areas are the remnants of the initial arterial and venous poles formed during development (see Chapter 2). The ***arterial component*** is located superiorly, with

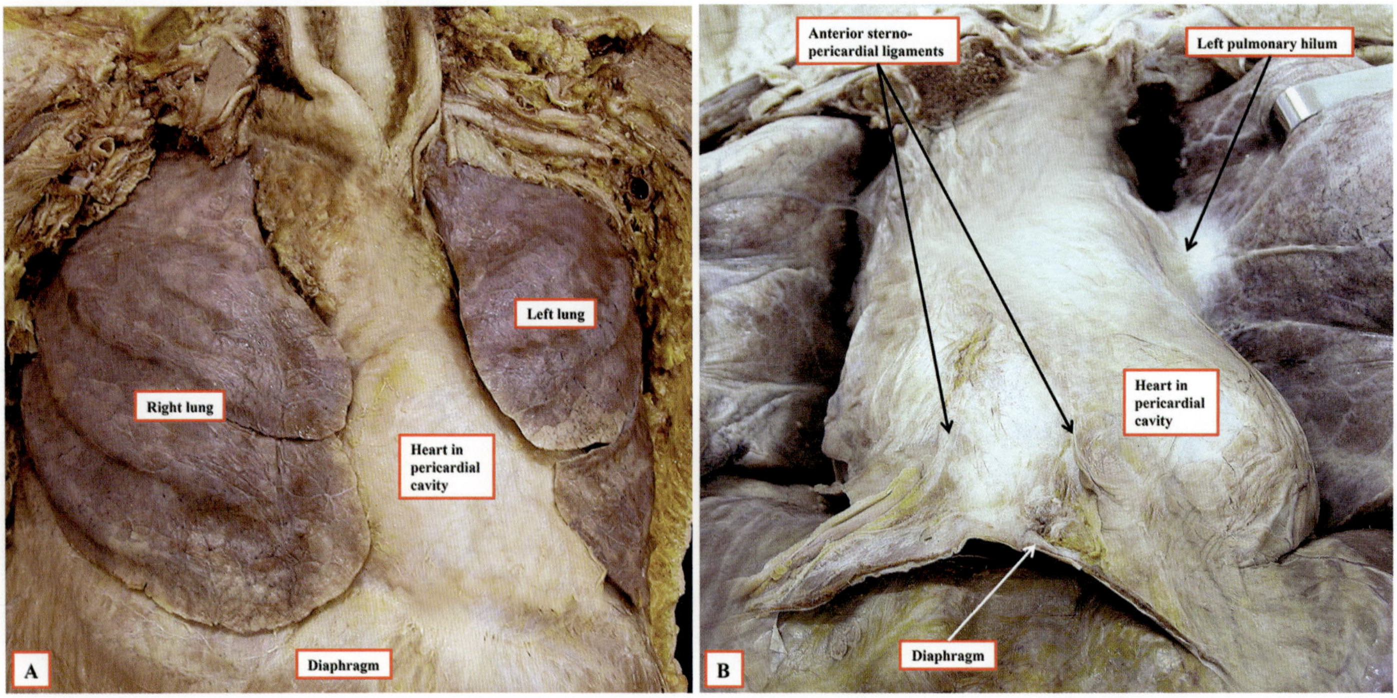

Figure 3.1. Panel A is an anterior view of the thorax, having removed the sternocostal rib cage. It shows the heart within its pericardial sac occupying the larger part of the mediastinum. In panel B, the left lung has been retracted to show the left pulmonary hilum. It is possible to recognize the anterior sterno-pericardial ligaments, which bind the pericardium to the posterior surface of the sternum, and the dense connection of the pericardium with the diaphragm.

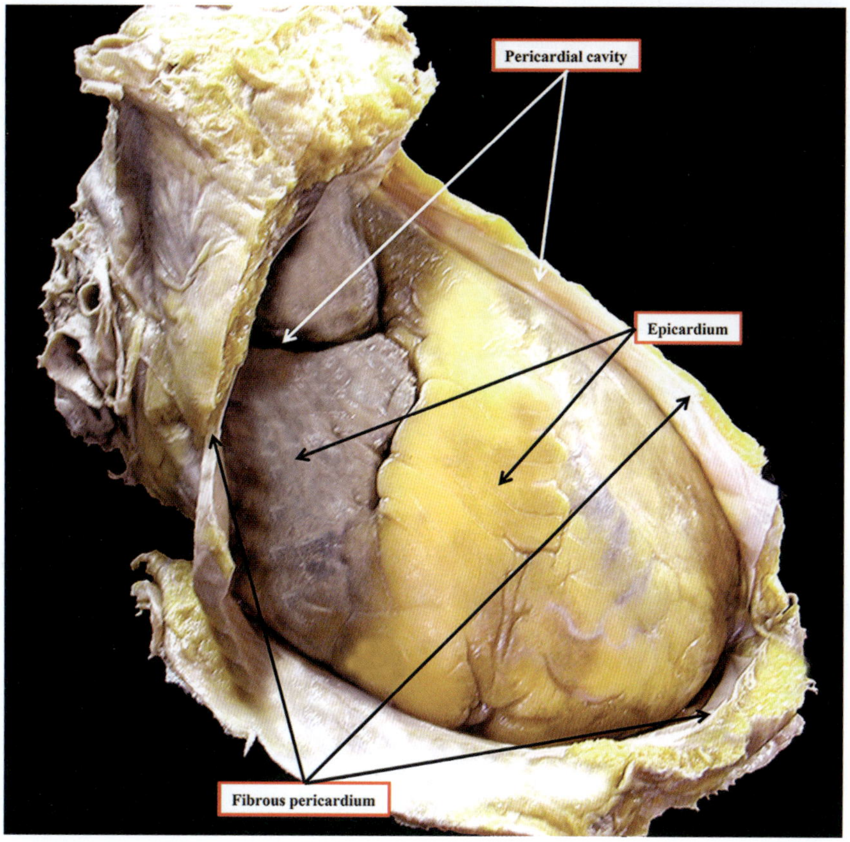

Figure 3.2. The fibrous pericardial sac has been opened to show how it wraps itself in tube-like fashion around the right atrial appendage and the ventricular mass.

the reflections enclosing the exits of the intrapericardial aorta and the pulmonary trunk within a common hilum. The boundaries of the ***venous hilum*** are much more complex. The complexity reflects the asymmetry during embryonic development of the sinus horns, along with the manner of integration of the pulmonary veins into the roof of the left atrium during early fetal life. Subsequent to the changes, the entrances of the right pulmonary veins, together with those of the superior and inferior caval veins, produce the extensive right boundary of the venous hilum.

The left border of the hilum is much shorter, being formed by the reflections round the orifices of the left pulmonary veins (Figure 3.3). The space between the right and left boundaries of the venous hilum is the ***oblique sinus*** of the pericardial cavity, which makes up the base of the overall pericardial cavity posterior to the wall of the left atrium (Figure 3.4).

There is then a second sinus found within the cavity, with this space separating the reflections around the arterial and venous hilums. This is the ***transverse sinus*** (Figure 3.5). It lines the initial inner heart curvature seen during development (see Chapter 2).

The sinus, itself lined by the serous layer of the pericardium, is bounded anteriorly by the posterior walls of the arterial trunks within the superior hilum and posteriorly by the interatrial groove (Figure 3.3). It opens on the right side to the space between the aorta and the superior caval vein. This is known as the ***aorto-caval recess*** (Figure 3.6 panel A).[5] On the left side, the sinus opens between the origin of the left pulmonary artery from the pulmonary trunk and the left atrial appendage (Figure 3.6 panel B). The floor of this area is the left ventricular summit. Further recesses can then be found at the base of the heart between the entrances of the pulmonary veins. These are known as the ***lateral pulmonary recesses*** (Figure 3.6). An additional fold is present within the leftward border of the venous hilum (Figure 3.7). This encloses the ***ligament of Marshall*** in consequence of the attenuation of the left superior caval vein during normal embryonic development.

The fibrous pericardium functions as the cardiac seatbelt in that it restrains the cardiac chambers during the cardiac cycle. In addition, the sac, by limiting chamber dilation, is an important determinant of cardiac filling, also serving to equalize compliance between the right and left ventricles. In terms of its lymphatic drainage, the pericardial cavity drains to both the thoracic duct and the right lymphatic duct.[6]

Several key extracardiac structures are directly related to the pericardium. Running posterior to the arterial and venous hilums is the ***oesophagus***, with the ***trachea*** bifurcating in the middle mediastinum to give rise to the right and left bronchuses as they enter the pulmonary hilums (Figure 3.8). The vagus and phrenic nerves

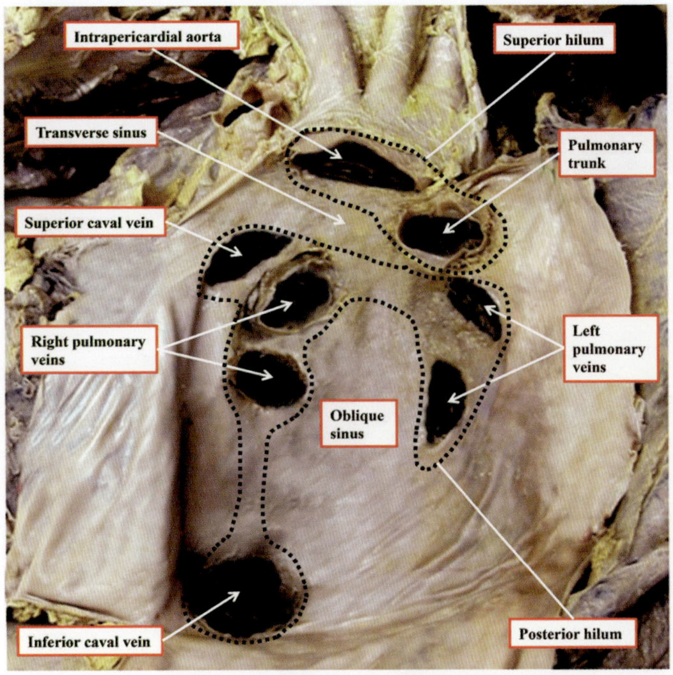

Figure 3.3. The heart has been removed from its pericardial cradle, revealing the entrances of the great veins and the exits of the arterial trunks. The reflections have been superimposed to show the boundaries of the cardiac hilums and the locations of the oblique and transverse sinuses.

are directly related to both of the pulmonary hilums, with the ***vagus nerve*** giving rise to its recurrent laryngeal nerve on both sides before continuing on to join the oesophagus (Figure 3.8). The ***phrenic nerves*** are more directly related to the pericardial sac, accompanied by the arteries and veins which directly supply the fibrous pericardium itself (Figure 3.9), the arteries being branches of the internal thoracic arteries.

Lubricating the space between the visceral and parietal layers of the serous pericardium is the ***pericardial fluid***. In healthy individuals, the fluid is between 15 and 50 ml of a plasma ultrafiltrate.[7,8] Pressure within the cavity is normally similar to pleural pressure, varying from around 6 mm of mercury at the end of inspiration to around 3 mm at the end of expiration.

Pericardiocentesis may be necessary for the resolution of large idiopathic pericardial effusions, particularly when recurrent, and especially in the presence of haemodynamic compromise should there be cardiac tamponade.[9] It is easiest to enter the space towards the cardiac apex, where the pericardial layers simply enclose the ventricular mass, having none of the complexities found at the cardiac base. The usual approach is through the left sternocostal triangle (Figure 3.10). Known also as Larrey's space, the triangle is bordered anteriorly by the left inferior sternocostal joints, by the diaphragm inferiorly, and by the apical layer of the pericardium superiorly.[10] The space itself is relatively avascular, but several arteries are found at its borders, of which the most vulnerable is probably the ***left superior epigastric artery***, which runs along its inferior and leftward border.

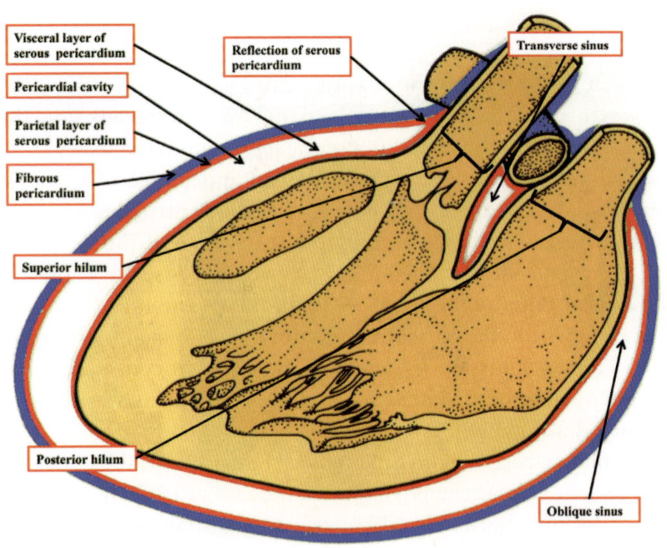

Figure 3.4. The drawing shows how the pericardial cavity is the space between the two layers of the serous pericardium, shown in red. The visceral layer of the serous pericardium is the epicardium, while the parietal layer lines the fibrous pericardial sac, which is shown in blue. The serous pericardium is reflected on itself at the exits of the arterial trunks, forming the superior cardiac hilum, and around the entrances of the systemic and pulmonary veins, forming the posterior cardiac hilum. There are two sinuses within the cavity: the oblique and transverse sinuses. The original drawing was made by Mrs Gemma Price and has been modified with her permission.

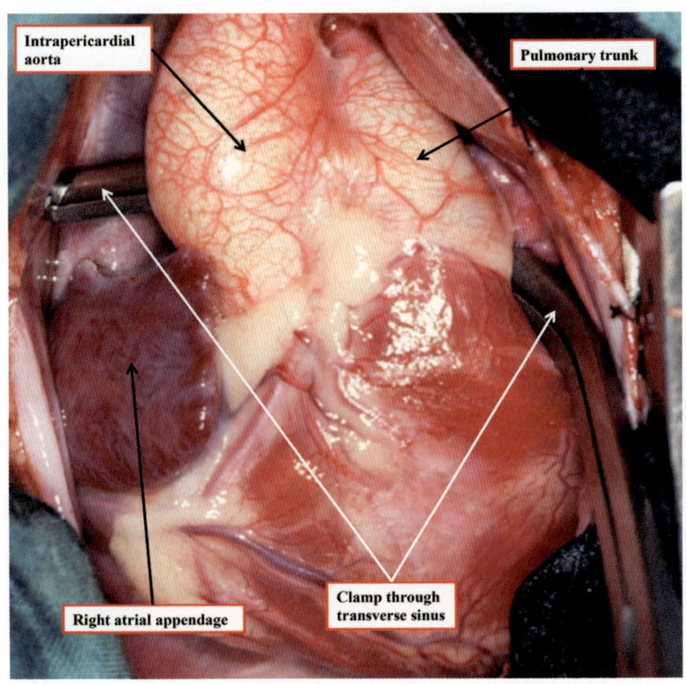

Figure 3.5. The picture was taken in the operating room by the late Benson R. Wilcox. It shows how a right-angled clamp has been passed through the transverse sinus of the pericardial cavity.

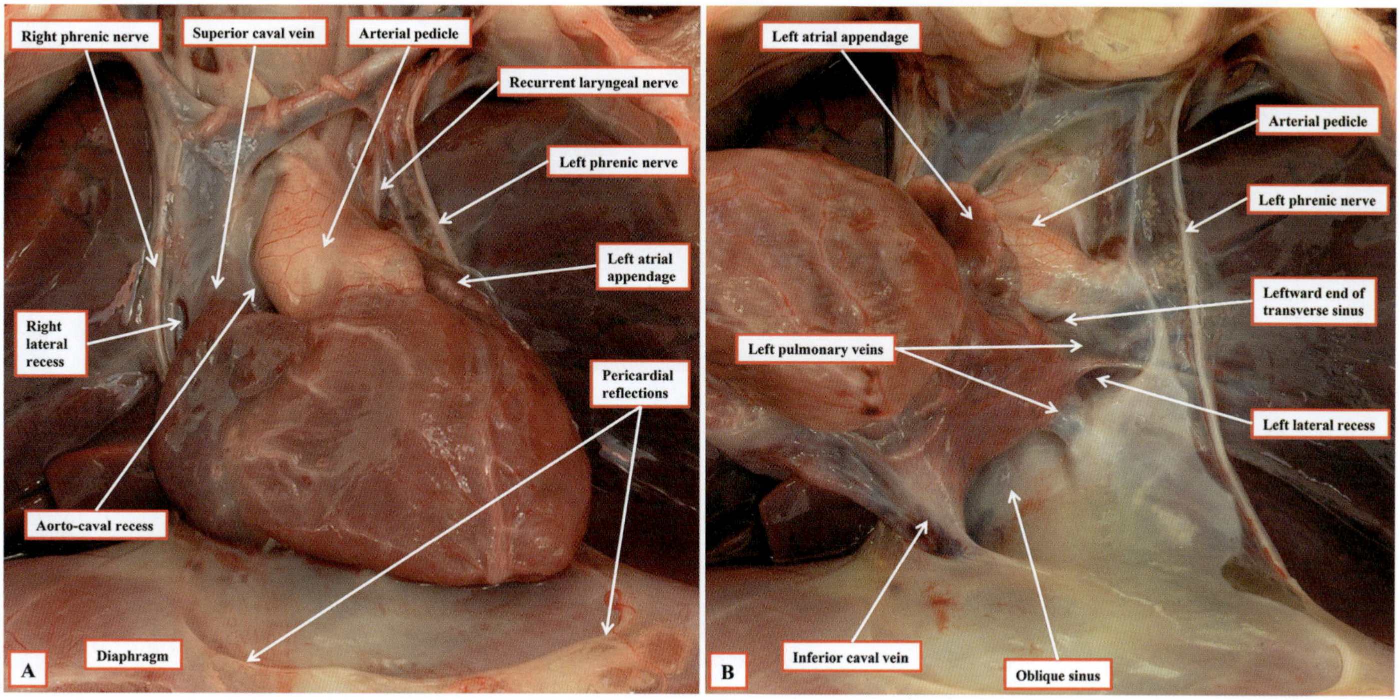

Figure 3.6. In this heart, the fibrous pericardium has been dissected away from its anterior surface. In panel A, which shows the heart as it lies in its pericardial cradle, it is possible to recognize the aorto-caval and right lateral recesses at the cardiac base. In panel B, the apex has been retracted superiorly to show the entrance to the oblique sinus and the left lateral recess. Note also the locations of the phrenic nerves.

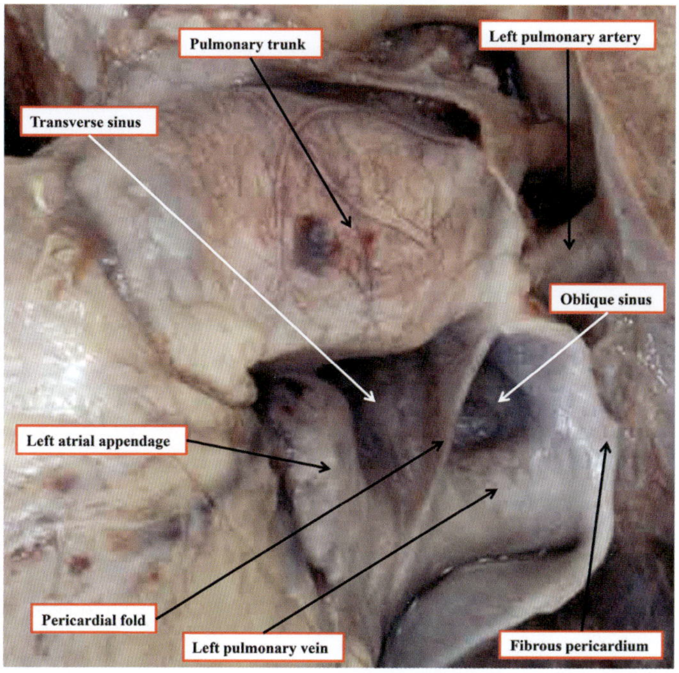

Figure 3.7. This view of the left side of the ventriculo-arterial and atrioventricular junctions shows the location of the oblique sinus and the pericardial fold that wraps itself around the ligament of Marshall. It is also possible to recognize the leftward end of the transverse sinus.

Entering the pericardial cavity has also now been used to carry out multiple ***electrophysiological*** and ***interventional procedures***.[11] In approximately one-tenth of patients with left ventricular non-ischaemic cardiomyopathies and ventricular tachycardia, the scar substrate is confined to the subepicardial and epicardial layers, predominantly in the basal lateral aspect of the left ventricle. Epicardial catheter ablation is indicated in this setting.[12,13] Ventricular tachycardia circuits in postmyocardial infarction patients are usually subendocardial, but in up to three-tenths of patients, when mid-myocardial or subepicardial, they too may require epicardial ablation.[14] For pericardial access, an anterior approach or a posterior approach can be used.[15] The anterior approach involves a shallow angle, of less than 45 degrees, to the skin, while the posterior approach involves a deeper angle, greater than 45 degrees. The anterior approach allows easier access to the anterior surface of the heart and ventricles and is the safer option. It is, nonetheless, associated with an increased risk of puncture of the superior epigastric artery or left internal thoracic artery. In certain situations, therefore, such as previous history of cardiac surgery involving a sternotomy, a posterior puncture approach is preferred. The posterior approach allows easier access to the inferior ventricular walls and posterior left atrial walls but has the potential for causing intra-abdominal bleeding through inadvertent puncture of the diaphragm and the subdiaphragmatic structures.[3] Epicardial access is also used for percutaneous closure of the left atrial appendage.[16]

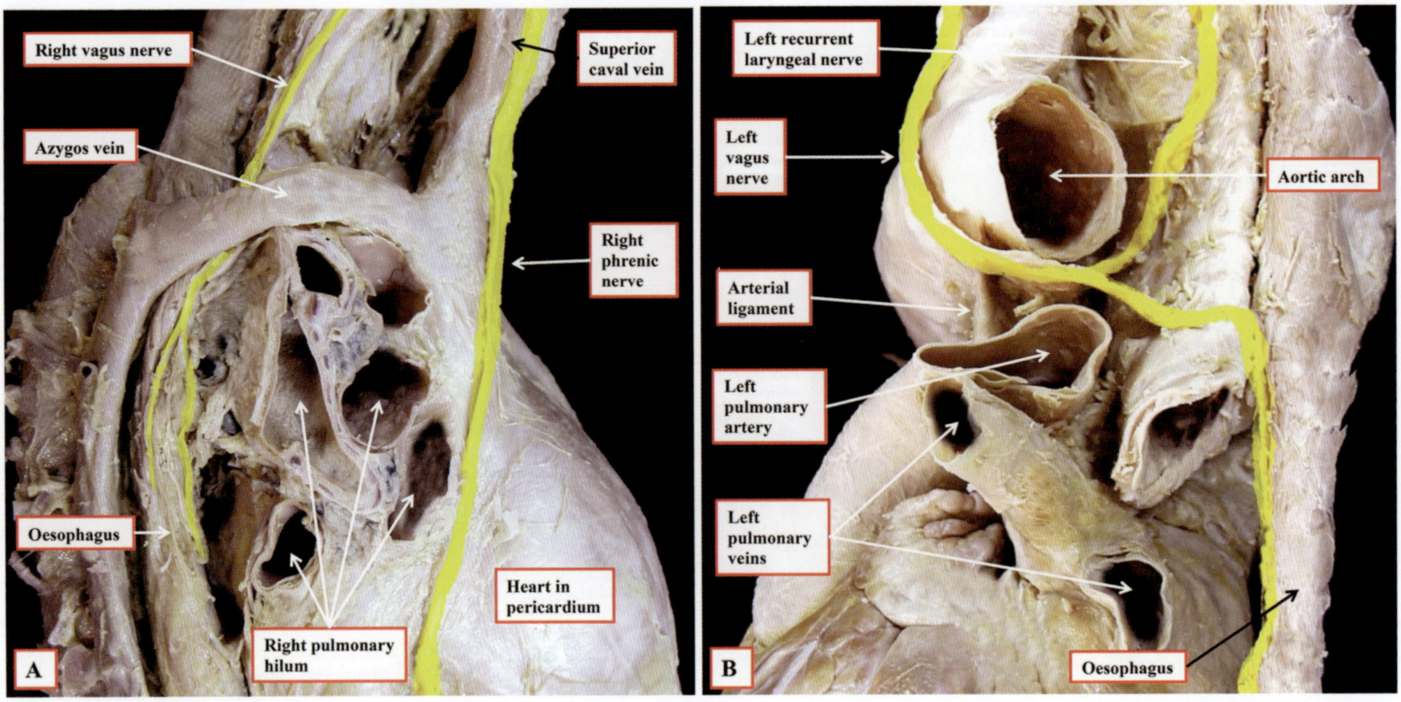

Figure 3.8. In these images, the right (panel A) and left (panel B) pulmonary hilums have been dissected to show the locations of, in panel A, of the right vagus and phrenic nerves, and, in panel B, the left vagus nerve giving off its recurrent laryngeal branch. Note how, on both sides, the vagus continues to accompany the oesophagus.

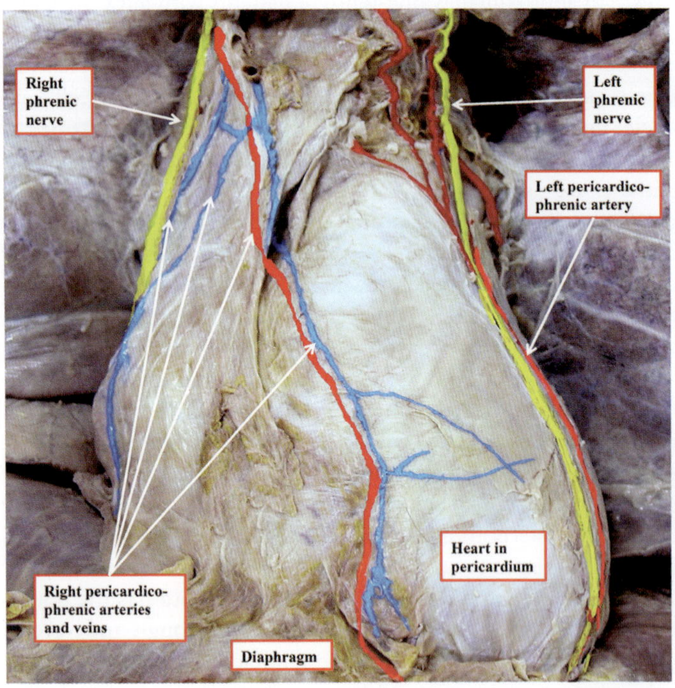

Figure 3.9. In this view of the heart also shown in Figure 3.1, the phrenic nerves have been marked in yellow, with the accompanying branches of the pericardiaco-phrenic arteries and veins coloured in red and blue, respectively.

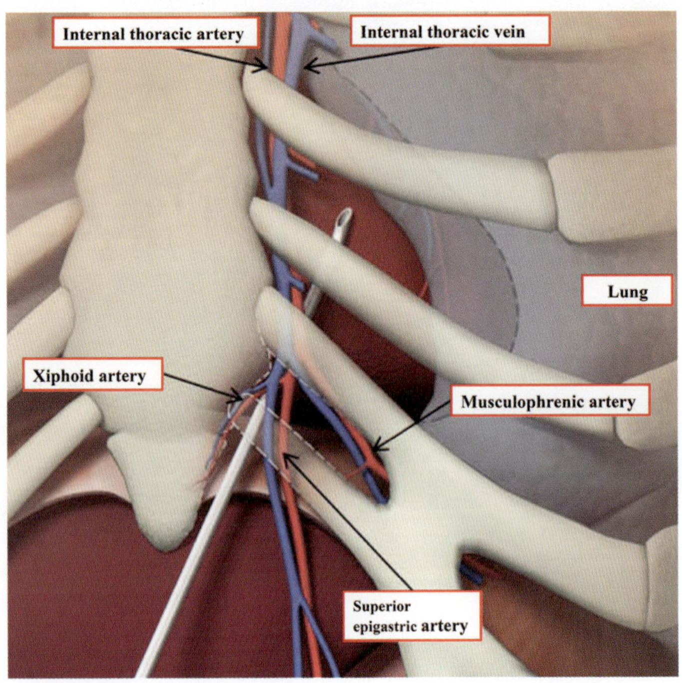

Figure 3.10. The drawing shows the location of the left inferior sternocostal triangle, also known as Larrey's triangle, and the potential dangers of those using the triangle to access the pericardial space due to the proximity of vascular structures.

REFERENCES

1. Mori S, Bradfield JS, Peacock WJ, Anderson RH, Shivkumar K. Living anatomy of the pericardial space: a guide for imaging and interventions. *JACC Clin Electrophysiol*. 2021;**7**:1628–1644. doi: 10.1016/j.jacep.2021.09.008
2. Mori S, Hanna P, Dacey MJ, Temma T, Hadaya J, Zhu C, Chang G, Peacock WJ, Fishbein MC, Shivkumar K. Comprehensive anatomy of the pericardial space and the cardiac hilum: anatomical dissections with intact pericardium. *JACC Cardiovasc Imaging*. 2022;**15**:927–942. doi: 10.1016/j.jcmg.2021.04.016
3. Aryana A, Tung R, d'Avila A. Percutaneous epicardial approach to catheter ablation of cardiac arrhythmias. *JACC Clin Electrophysiol*. 2020;**6**:1–20. doi: 10.1016/j.jacep.2019.10.016
4. Pauza DH, Pauziene N, Tamasauskas KA, Stropus R. Hilum of the heart. *Anat Rec*. 1997;**248**:322–324. doi: 10.1002/(SICI)1097-0185(199707)248:3<322::AID-AR3>3.0.CO;2-R
5. McAlpine WA. *Heart and Coronary Arteries: An Anatomical Atlas for Clinical Diagnosis, Radiological Investigation, and Surgical Treatment*. New York: Springer; 1975.
6. Bogaert J, Francone M. Cardiovascular magnetic resonance in pericardial diseases. *J Cardiovasc Magn Reson*. 2009;**11**:14. doi: 10.1186/1532-429X-11-14
7. Khandaker MH, Espinosa RE, Nishimura RA, Sinak LJ, Hayes SN, Melduni RM, Oh JK. Pericardial disease: diagnosis and management. *Mayo Clin Proc*. 2010;**85**:572–593. doi: 10.4065/mcp.2010.0046 S0025-6196(11)60350-9 [pii]
8. Troughton RW, Asher CR, Klein AL. Pericarditis. *Lancet*. 2004;**363**:717–727. doi: 10.1016/S0140-6736(04)15648-1 S0140-6736(04)15648-1 [pii]
9. Ristic AD, Imazio M, Adler Y, Anastasakis A, Badano LP, Brucato A, Caforio AL, Dubourg O, Elliott P, Gimeno J, et al. Triage strategy for urgent management of cardiac tamponade: a position statement of the European Society of Cardiology Working Group on Myocardial and Pericardial Diseases. *Eur Heart J*. 2014;**35**:2279–2284. doi: 10.1093/eurheartj/ehu217
10. Toth I, Rami-Porta R, Rendeki S, Molnar TF. First steps in the management of pericardial effusion: who was first to relieve the pericardial sac—Larrey or Romero? *World J Surg*. 2013;**37**:2242–2245. doi: 10.1007/s00268-013-2115-5
11. Sosa E, Scanavacca M, d'Avila A, Pilleggi F. A new technique to perform epicardial mapping in the electrophysiology laboratory. *J Cardiovasc Electrophysiol*. 1996;**7**:531–536. doi: 10.1111/j.1540-8167.1996.tb00559.x
12. Liuba I, Muser D, Chahal A, Tschabrunn C, Santangeli P, Kuo L, Frankel DS, Callans DJ, Garcia F, Supple GE, et al. Substrate characterization and outcome of catheter ablation of ventricular tachycardia in patients with nonischemic cardiomyopathy and isolated epicardial scar. *Circ Arrhythm Electrophysiol*. 2021;**14**:e010279. doi: 10.1161/CIRCEP.121.010279
13. Darma A, Bertagnolli L, Weber A, Dinov B, Torri F, Lurz JA, Shamloo AS, Dagres N, Bollmann A, Hindricks G, et al. Epicardial ablation of ventricular tachycardia in patients with structural heart disease: a single-centre experience over 12 years. *Europace*. 2021;**23**:1980–1988. doi: 10.1093/europace/euab194
14. Di Biase L, Santangeli P, Burkhardt DJ, Bai R, Mohanty P, Carbucicchio C, Dello Russo A, Casella M, Mohanty S, Pump A, et al. Endo-epicardial homogenization of the scar versus limited substrate ablation for the treatment of electrical storms in patients with ischemic cardiomyopathy. *J Am Coll Cardiol*. 2012;**60**:132–141. doi: 10.1016/j.jacc.2012.03.044
15. Kumareswaran R, Marchlinski FE. Practical guide to ablation for epicardial ventricular tachycardia: when to get access, how to deal with anticoagulation and how to prevent complications. *Arrhythm Electrophysiol Rev*. 2018;**7**:159–164. doi: 10.15420/aer.2018.10.2
16. Abibe Goia A, Xu M, Qiuming H. Long-term outcomes of left atrial appendage closure techniques on stroke prevention of recurrent atrial fibrillation patients: epicardial excision versus percutaneous occlusion. *Front Cardiovasc Med*. 2025;**12**:1601303. doi: 10.3389/fcvm.2025.1601303

4

The Right Atrium

When assessed in terms of their development, each atrial chamber is derived initially from the atrial component of the primary heart tube. This provides their bodies, but the larger part is committed to the left atrium. Very little of the body, therefore, is seen in the morphologically right atrium. Each atrium also possesses an appendage, which balloons from the body, a vestibule, derived from the atrioventricular canal myocardium, and a venous component. The two chambers are then separated one from the other by the septal components (Figure 4.1).[1] Opening the right atrium through a long incision along its extensive lateral wall and folding back the wall reveals the postnatal arrangement of these developmental components (Figure 4.2).

The large part is occupied by the ***appendage***. Its extent is revealed by the pectinate muscles observed on its endocardial surface. Its triangular shape is immediately recognizable when viewed from the epicardial aspect (Figure 4.3). When viewed from this perspective, the appendage can be seen to form almost the entirety of the lateral wall of the chamber, extending anteriorly from

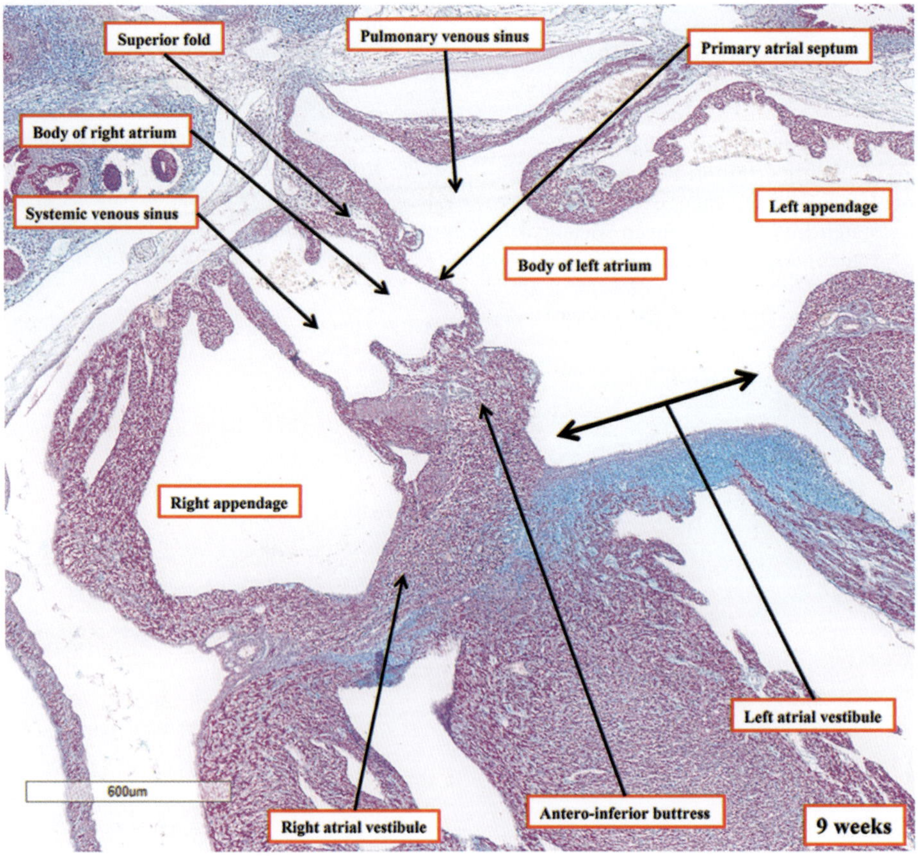

Figure 4.1. The image shows a frontal section from a human fetus at 9 weeks of gestation. It is possible to recognize all the developmental components of the atrial chambers, namely a body, most of which is committed to the left atrium, a venous component, a vestibule, and an appendage. The chambers are separated by the atrial septum, which is largely formed by the component derived from the primary septum, but reinforced by an antero-inferior buttress. The superior margin of the oval fossa, often described as the "septum secundum", can be seen to be no more than a deep interatrial fold.

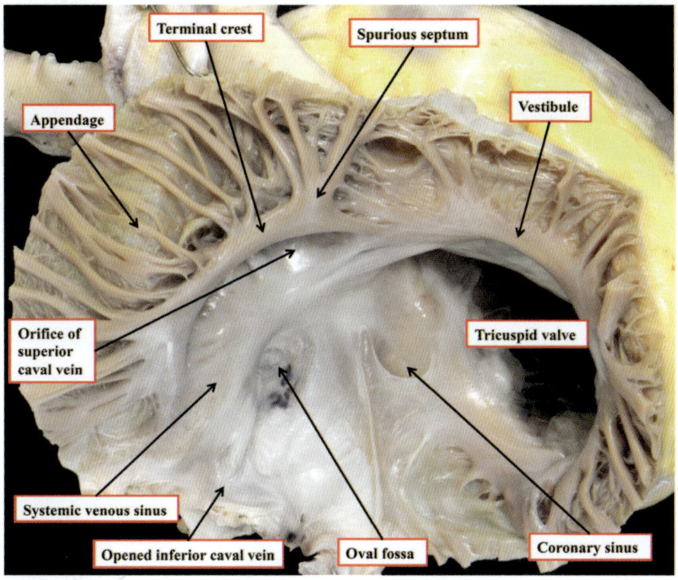

Figure 4.2. The morphologically right atrium has been opened by making a long incision parallel to the terminal groove marking the boundary between the appendage and the systemic venous sinus, with this being marked internally by the terminal crest. The pectinate muscles within the appendage are separated from the hinges of the antero-superior and -inferior leaflets of the tricuspid valve by the smooth-walled vestibule. The opening of the inferior caval vein is guarded by the Eustachian valve, with the Thebesian valve guarding the opening of the coronary sinus.

the terminal groove, which marks its boundary with the systemic venous sinus.

The groove corresponds internally with the location of the ***terminal crest***, or ***crista terminalis*** (Figure 4.4). The ***pectinate muscles*** extend at right angles from the terminal crest, which runs vertically, onto the wall of the appendage. One of the muscles is particularly prominent superiorly and anteriorly. It spans the cavity as the spurious septum, or ***septum spurium*** (Figure 4.2).

The ***sinus node*** is located within the terminal crest. It extends subepicardially in a cigar-like fashion for around 2–3 cm (Figures 4.3, 4.4, 4.5). It has irregular margins and is not insulated by a sheath of fibrous tissue.[2] Instead, its histologically specialized cardiomyocytes merge at the margins of the node with the muscular sleeve of the superior caval vein and with the working myocardium of the terminal crest.

The node, in most individuals, is located with its head just inferior to the crest of the appendage, with its tail running within the groove towards the orifice of the inferior caval vein.[2] In around one-tenth of individuals, however, the node extends across the appendage to merge with the working myocardium of the interatrial groove.[3] In its more usual position, the nodal cells merge at the margins of the node with the working cardiomyocytes of the terminal crest. These cells of the crest are themselves aggregated together in parallel fashion, underscoring the preferential conduction known to occur along its long axis inferiorly towards the cavotricuspid isthmus.

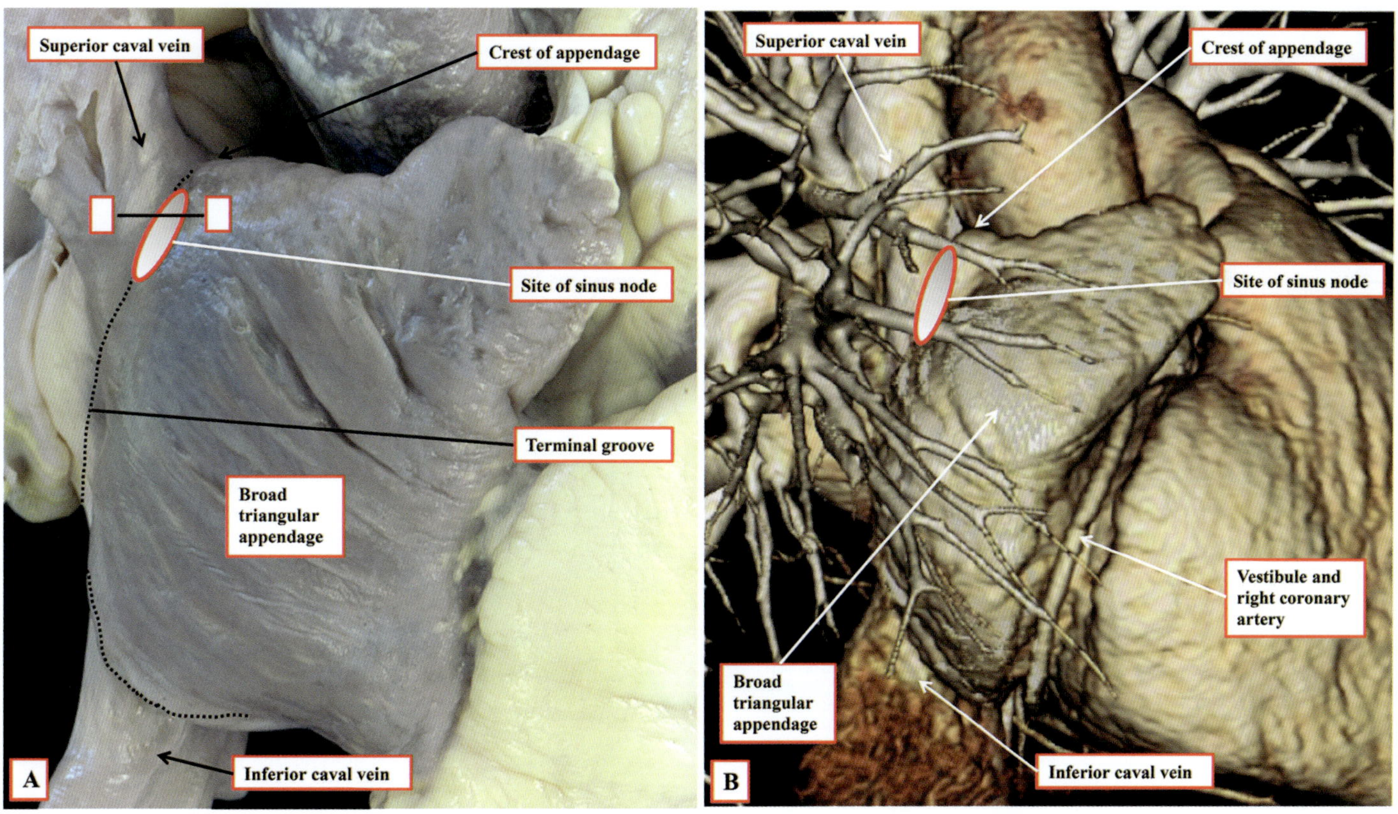

Figure 4.3. Panel A shows a photograph of the heart taken from the right side. It reveals how the appendage forms the entirety of the lateral wall of the right atrial chamber, with the terminal groove marking its posterior boundary with the systemic venous sinus. The anticipated location of the sinus node, which lies subepicardially within the groove, is marked by the oval. The line connecting the two boxes shows the plane of a section taken to reveal the arrangement of the node, as portrayed in the histological image shown in Figure 4.5. Note that the plane of section is horizontal when making comparisons with Figure 4.5. Panel B is a reconstruction from a computed tomographic dataset in comparable orientation to panel A. It shows how the anatomy can now be displayed with just as much accuracy during life as when the morphologist holds the heart in their hands.

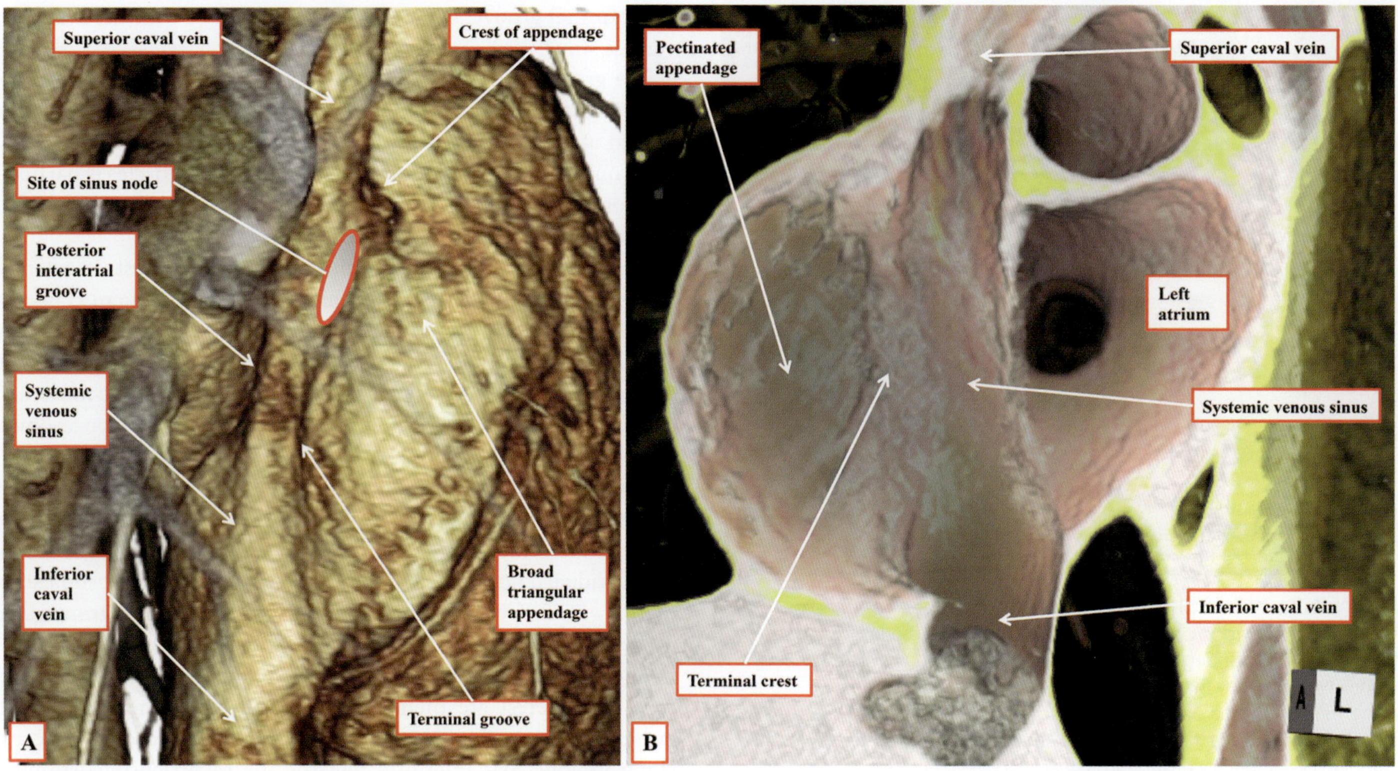

Figure 4.4. The images, as with Figure 4.3B, are prepared from computed tomographic datasets obtained from living patients. They show the boundaries of the systemic venous sinus, with panel A showing a reconstruction of the cavities viewed from the right side and panel B showing a virtual dissection seen in left lateral projection.

When traced superiorly, the crest, retaining the parallel aggregation of its cardiomyocytes, passes in front of the orifice of the superior caval vein as the ***precaval band***. This part of the crest then merges with the anterior part of the superior interatrial groove, still with the cardiomyocytes aggregated in parallel fashion, to produce the preferential pathway for conduction from the sinus node to the left atrium known as ***Bachmann's bundle*** (Figures 4.6, 4.7).[4] Changes in orientation and thickness at the boundary of these bundles may lead

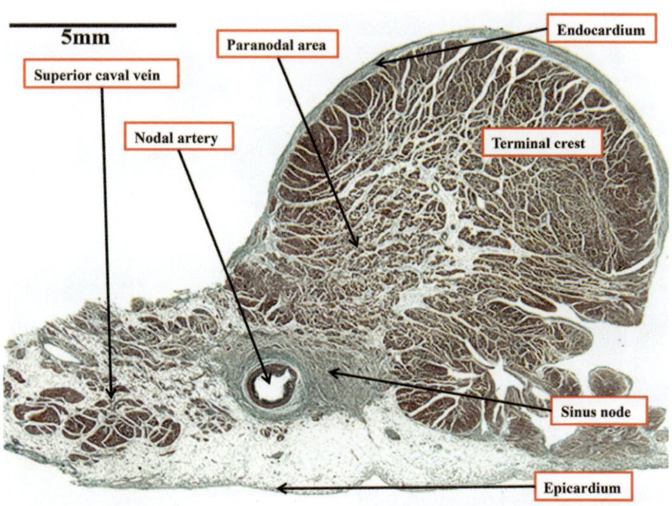

Figure 4.5. The image shows a histological section taken along the plane shown by the two boxes in Figure 4.3. The section comes from a different heart. It reveals the location of the body of the sinus node and its junctions with the working myocardium of the terminal crest and the superior caval vein. Note the paranodal area within the myocardium of the terminal crest. The potential significance of this area will be discussed in the chapter devoted specifically to the conduction system (Chapter 12).

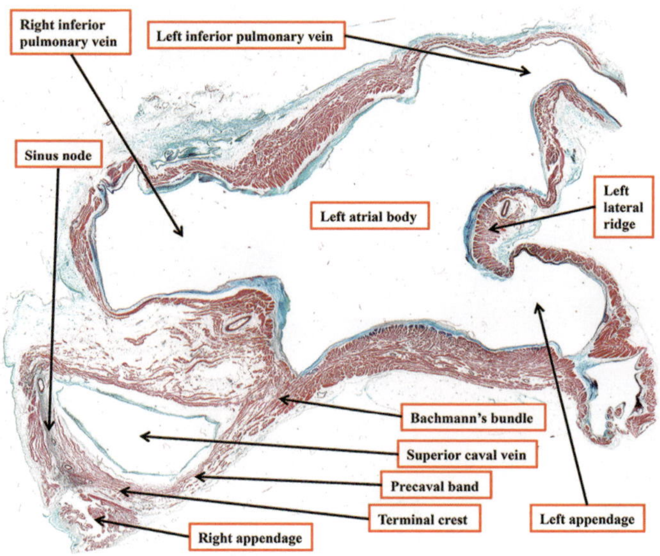

Figure 4.6. The image shows a transverse histological section taken through both atrial chambers at the level of the superior cavoatrial junction. It shows how the terminal crest continues in front of the orifice of the superior caval vein, with its cardiomyocytes aggregated together in parallel fashion, continuing into the walls of the left atrium as Bachmann's bundle.

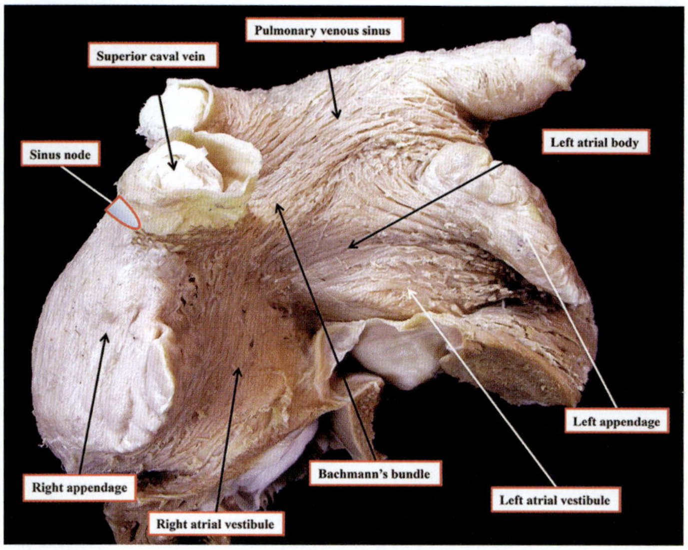

Figure 4.7. The dissection, made by removing the epicardium from the anterior interatrial groove and the walls of the left atrium, shows how the aggregated working atrial cardiomyocytes provide a direct path from the location of the sinus node in the terminal groove to the body, vestibule, and pulmonary venous component of the left atrium.

to conduction block during the propagation of sinus rhythm or provide the substrate for atrial arrhythmias.[5] Traditionally, atrial pacing has been conducted by placing the lead in the right atrial appendage. This produces an increase in the interatrial delay, as indicated by a wider P wave than observed during sinus rhythm. This approach is recognized as being associated with an increased risk of developing atrial fibrillation.[6]

Specific pacing of Bachmann's bundle has now become recognized as a promising modality, which theoretically might restore biatrial resynchronization and reduce atrial arrhythmias.[7,8] This is achieved, when pacing from the right atrium, by placing the lead within the infero-septal superior cavoatrial junction (Figure 4.8). If the lead is placed low within the anterior interatrial groove, there is the danger of impacting the aortic root. Placing the lead more cranially and posteriorly should avoid the danger of entering the ascending aorta (Figure 4.8 panel B). The technique is particularly attractive when pacing is required subsequent to cardiac surgery, should the right atrial appendage have been partially excised for implementation of cardiopulmonary bypass.

At the caudal end of the sinus node, within the adipose tissues occupying the terminal groove, is located the ***anterior right ganglionated plexus***. As part of the intrinsic cardiac autonomic nervous system, the plexus may modulate the sinus rate.[9] Specific ablation of the ganglionated plexuses has been used as an adjunct to ablation

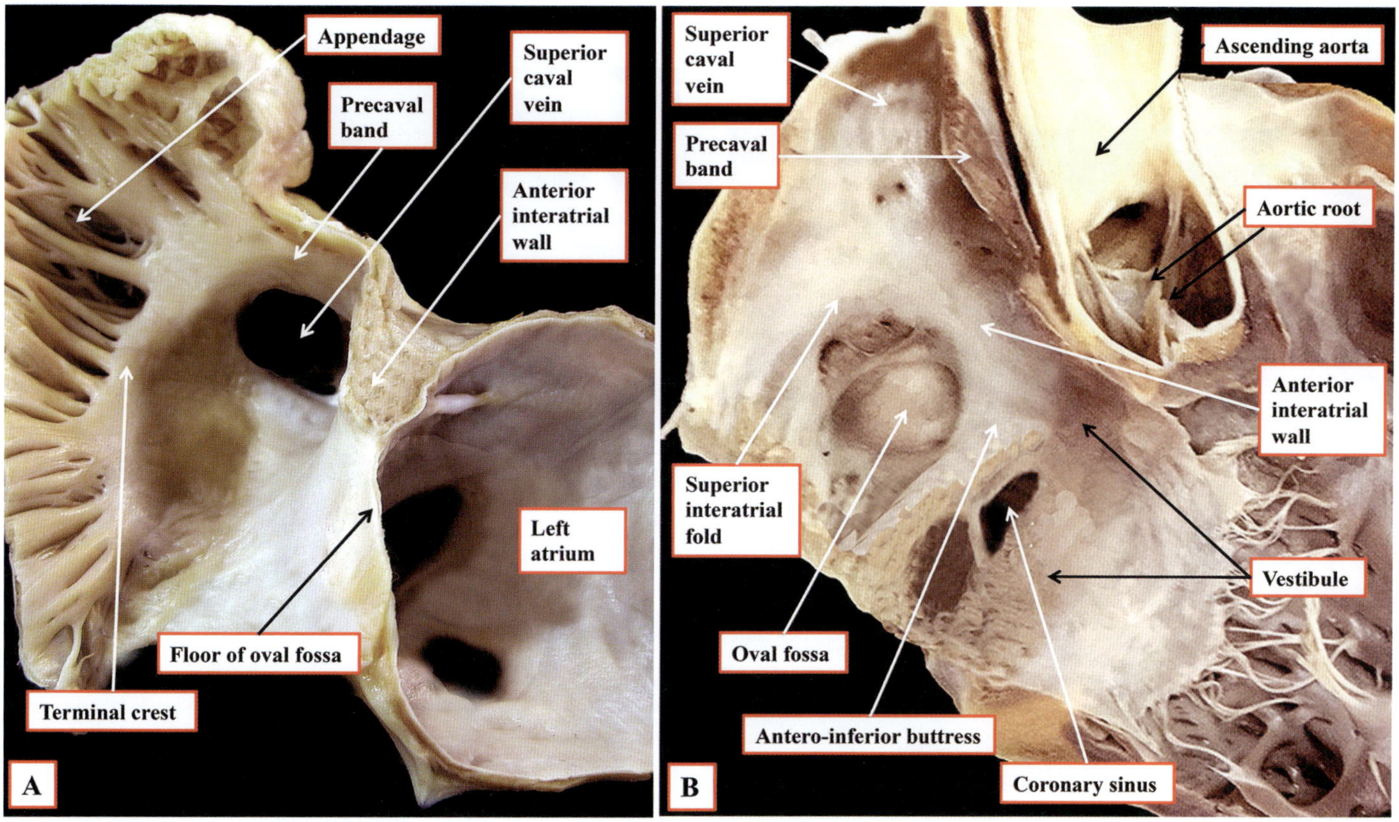

Figure 4.8. Panel A, which is a view of the superior cavoatrial junction taken from beneath looking towards the head, shows how the terminal crest continues in front of the orifice of the superior caval vein, merging with the anterior interatrial wall. As was shown in Figures 4.6 and 4.7, it is the parallel aggregation of the cardiomyocytes within the anterior interatrial wall that produces Bachmann's bundle. Panel B shows the septal surface of the right atrium, emphasizing the close relationship between the anterior interatrial wall to the aortic root and the ascending aorta. It is the vestibular component of the anterior wall, however, that is most closely related to the aortic components. Pacing leads placed more posteriorly around the superior cavoatrial junction in attempts to capture Bachmann's bundle would be less likely to engage the ascending aorta.

of the pulmonary veins during treatment of atrial fibrillation.[10] Circumferential isolation of the pulmonary veins itself may also result in coincidental modification of the plexuses.[11] Ablation of the anterior right ganglionated plexus, however, has been shown to have short-term, rather than long-term, effects on the structure and function of the sinus node. The ablative approaches to atrial fibrillation, therefore, are safe in this respect.[12] The electrical activity of the sinus node itself, and its related arrhythmias, are discussed in detail in Chapter 12 devoted specifically to the conduction system.

Throughout its length, the terminal crest, also known as the ***crista terminalis***, marks the border between the pectinated wall of the appendage and the extensive systemic venous component spanning between the caval veins, with the latter part being smooth-walled (**Figures 4.2, 4.4**).[13] As already emphasized, the most prominent pectinate muscle, known as the spurious septum or ***septum spurium*** (**Figures 4.2, 4.9**), takes its origin from the precaval component of the crest. When traced inferiorly, the crest supports the remnant of the embryonic right venous valve. This is the ***Eustachian valve***, which guards in part the orifice of the inferior caval vein as it, too, enters the systemic venous sinus (**Figure 4.10**). Although the working cardiomyocytes within the terminal crest are aggregated together in parallel fashion, thus favouring preferential conduction,[4,9] the poor transverse cell-to-cell coupling means that the crest, at the sites of origin of the pectinate muscles, is also an area of marked electrical anisotropy.[14] Most *right atrial arrhythmias* arise along the crest. Less commonly, arrhythmias can originate from sites along the tricuspid vestibule in substrates with a scar or previous incisional atrial lesions, but particularly in older people when they can occur in the absence of apparent abnormalities.[15] Other possible right atrial sites of arrhythmic origin include the orifice of the coronary sinus and the perinodal or para-Hisian region. Atrial tachycardias arising near the atrioventricular node, which itself cannot currently be identified by available mapping technology in the human, are of particular interest. They are usually re-entrant and sensitive to adenosine or verapamil. This makes it difficult to differentiate them from junctional tachycardias.[16,17] Their attempted catheter ablation may produce inadvertent complete heart block, since the distance of the mapped tachycardia from the His bundle electrograms may convey an illusionary sense of safety.[18]

Assessment of the right atrial cavity from the endocardial aspect reveals that, although the pectinate muscles encircle the entirety of the parietal margins of the right atrioventricular junction, they do not reach to the hinge of the valvar leaflets. This is because the smooth-walled ***vestibule*** interposes between the pectinated area and the valvar hinges (**Figures 4.2, 4.9, 4.10**). It is the extent of the pectinate muscles relative to the vestibules that serves to distinguish morphologically between the right and left atriums when the heart is congenitally malformed. The extent of the vestibule itself is well seen anteriorly (**Figure 4.11**). When traced posteriorly and inferiorly, the pectinate muscles reach to the orifice of the inferior caval vein (**Figure 4.2, 4.10**). They then continue further onto the septal aspect, where they run into the sub-Thebesian sinus (**Figure 4.12**). This pectinated inferior area of the septal aspect of the right atrium is an integral part of the ***cavotricuspid isthmus*** (**Figures 4.11, 4.12**).

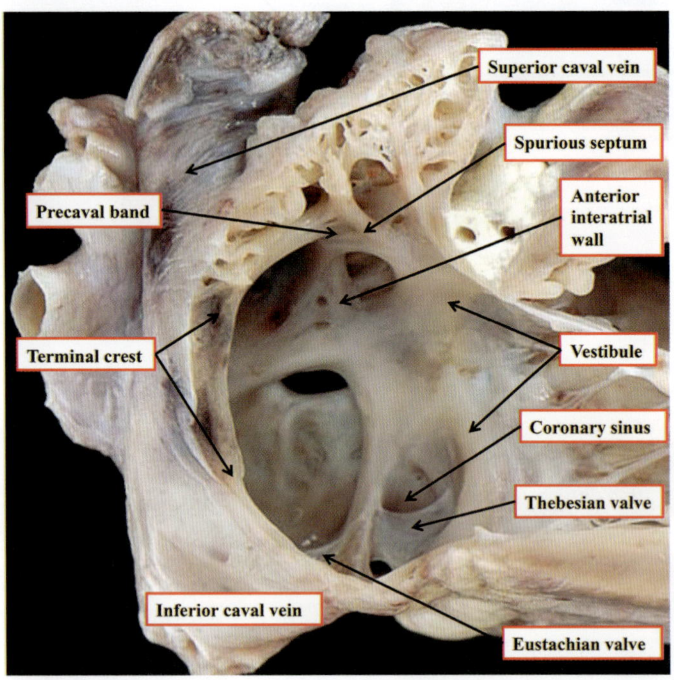

Figure 4.9. The image shows again how the terminal crest, marking the border between the appendage and the smooth-walled systemic venous component, continues cranially in front of the orifice of the superior caval vein as the precaval band to reach, and merge with, the anterior interatrial fold. As it passes in front of the cavoatrial junction, it also gives rise to the prominent pectinate muscle known as the "septum spurium" or the spurious septum.

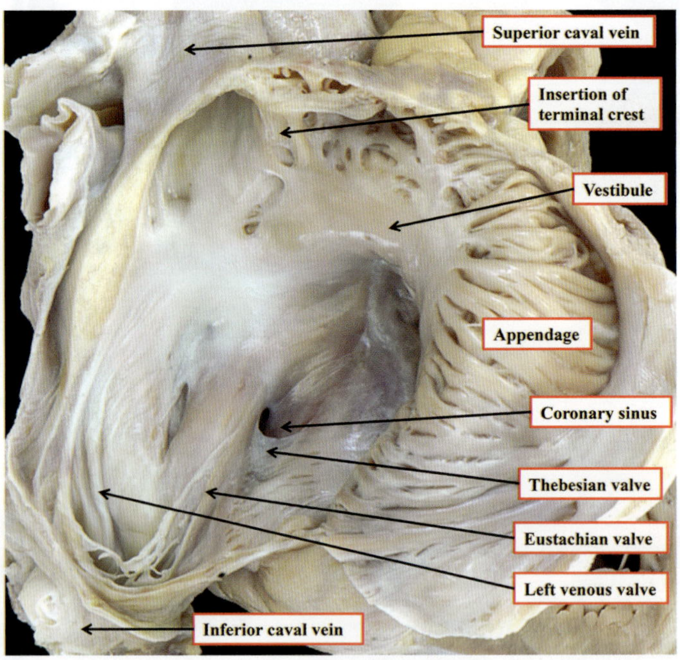

Figure 4.10. In this heart, the right atrium has been opened by making a cut through the terminal crest. The dissection shows that, when traced caudally, the crest supports the Eustachian valve, which guards the orifice of the inferior caval vein. When traced leftward in from the orifice of the superior caval vein, the crest inserts into the anterior interatrial groove, where it continues into the walls of the left atrium as Bachmann's bundle (see Figures 4.6 and 4.7). In this heart it is also possible to recognize the left venous valve, permitting recognition of the small part of the body that extends between the valve and the septum.

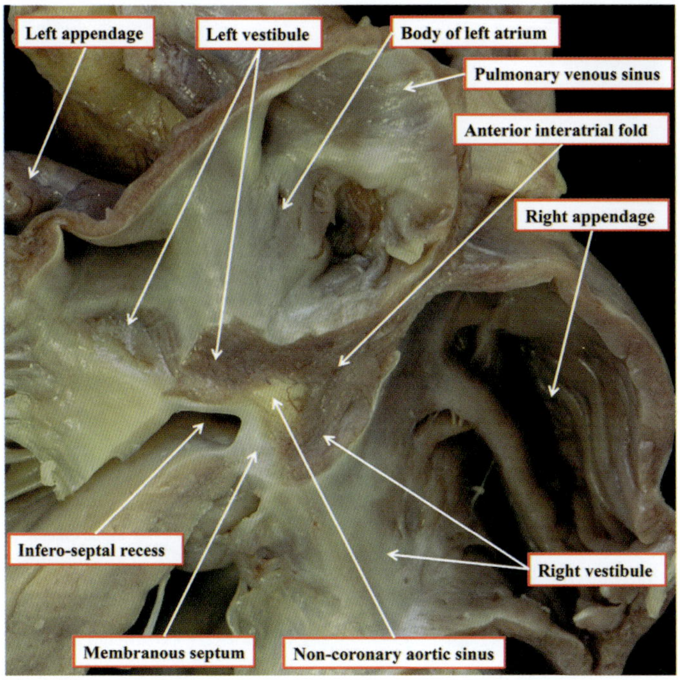

Figure 4.11. The heart has been sectioned in the frontal plane and the anterior part photographed from behind. The image shows how the vestibular myocardium on both sides inserts into the atrioventricular junctions, separating on the right side the pectinate muscles of the appendage from the hinge of the antero-superior leaflet of the tricuspid valve.

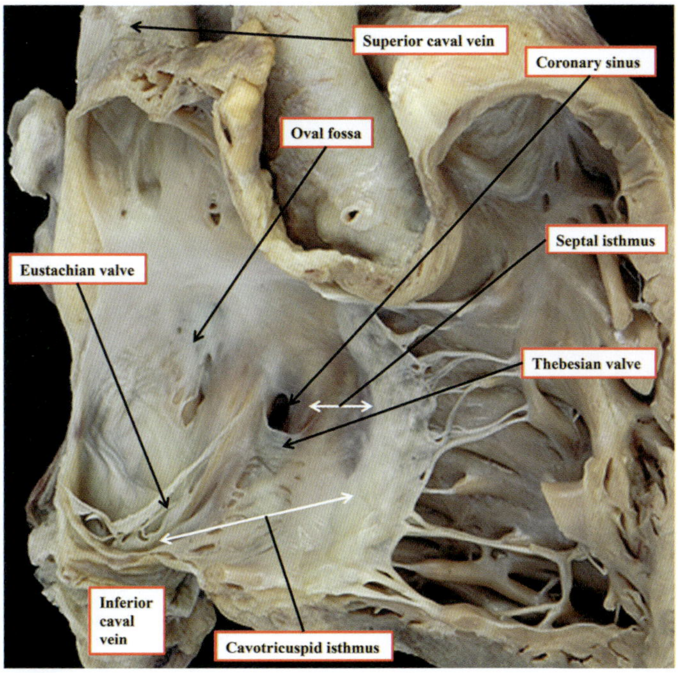

Figure 4.12. The septal surface of the right atrium has been revealed by removing the parietal wall. This shows the location of the cavotricuspid isthmus, between the orifice of the inferior caval vein and the hinge of the septal leaflet of the tricuspid valve. Note also the presence of a second septal isthmus between the orifice of the coronary sinus and the hinge of the septal leaflet.

The non-uniform arrangement of the terminal ramifications of the terminal crest may account for delay and discontinuity in the spread of the excitatory wavefront that uses the isthmus as part of the circuit for atrial flutter.[19] The pectinated area makes up the largest middle part of the isthmus, but it also has a smooth anterior myocardial component, which is part of the atrial vestibule, and a posterior fibrous part, where the isthmus abuts the wall of the inferior caval vein (Figure 4.13).[20,21]

The typical form of *cavotricuspid isthmus-dependent flutter* can run in counter-clockwise or clockwise fashion (Figure 4.14).[22] The circuit has a strong reproducible anatomical dependence, rotating around the orifice of the inferior caval vein instead of around the right atrioventricular junction,[23] and in turn providing the morphological electrocardiographic reproducibility.[24,25] The finding of an atypical electrocardiogram, nonetheless, does not exclude cavotricuspid isthmus-dependent flutter, especially after extensive left atrial ablation.[26] When considering the circuits themselves, in the *lower-loop re-entry* variant the pathway rotates around the orifice of the inferior caval vein. In the *figure-of-eight double-loop re-entry* variant, the circuit also includes the orifice of the tricuspid valve, mimicking the typical clockwise atrial flutter, as well as other circuits which use parts of the cavotricuspid isthmus.[27–29] Cavotricuspid isthmus-dependent flutter is also the most common arrhythmia in patients with transposition treated using the atrial switch operation.[30] All these arrhythmias respond to ablation of the isthmus with resultant bidirectional conduction block. It follows that a clear understanding of the underlying anatomy (Figures 4.12, 4.13) is required if the ablation is to be successful, and also to avoid the inferior extensions of the atrioventricular node.

The need to avoid the nodal extensions focuses attention on a second significant isthmus, discrete from the cavotricuspid isthmus, which is found on the septal aspect of the right atrium (Figure 4.12). This ***septal isthmus*** is the area between the orifice of the coronary sinus and the hinge of the septal leaflet of the tricuspid valve. It represents the optimal site for ablation of atrioventricular nodal re-entrant tachycardia.[31,32] Although the vestibular myocardium is composed of working rather than specialized cardiomyocytes, the area in question forms part of the base of the ***triangle of Koch*** (Figure 4.15), with this crucial area containing both the atrioventricular node (Figure 4.16) and its extensions, which are made up of specialized cardiomyocytes.

The triangle itself is the right atrial wall of a pyramidal superior extension of the inferior atrioventricular groove known as the inferior pyramidal space.[33,34] The right atrial wall, which provides the

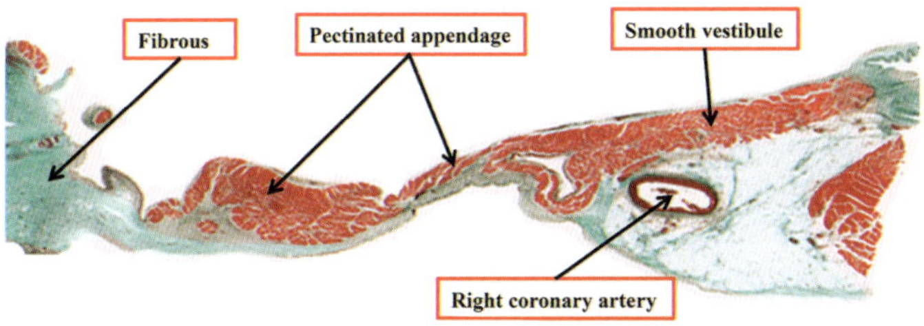

Figure 4.13. This histological section through the cavotricuspid isthmus reveals that it is made up of a posterior fibrous component, a middle pectinated part, and an anterior smooth part, with the latter being part of the septal component of the atrial vestibule.

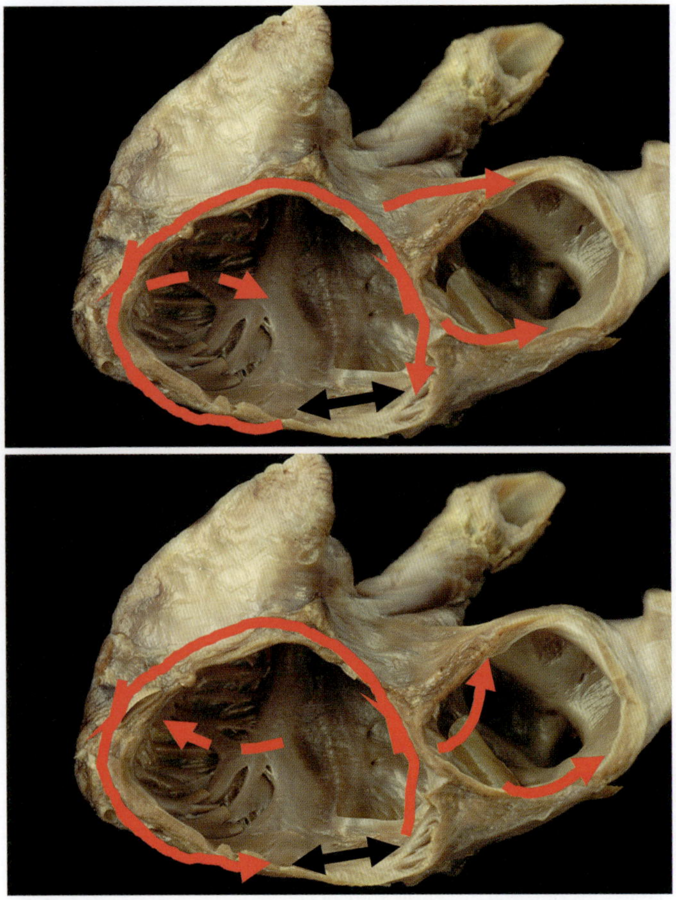

Figure 4.14. The drawings show the usual anticlockwise and the reverse circuits for atrial flutter (red arrows) depending on involvement of the cavotricuspid isthmus (double-headed black arrows). The lower panel shows the common anticlockwise variant, with the upper panel showing the clockwise version. The atrioventricular junctions are shown in the left anterior oblique view.

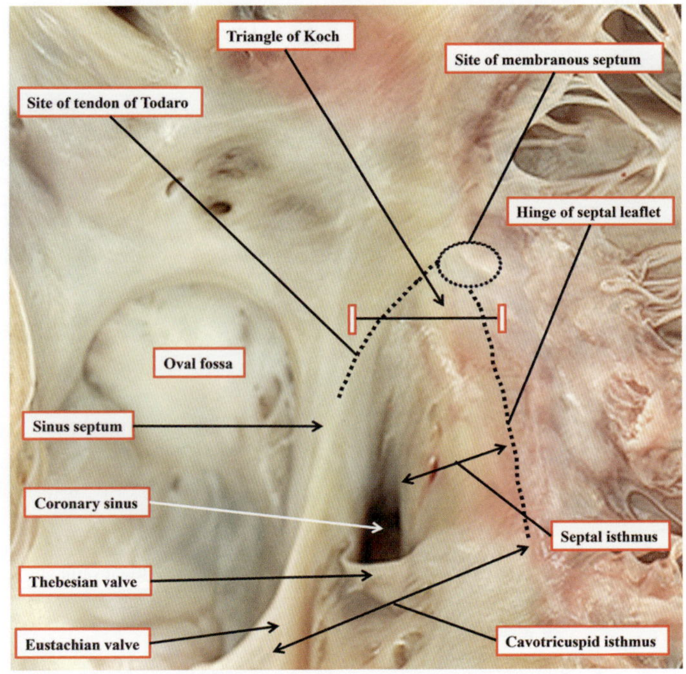

Figure 4.15. The image shows the location of the triangle of Koch on the septal aspect of the right atrial cavity. The line between the two white columns with red borders shows the site of a section through the atrioventricular node (see Figure 4.16). Note the location of the cavotricuspid and septal isthmuses.

anatomical landmark for the location of the atrioventricular node, includes not only that part of the vestibule that is located anterior-superior to the orifice of the coronary sinus, but also the myocardium of the antero-inferior buttress of the atrial septum (Figure 4.15). The posterior border of the triangle of Koch is the ***tendon of Todaro***, which forms its hypotenuse. The tendon is a fibrous structure (Figure 4.17). It is the continuation of the commissure between the ***Eustachian*** and ***Thebesian valves***. It buries itself within the so-called ***Eustachian ridge***, which is the fold of myocardium between the orifices of the inferior caval vein and the coronary sinus. Having buried itself within the myocardium, the tendon extends superiorly to insert into the ***membranous septum*** (Figure 4.17).

The anterior border of the triangle is formed by the hinge of the septal leaflet of the tricuspid valve, with the orifice of the coronary sinus marking its base (Figures 4.15, 4.18). The apex of the triangle is formed by the membranous septum. It used to be thought that the floor of the triangle was an atrioventricular muscular septum, but the epicardial fat of the inferior pyramidal space is interposed between the atrial wall and the underlying ventricular myocardium at its base. The ***compact atrioventricular node***, located towards the apex of the triangle within the antero-inferior buttress of the atrial septum, is supported by the insulating atrioventricular fibrous tissues of the central fibrous body (Figure 4.16). As will be discussed further in Chapter 6, devoted to the atrioventricular junctions, this part of the central fibrous body is an area of continuity between the leaflets of the mitral and tricuspid valves. The superior apex of the inferior pyramidal space, formed by this area of fibrous tissue, is

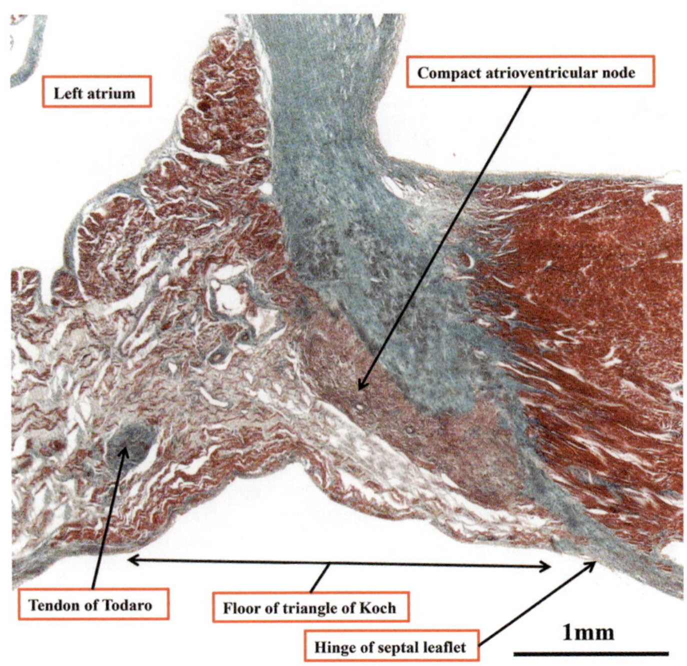

Figure 4.16. The image shows the location of the compact atrioventricular node at the level of the line shown in Figure 4.15.

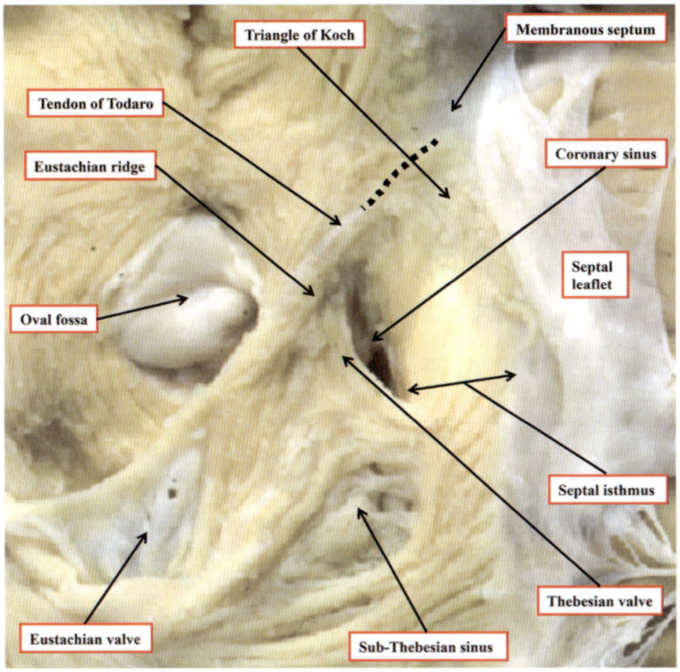

Figure 4.17. The right atrial endocardium has been removed in this heart to show the aggregation of the working cardiomyocytes. It also shows how the commissure of the Eustachian and Thebesian valves becomes the tendon of Todaro (black dotted line), which embeds itself into the myocardium of the Eustachian ridge before inserting into the membranous septum.

juxtaposed on the other side of the septum with the inferior extent of the infero-septal recess of the left ventricular outflow tract (Figure 4.18). The atrioventricular conduction axis traverses between the two spaces as it becomes insulated by the fibrous tissues of the atrioventricular junctions to become the ***non-branching bundle***, which is usually described as the bundle of His (Figure 4.19). The electrical activity of the atrioventricular node and its related arrhythmias are discussed in detail Chapter 12, devoted specifically to the conduction system.

When viewed from the atrial cavity, it seems that an extensive posterior part of the right atrial walls borders on the cavity of the left atrium (Figure 4.9). The ***true septum*** between the two cavities, however, is not nearly as extensive as generally believed.[35] Only the floor of the oval fossa, derived from the ***primary atrial septum***, or "***septum primum***", and its ***antero-inferior buttress***, which then represents a true ***second atrial septum***, are made up of walls that directly separate the atrial cavities (Figure 4.20). The superior margin of the oval fossa, previously described incorrectly as the "septum secundum", can be seen to be no more than a deep interatrial fold (Figure 4.1). Along with the remainder of the rims of the oval fossa, it is filled with extracavitary adipose tissue (Figure 4.21). Apart from the antero-inferior buttress, the remainder of the rims of the oval fossa are infoldings of the atrial walls, with the folds filled with extracavitary adipose tissue (Figure 4.21). The area between the mouth of the inferior caval vein and the orifice of the coronary sinus, often described as the ***sinus septum***, is likewise an infolding of the atrial walls. The atrial vestibule, as it extends from the inferior part of the atrioventricular junction, seemingly to become

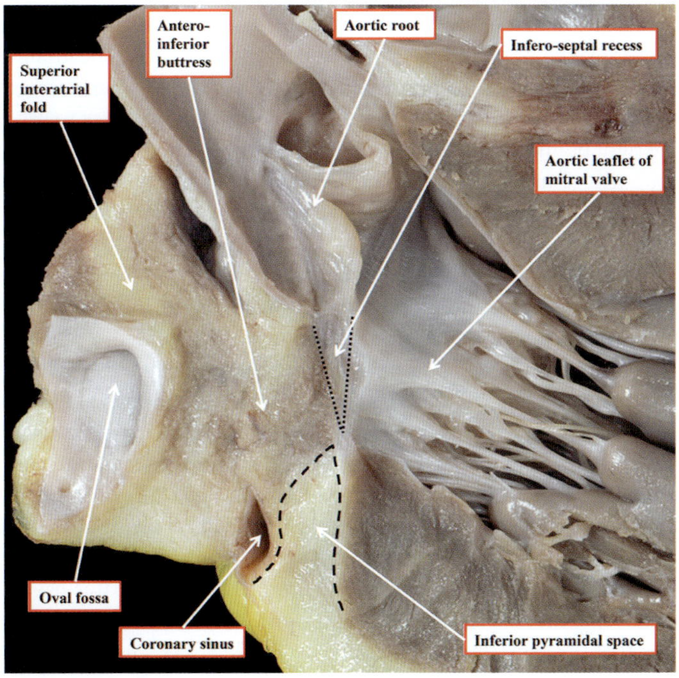

Figure 4.18. The image is a section taken through the triangle of Koch, cutting through into the cavity of the left ventricle. It shows how the superior apex of the inferior pyramidal space meets the inferiorly directed apex of the infero-septal recess of the left ventricular outflow tract.

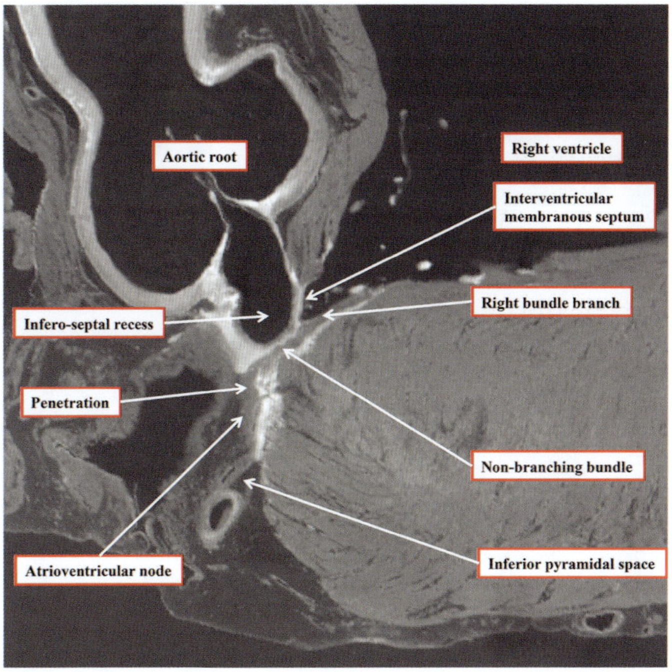

Figure 4.19. The image is taken from a human heart scanned using hierarchical phase contrast computed tomographic (Hip-CT) technology. The heart is sectioned in the sagittal plane, such that the apex of the inferior pyramidal space is pointing superiorly, with the cut passing through the inferior part of the muscular ventricular septum. The section shows how the conduction axis becomes insulated by the atrioventricular fibrous tissues as it transitions from the atrioventricular node to become the non-branching bundle, with the latter component forming the so-called bundle of His. In this section, the axis continues as the right bundle branch.

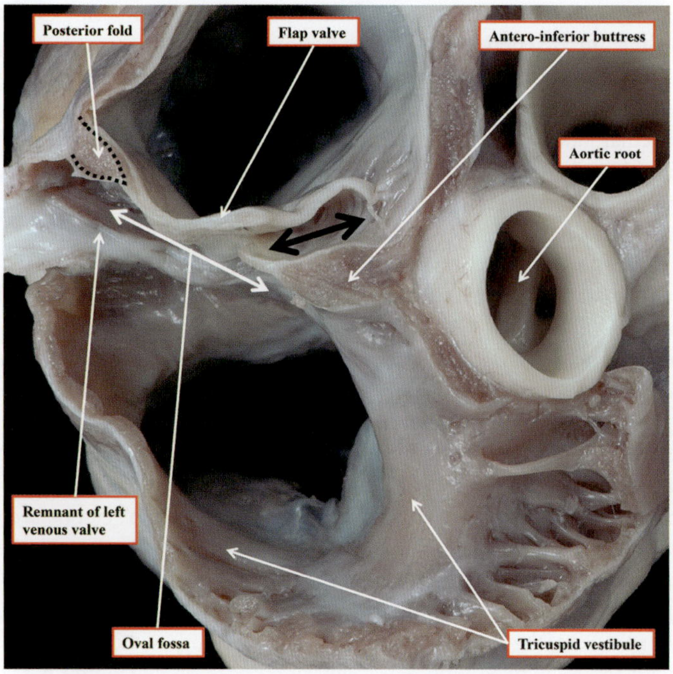

Figure 4.20. The heart has been sectioned in its short axis through the middle of the oval fossa. The section shows how the antero-inferior buttress and the floor of the fossa are true septal structures. The posterior rim, along with the superior rim, is a fold between the atrial walls. Note the remnant of the left venous valve. Note also that, in this heart, the oval foramen is persistently patent (double-headed black arrow).

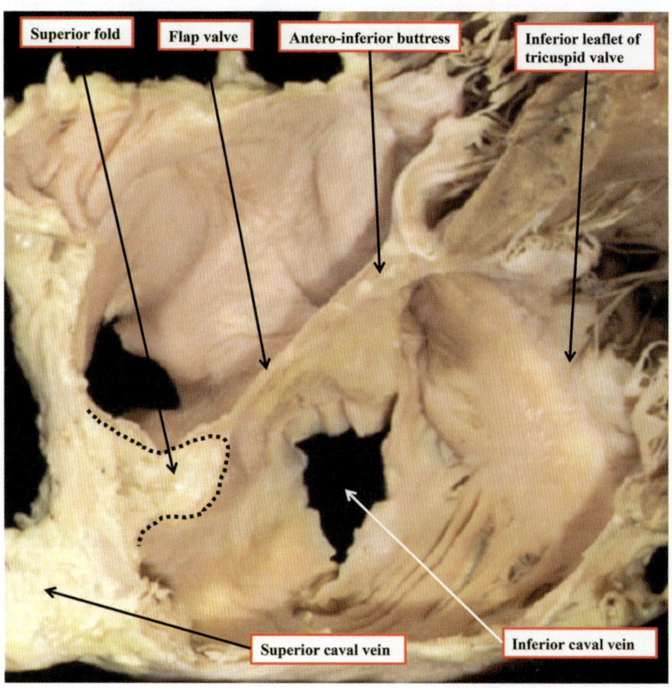

Figure 4.21. The heart has been sectioned obliquely from the superior caval vein down through the oval fossa, cutting inferiorly into the ventricular septum. The section shows how the superior rim of the fossa is a deep infolding between the atrial walls, filled with extracavitary adipose tissue.

part of the septal surface, then overlies another extracavitary area. As already explained, this superior extension of the inferior atrioventricular groove, which extends superiorly to reach the area of mitral-to-tricuspid fibrous continuity and the membranous septum, is the ***inferior pyramidal space***.[33,34] The atrial vestibules form its rightward and leftward walls. Its roof is formed by the antero-inferior buttress of the atrial septum, with the floor formed by the crest of the inferior part of the diverging right ventricular wall. As also shown, the superior apex of the inferior pyramidal space is juxtaposed, on the other side of the septum, with the inferior extent of the infero-septal recess of the left ventricular outflow tract (Figure 4.18). It is the relationship of these two areas that permits the atrioventricular conduction axis to transition from the atrial to the ventricular myocardial components, penetrating the insulating tissues to become the bundle of His (Figure 4.19).

A proper understanding of the anatomy of the septum is crucial for the safe accomplishment of ***trans-septal puncture***, especially when trans-oesophageal or intracardiac echocardiography assistance is not available and anatomical landmarks are being used.[19] When seeking to puncture the septum, having accessed the heart through the inferior caval vein and having passed the trans-septal sheath into the superior caval vein, the operator should withdraw the sheath, with the needle inside it, albeit without protruding, until it drops into the oval fossa. Tenting of the fossa by the sheath should then be confirmed, optimally by ultrasound or by injection of contrast. The needle can then be advanced into the left atrium, ideally with continuous pressure monitoring. If the puncture is made through the floor of the fossa, or its antero-inferior buttress, the needle will enter the left atrial cavity directly. Should the needle be advanced through the superior or posterior rims of the fossa, or directly anteriorly, entrance into the pericardial space is likely, or even into the non-coronary sinus of the aortic root. Puncturing too anteriorly risks entrance into the aorta, while too posterior or superior a puncture risks entry into the pericardial space. If the needle inadvertently punctures the aorta, it can usually simply be withdrawn without adverse effects, unless the dilator and sheath have been advanced over the needle and into the aorta.[19] A superior puncture may also restrict manoeuvring of the ablation catheter towards the right pulmonary veins, especially the inferior one. The trans-septal approach is necessary for *atrial fibrillation* ablation procedures and ablation of atypical forms of *atrioventricular nodal re-entrant tachycardia*,[36] and is the access of choice for ablation of left-sided *accessory pathways*.[37] For trans-catheter procedures designed to repair *mitral regurgitation*, such as those using the Mitraclip device, the suitable site for the trans-septal puncture is chosen under the guidance of three-dimensional trans-oesophageal echocardiography. In up to one-third of individuals the oval foramen remains persistently patent (Figures 4.20).[38] In these circumstances, it should be feasible to pass the sheath directly into the left atrium, without having to resort to septal puncture. This is the case during procedures designed to close the ***persistent patent foramen*** using dedicated devices.[39] The left atrial cavity is accessed directly when devices are used to close ***atrial septal defects*** of moderate size in the floor of the oval fossa (Figure 4.22). In adults, this usually means that they are sized at less than 35 mm. It is also necessary to ensure that the rims are suitable to anchor the device (Figure 4.22 panel A), ideally measured at greater than 5 mm, and that, when placed, the device is not impinging on the leaflets of the atrioventricular valve, the coronary sinus, or the orifices of the caval veins.[40,41]

Of note, the interatrial channels closed in this fashion (Figure 4.22) are usually described as being "secundum atrial septal" defects. It is

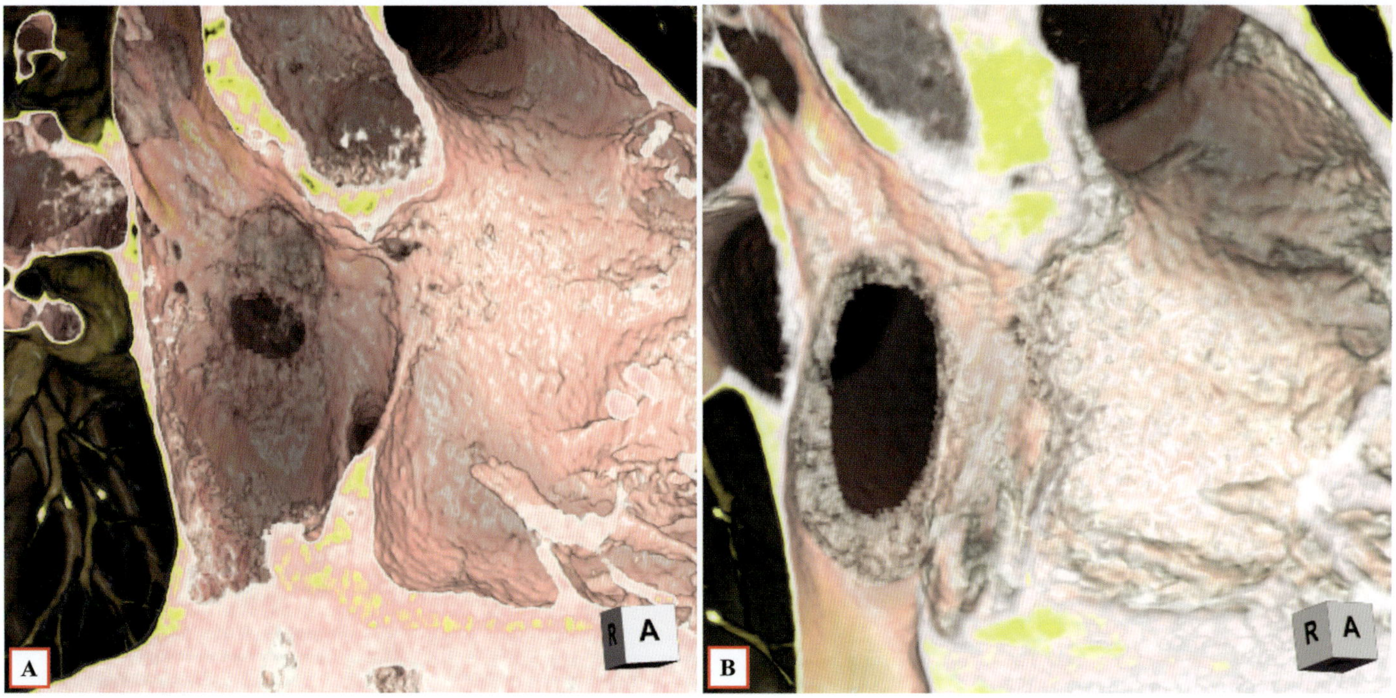

Figure 4.22. The panels show two defects in the floor of the oval fossa as revealed by virtual dissection of computed tomographic datasets. In panel A, the defect, of moderate size, is less than 3.5 cm in diameter and has well-formed rims. It is an ideal lesion for interventional closure. In contrast, the defect shown in panel B is larger than 3.5 cm, essentially occupying the entirety of the floor of the oval fossa, and without any well-formed rims. Note in particular the proximity of the anterior rim of the defect to the aortic root. The case would not be suitable for interventional closure.

true, as explained in Chapter 2, that they represent the secondary interatrial foramen as formed during cardiac development.[35] They are, therefore, a consequence of a deficiency of the primary atrial septum, with the channels being ostium secundum defects, rather than defects of the superior interatrial fold, which was previously described incorrectly as the "septum secundum". It is possible, however, for defects to exist in the true second atrial septum, which is the antero-inferior buttress of the fossa. Such defects are more intimately positioned near the atrioventricular node and its inputs, potentially increasing the risk of disturbing the conduction system. These are the ***vestibular defects***, which can co-exist with defects within the fossa (Figure 4.23).[42]

It is also necessary to distinguish the true septal defects, be they vestibular or within the oval fossa, from the other channels which permit interatrial shunting, but which are outside the confines of the oval fossa and its rims. Of these defects, it has now become recognized that the sinus venosus variant (Figure 4.24 panel A) can also be closed interventionally.[37] This involves insertion of a long, covered stent across the junction between the superior caval vein and right atrium so as to divert the caval venous flow to the right atrium and redirect the pulmonary venous flow around the stent into the left atrium.[43] The ***"ostium primum" defect***, in contrast, is an atrioventricular septal defect. It is found in the setting of a common atrioventricular junction, but with shunting confined at atrial level. This is because the bridging leaflets of the common atrioventricular valve are fused with each other and also with the scooped-out crest of the muscular ventricular septum (Figure 4.24 panel B).[44]

As has been emphasized, only a small part of the body of the primary atrial component of the developing heart is committed to the morphologically right atrium. This part is well recognized during early fetal life as the space between the left venous valves and the

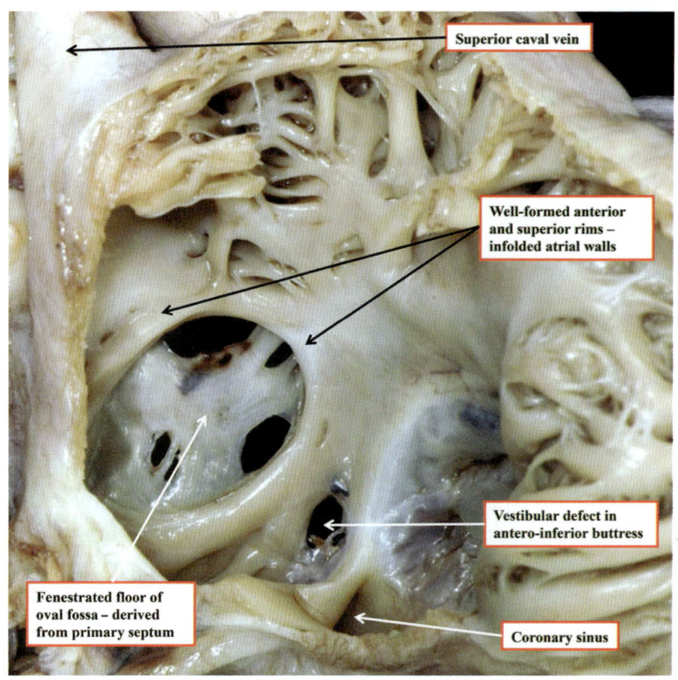

Figure 4.23. The figure shows how defects can exist within the oval fossa due to the fenestration of its floor, which is derived from the primary atrial septum. Such defects, therefore, are "ostium secundum" defects, rather than defects of the secondary atrial septum. In this heart, however, there is also a defect in the true second atrial septum, which is the antero-inferior buttress of the fossa. This produced a vestibular defect.

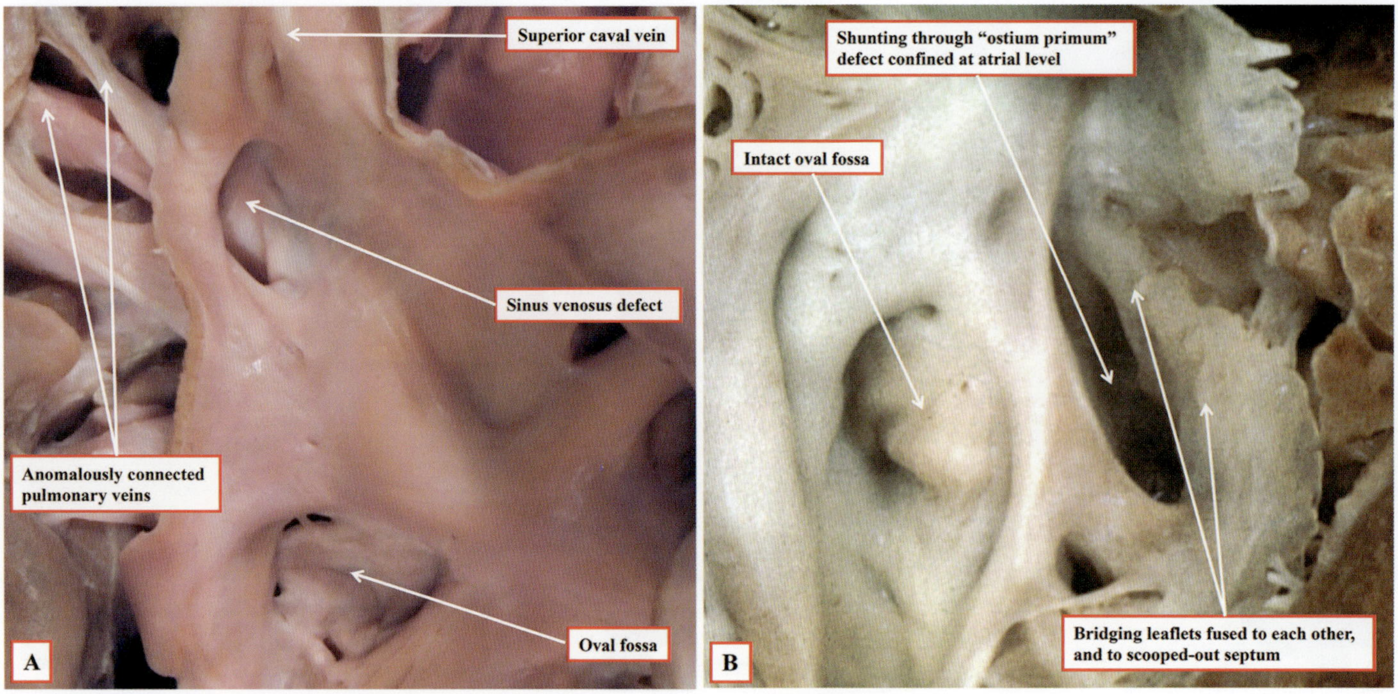

Figure 4.24. The images show how not all the channels that permit atrial shunting are within the confines of the oval fossa. Panel A shows a superior sinus venosus defect, which in this heart is the consequence of anomalous connection of two right pulmonary veins to the superior caval vein, albeit with the pulmonary veins retaining their left atrial connections. Panel B shows the "ostium primum", which exists because of failure to close, during development, the primary interatrial foramen. This defect is an atrioventricular septal defect, but with shunting confined at atrial level because the bridging leaflets of the common atrioventricular valve are fused to each other, but also to the crest of the muscular ventricular septum.

floor of the oval fossa (Figure 4.1). The left venous valve, however, usually regresses almost in its entirety, sometimes with remnants found on the inferior rim of the oval fossa (Figure 4.20). In a minority of individuals, nonetheless, the valve can persist so as to produce a fenestrated shelf across the right atrial aspect of the oval fossa (Figure 4.25). This arrangement might prevent the tenting ideally required during attempted septal puncture.

The remaining component of the right atrium is the ***systemic venous sinus***. This part, again with smooth walls, makes up the most posterior part of the atrial cavity, with its lateral and superior border marked by the terminal crest (Figure 4.10). Its leftward border is seemingly the atrial septum, but the small part of the cavity made up by the developmental body is also part of the leftward border. This component can be recognized when there is persistence of the left venous valve (Figure 4.25). The venous sinus receives the ***superior caval vein*** at the superior aspect of the right atrium, in close relation to the right superior pulmonary vein posteriorly and the ascending aorta medially.[45,46] The ***inferior caval vein***, the largest vein in the body, enters its inferior aspect.[47] The myocardium of the walls of the venous sinus extends well into the intrapericardial component of the superior caval vein in three-quarters of individuals, with the extensions often being circumferential. Myocardial extensions into the walls of the inferior caval vein, in contrast, are most unusual.[4]

The ***coronary sinus*** is the third tributary entering the venous sinus. This channel, which normally serves to return the venous blood from the heart itself, seems at first sight to be a septal structure (Figure 4.2). In reality, it occupies the left atrioventricular groove (Figure 4.26), opening to the right atrium inferiorly to the orifice of the oval fossa. It is formed by union between the left anterior

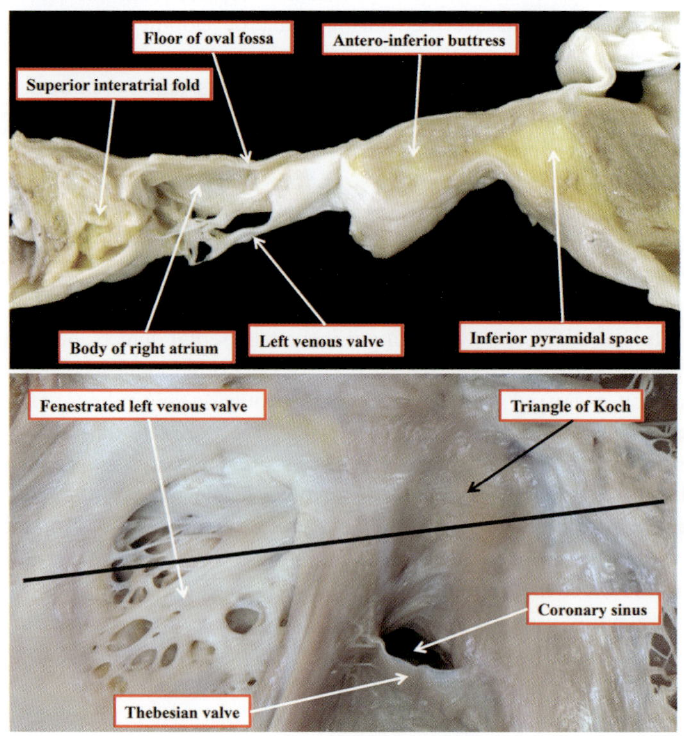

Figure 4.25. The lower panel shows a view of the oval fossa in the heart obtained from an individual retaining a fenestrated left venous valve. The upper panel, which is a section taken along the line shown in the lower panel, shows how this arrangement reveals the location of the body of the right atrium. It is feasible that this arrangement could prevent the tenting ideally required during attempted septal puncture.

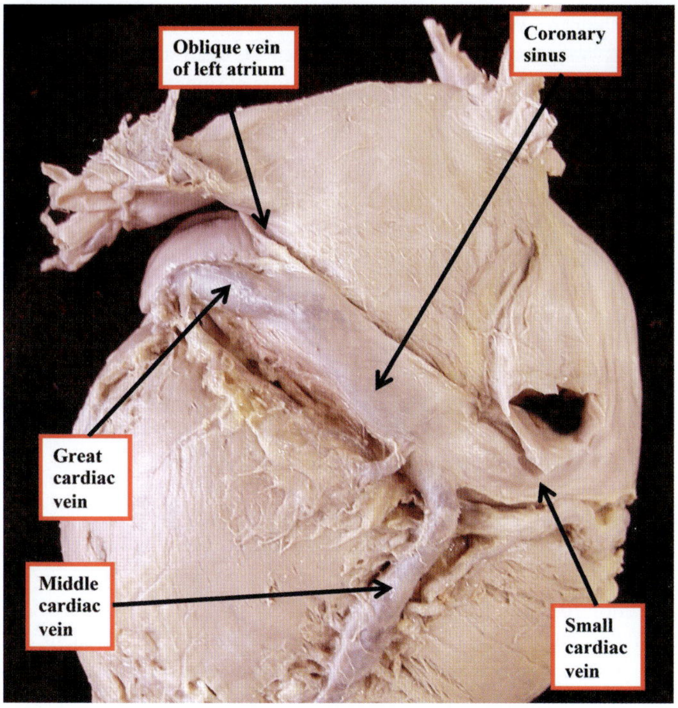

Figure 4.26. The image shows the diaphragmatic surface of an adult heart. The venous tributaries returning blood from the heart itself are dilated, but the image shows well the location of the coronary sinus in the left atrioventricular groove. The sinus is formed by the union of the left anterior interventricular vein, also known as the great cardiac vein, with the oblique vein of the left atrium. The oblique vein is the remnant of the embryonic left superior caval vein, which also persists as the ligament of Marshall, which can be seen in this heart.

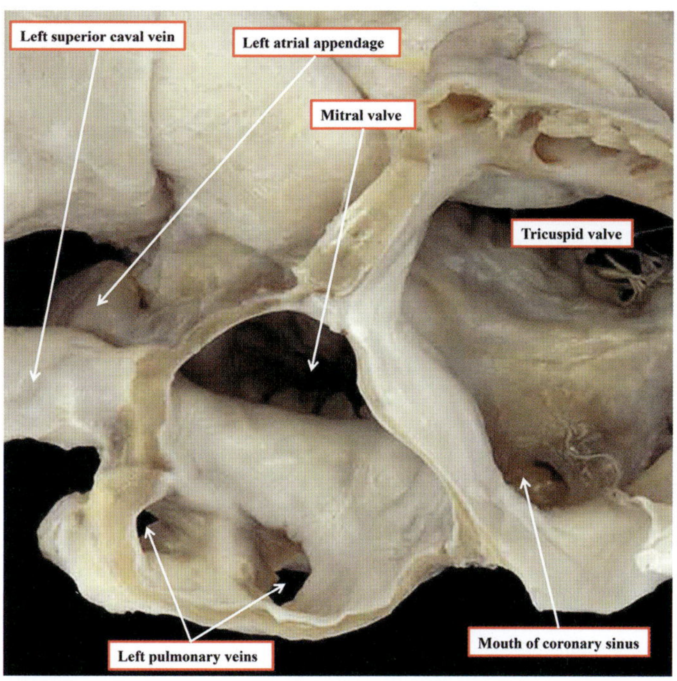

Figure 4.27. The image has been prepared by removing the atrial walls and photographing the base of the ventricular mass from above. There is a persistent left superior caval vein, which produces a tumulus in the posterior wall of the left atrium, even though the caval vein and the atrium have their own walls. The persistent caval vein is in the left atrioventricular groove, which it enters by passing between the left atrial appendage and the left pulmonary veins (compare with the location of the oblique vein of the left atrium as shown in Figure 4.26). The vein drains into the right atrium through the mouth of the coronary sinus.

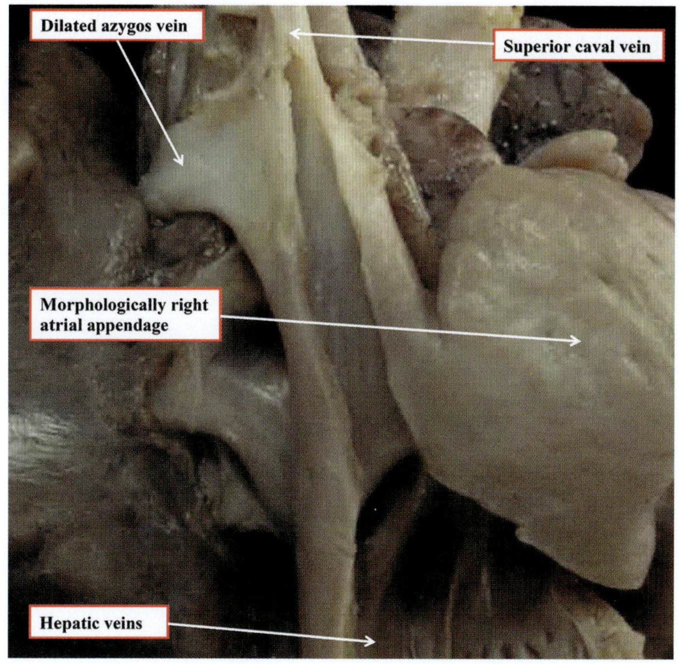

Figure 4.28. The right atrium is photographed from the right side in an individual with interruption of the inferior caval vein. The veins draining inferiorly to the systemic venous sinus carry only the venous return from the liver. The remainder of the venous return from the abdomen is carried through a dilated azygos vein, which opens into the superior caval vein.

interventricular vein, also known as the great cardiac vein, and the oblique vein of the left atrium, with the latter channel being the remnant of the embryonic left superior caval vein (see Chapter 2). The cranial part of the left caval vein can be recognized as the ***ligament of Marshall***, which passes between the left pulmonary veins and the left atrial appendage (Figure 4.26). The myocardium between the atrial orifice of the coronary sinus and that of the inferior caval vein is often described as the "sinus septum". Like many of the other myocardial areas surrounding the oval fossa, it is a myocardial fold. The coronary sinus is further discussed in Chapter 11, devoted to the coronary circulation.

Each of the venous tributaries can present with anatomical variants. The most common variant is ***persistence of the left superior caval vein***, which then opens to the right atrium through the orifice of the coronary sinus (Figure 4.27). This variant is seen in around 1% of the general population but is found more frequently in patients with congenitally malformed hearts. When found as a simple variant, it co-exists with the right superior caval vein, with an intercommunicating bridge found in around one-third of the cases.[46] When additionally malformed, the left caval vein can open directly to the roof of the left atrium, or serve as a conduit for partial or totally anomalous drainage of the pulmonary veins.

The inferior caval vein can be duplicated, but the most significant variant is found when there is ***interruption of the inferior caval vein***. The venous return from the abdomen then passes through the azygos venous system, draining into the superior caval vein (Figure 4.28). The lesion is an anticipated finding when there is left isomerism, but, as shown in Figure 4.28, it can also be found as an anatomical variant in the setting of usual atrial arrangement. Although most variations do not produce symptoms, they can complicate procedures such as insertion of pacemaker leads through the superior caval vein, trans-septal puncture, or percutaneous closure of the interatrial communications through the inferior caval vein.

The superior caval vein, and especially the variant of persistent left superior caval vein, has been considered a potential source of atrial arrhythmias triggering atrial fibrillation. In this setting, therefore, isolation of the superior caval vein has been advocated in addition to ablation of the pulmonary veins.[48,49] Recent randomized studies, however, have produced controversial findings in terms of the efficacy of the approach and have raised the possibility of increased complications.[50,51]

REFERENCES

1. Crucean A, Spicer DE, Tretter JT, Mohun TJ, Cook AC, Sanchez-Quintana D, Lamers WH, Anderson RH. Revisiting the anatomy of the atrial chambers in the light of knowledge of their development. *J Anat*. 2025 (in press).
2. Sanchez-Quintana D, Cabrera JA, Farre J, Climent V, Anderson RH, Ho SY. Sinus node revisited in the era of electroanatomical mapping and catheter ablation. *Heart*. 2005;**91**:189–194. doi: 91/2/189 [pii]10.1136/hrt.2003.031542
3. Anderson KR, Ho SY, Anderson RH. Location and vascular supply of sinus node in human heart. *Br Heart J*. 1979;**41**:28–32. doi: 10.1136/hrt.41.1.28
4. Saremi F, Channual S, Krishnan S, Gurudevan SV, Narula J, Abolhoda A. Bachmann bundle and its arterial supply: imaging with multidetector CT—implications for interatrial conduction abnormalities and arrhythmias. *Radiology*. 2008;**248**:447–457. doi: 10.1148/radiol.2482071908
5. Ariyarajah V, Spodick DH. The Bachmann bundle and interatrial conduction. *Cardiol Rev*. 2006;**14**:194–199. doi: 10.1097/01.crd.0000195221.26979.2b
6. Yoshimoto D, Sakamoto Y, Uemura Y, Yamaguchi R, Naganawa H, Suzuki T. Comparative assessment of interatrial conduction delay during Bachmann's bundle pacing and right atrial appendage pacing using biatrial strain rate echocardiography. *Heart Rhythm*. 2025;**22**:2753–2754. doi: 10.1016/j.hrthm.2024.12.016
7. Lustgarten DL, Habel N, Sanchez-Quintana D, Winget J, Correa de Sa D, Lobel R, Thompson N, Infeld M, Meyer M. Bachmann bundle pacing. *Heart Rhythm*. 2024;**21**:1711–1717. doi: 10.1016/j.hrthm.2024.03.1786
8. Infeld M, Lobel R, Hopper M, Habel N, Winget J, Correa de Sa D, Thompson N, Sanchez-Quintana D, Lustgarten D. Biatrial resynchronization with electrogram-guided Bachmann bundle pacing. *JACC Clin Electrophysiol*. 2024;**10**:2103–2107. doi: 10.1016/j.jacep.2024.04.030
9. Hou Y, Scherlag BJ, Lin J, Zhou J, Song J, Zhang Y, Patterson E, Lazzara R, Jackman WM, Po SS. Interactive atrial neural network: determining the connections between ganglionated plexi. *Heart Rhythm*. 2007;**4**:56–63. doi: 10.1016/j.hrthm.2006.09.020
10. Katritsis DG, Pokushalov E, Romanov A, Giazitzoglou E, Siontis GC, Po SS, Camm AJ, Ioannidis JP. Autonomic denervation added to pulmonary vein isolation for paroxysmal atrial fibrillation: a randomized clinical trial. *J Am Coll Cardiol*. 2013;**62**:2318–2325. doi: 10.1016/j.jacc.2013.06.053
11. Hu F, Zheng L, Liu S, Shen L, Liang E, Ding L, Wu L, Chen G, Fan X, Yao Y. Avoidance of vagal response during circumferential pulmonary vein isolation: effect of initiating isolation from right anterior ganglionated plexi. *Circ Arrhythm Electrophysiol*. 2019;**12**:e007811. doi: 10.1161/CIRCEP.119.007811
12. Zhang M, Wang X, Xie X, Wang Z, Liu X, Guan J, Wang W, Li Z, Wang J, Gao M, et al. Long-term effects of atrial ganglionated plexi ablation on function and structure of sinoatrial and atrioventricular node in canine. *Pacing Clin Electrophysiol*. 2015;**38**:1181–1191. doi: 10.1111/pace.12689
13. Ho SY, Anderson RH, Sánchez-Quintana D. Atrial structure and fibres: morphologic bases of atrial conduction. *Cardiovasc Res*. 2002;**54**:325–336. doi: 10.1016/S0008-6363(02)00226-2
14. Kalman JM, Olgin JE, Karch MR, Hamdan M, Lee RJ, Lesh MD. "Cristal tachycardias": origin of right atrial tachycardias from the crista terminalis identified by intracardiac echocardiography. *J Am Coll Cardiol*. 1998;**31**:451–459. doi: 10.1016/s0735-1097(97)00492-0
15. Rosso R, Kistler PM. Focal atrial tachycardia. *Heart*. 2010;**96**:181–185. doi: 10.1136/hrt.2008.143552hrt.2008.143552 [pii]
16. Yamabe H, Soejima T, Kajiyama K, Fukami Y, Haraguchi K, Okonogi T, Hirai K, Fukuoka R, Umeji K, Orita Y, et al. Efficacy of catheter ablation from the noncoronary aortic cusp of verapamil-sensitive atrial tachycardia arising near the atrioventricular node. *Heart Rhythm*. 2022;**19**:719–727. doi: 10.1016/j.hrthm.2021.12.021
17. Bohora S, Lokhandwala Y, Sternick EB, Anderson RH, Wellens HJJ. Reappraisal and new observations on atrial tachycardia ablated from the non-coronary aortic sinus of Valsalva. *Europace*. 2018;**20**:124–133. doi: 10.1093/europace/euw324
18. Katritsis DG, Siontis KC, Agarwal S, Stavrakis S, Giazitzoglou E, Amin H, Marine JE, Tretter JT, Sanchez-Quintana D, Anderson RH, et al. Anatomical ablation of the atrioventricular node. *Arrhythm Electrophysiol Rev*. 2024;**13**:e12. doi: 10.15420/aer.2024.13
19. Katritsis DG, Morady F. *Clinical Cardiac Electrophysiology. A Practical Guide*. Philadelphia: Elsevier; 2021.
20. Cabrera JA, Sanchez-Quintana D, Farre J, Rubio JM, Ho SY. The inferior right atrial isthmus: further architectural insights for current and coming ablation technologies. *J Cardiovasc Electrophysiol*. 2005;**16**:402–408. doi: doi:10.1046/j.1540-8167.2005.40709.x
21. Baccillieri MS, Rizzo S, De Gaspari M, Paradiso B, Thiene G, Verlato R, Basso C. Anatomy of the cavotricuspid isthmus for radiofrequency ablation in typical atrial flutter. *Heart Rhythm*. 2019;**16**:1611–1618. doi: 10.1016/j.hrthm.2019.05.030
22. Brugada J, Katritsis DG, Arbelo E, Arribas F, Bax JJ, Blomström-Lundqvist C, Calkins H, Corrado D, Deftereos SG, Diller G-P, et al. 2019 ESC Guidelines for the management of patients with supraventricular tachycardias. *Eur Heart J*. 2020;**41**:655–720. doi: https://doi.org/10.1093/eurheartj/ehz467
23. Olgin JE, Kalman JM, Fitzpatrick AP, Lesh MD. Role of right atrial endocardial structures as barriers to conduction during human type I atrial flutter: activation and entrainment mapping guided by intracardiac echocardiography. *Circulation*. 1995;**92**:1839–1848. doi: 10.1161/01.cir.92.7.1839
24. Baccillieri MS, Rizzo S, De Gaspari M, Paradiso B, Thiene G, Verlato R, Basso C. Anatomy of the cavotricuspid isthmus for radiofrequency ablation in typical atrial flutter. *Heart Rhythm*. 2019;**16**:1611–1618. doi: 10.1016/j.hrthm.2019.05.030
25. Saoudi N, Cosio F, Waldo A, Chen S-A, Iesaka Y, Lesh M, Saksena S, Salerno J, Schoels W. Classification of atrial flutter and regular atrial tachycardia according to electrophysiologic mechanism and anatomic bases: a statement from a Joint Expert Group from the Working Group of Arrhythmias of the European Society of Cardiology and the North American Society of Pacing and Electrophysiology. *J Cardiovasc Electrophysiol*. 2001;**12**:852–866. doi: doi:10.1046/j.1540-8167.2001.00852.x

26. Bochoeyer A, Yang Y, Cheng J, Lee RJ, Keung EC, Marrouche NF, Natale A, Scheinman MM. Surface electrocardiographic characteristics of right and left atrial flutter. *Circulation*. 2003;**108**:60–66. doi: 10.1161/01.cir.0000079140.35025.1e
27. Zhang S, Younis G, Hariharan R, Ho J, Yang Y, Ip J, Thakur RK, Seger J, Scheinman MM, Cheng J. Lower loop reentry as a mechanism of clockwise right atrial flutter. *Circulation*. 2004;**109**:1630–1635. doi: 10.1161/01.cir.0000124221.84399.48
28. Yang Y, Cheng J, Bochoeyer A, Hamdan MH, Kowal RC, Page R, Lee RJ, Steiner PR, Saxon LA, Lesh MD, et al. Atypical right atrial flutter patterns. *Circulation*. 2001;**103**:3092–3098. doi: 10.1161/01.cir.103.25.3092
29. Yang Y, Varma N, Badhwar N, Tanel RE, Sundara S, Lee RJ, Lee BK, Tseng ZH, Marcus GM, Kim AM, et al. Prospective observations in the clinical and electrophysiological characteristics of intra-isthmus reentry. *J Cardiovasc Electrophysiol*. 2010;**21**:1099–1106. doi: 10.1111/j.1540-8167.2010.01778.x
30. Chiriac A, Cheema KP, Giardi D, Espinosa SM, Fitzgerald P, Perez-Downes JC, Umadat G, Hodge DO, Phillips SD, Madhavan M, et al. Atrial arrhythmia ablation in patients with D-transposition of the great arteries and atrial switch. *Circ Arrhythm Electrophysiol*. 2022;**15**:e010546. doi: 10.1161/CIRCEP.121.010546
31. Katritsis DG, Zografos T, Siontis KC, Giannopoulos G, Muthalaly RG, Liu Q, Latchamsetty R, Varga Z, Deftereos S, Swerdlow C, et al. End-points for successful slow pathway catheter ablation in typical and atypical atrioventricular nodal reentrant tachycardia: a contemporary, multicenter study. *JACC Clin Electrophysiol*. 2019;**5**:113–119. doi: 10.1016/j.jacep.2018.09.012
32. Katritsis DG, Anderson RH. New insights into the mechanisms of fast and slow conduction in the atrioventricular node. *Heart Rhythm*. 2023;**20**:627–630. doi: 10.1016/j.hrthm.2022.08.025
33. Sanchez-Quintana D, Ho SY, Cabrera JA, Farre J, Anderson RH. Topographic anatomy of the inferior pyramidal space: relevance to radiofrequency catheter ablation. *J Cardiovasc Electrophysiol*. 2001;**12**:210–217. doi: 10.1046/j.1540-8167.2001.00210.x
34. Tretter JT, Spicer DE, Sanchez-Quintana D, Back Sternick E, Farre J, Anderson RH. Miniseries 1—Part III: 'Behind the scenes' in the triangle of Koch. *Europace*. 2022;**24**:455–463. doi: 10.1093/europace/euab285
35. Jensen B, Spicer DE, Sheppard MN, Anderson RH. Development of the atrial septum in relation to postnatal anatomy and interatrial communications. *Heart*. 2017;**103**:456–462. doi: 10.1136/heartjnl-2016-310660
36. Katritsis DG, John RM, Latchamsetty R, Muthalaly RG, Zografos T, Katritsis GD, Stevenson WG, Efimov IR, Morady F. Left septal slow pathway ablation for atrioventricular nodal reentrant tachycardia. *Circ Arrhythm Electrophysiol*. 2018;**11**:e005907. doi: 10.1161/CIRCEP.117.005907
37. Katritsis D, Giazitzoglou E, Korovesis S, Zambartas C. Comparison of the transseptal approach to the transaortic approach for ablation of left-sided accessory pathways in patients with Wolff–Parkinson–White syndrome. *Am J Cardiol*. 2003;**91**:610–613. doi: https://doi.org/10.1016/S0002-9149(02)03321-0
38. Hagen PT, Scholz DG, Edwards WD. Incidence and size of patent foramen ovale during the first 10 decades of life: an autopsy study of 965 normal hearts. *Mayo Clin Proc*. 1984;**59**:17–20. doi: 10.1016/s0025-6196(12)60336-x
39. Stortecky S, da Costa BR, Mattle HP, Carroll J, Hornung M, Sievert H, Trelle S, Windecker S, Meier B, Juni P. Percutaneous closure of patent foramen ovale in patients with cryptogenic embolism: a network meta-analysis. *Eur Heart J*. 2015;**36**:120–128. doi: 10.1093/eurheartj/ehu292
40. Stout KK, Daniels CJ, Aboulhosn JA, Bozkurt B, Broberg CS, Colman JM, Crumb SR, Dearani JA, Fuller S, Gurvitz M, et al. AHA/ACC Guideline for the management of adults with congenital heart disease: executive summary: a report of the American College of Cardiology/American Heart Association Task Force on Clinical Practice Guidelines. *J Am Coll Cardiol*. 2019;**73**:1494–1563. doi: 10.1016/j.jacc.2018.08.1028
41. Baumgartner H, De Backer J, Babu-Narayan SV, Budts W, Chessa M, Diller GP, Lung B, Kluin J, Lang IM, Meijboom F, et al. ESC Guidelines for the management of adult congenital heart disease. *Eur Heart J*. 2021;**42**:563–645. doi: 10.1093/eurheartj/ehaa554
42. Loomba RS, Tretter JT, Mohun TJ, Anderson RH, Kramer S, Spicer DE. Identification and morphogenesis of vestibular atrial septal defects. *J Cardiovasc Dev Dis*. 2020;**7**:35. doi: 10.3390/jcdd7030035
43. Baruteau AE, Hascoet S, Malekzadeh-Milani S, Batteux C, Karsenty C, Ciobotaru V, Thambo JB, Fraisse A, Boudjemline Y, Jalal Z. Transcatheter closure of superior sinus venosus defects. *JACC Cardiovasc Interv*. 2023;**16**:2587–2599. doi: 10.1016/j.jcin.2023.07.024
44. Penkoske PA, Neches WH, Anderson RH, Zuberbuhler JR. Further observations on the morphology of atrioventricular septal defects. *J Thorac Cardiovasc Surg*. 1985;**90**:611–622.
45. Macedo PG, Kapa S, Mears JA, Fratianni A, Asirvatham SJ. Correlative anatomy for the electrophysiologist: ablation for atrial fibrillation. Part I: pulmonary vein ostia, superior vena cava, vein of Marshall. *J Cardiovasc Electrophysiol*. 2010;**21**:721–730. doi: 10.1111/j.1540-8167.2010.01728.x
46. Verma M, Pandey NN, Ojha V, Kumar S, Ramakrishnan S. Developmental anomalies of the superior vena cava and its tributaries: what the radiologist needs to know? *Br J Radiol*. 2021;**94**:20200856. doi: 10.1259/bjr.20200856
47. Li SJ, Lee J, Hall J, Sutherland TR. The inferior vena cava: anatomical variants and acquired pathologies. *Insights Imaging*. 2021;**12**:123. doi: 10.1186/s13244-021-01066-7
48. Liu H, Lim KT, Murray C, Weerasooriya R. Electrogram-guided isolation of the left superior vena cava for treatment of atrial fibrillation. *Europace*. 2007;**9**:775–780. doi: 10.1093/europace/eum118
49. Mariani MV, Palombi M, Jabbour JP, Pierucci N, Cipollone P, Piro A, Chimenti C, Miraldi F, Vizza CD, Lavalle C. Usefulness of empiric superior vena cava isolation in paroxysmal atrial fibrillation ablation: a meta-analysis of randomized clinical trials. *J Interv Card Electrophysiol*. 2024;**68**:93–100. doi: 10.1007/s10840-024-01867-y
50. Castro-Urda V, Segura-Dominguez M, Jimenez-Sanchez D, Aguilera-Agudo C, Vela-Martin P, Lorente-Ros A, Garcia-Rodriguez D, Sanchez-Ortiz D, Pham-Trung C, Garcia-Izquierdo E, et al. Superior vena cava isolation with cryoballoon in AF ablation: randomized CAVAC AF trial. *Circ Arrhythm Electrophysiol*. 2025:**18**:e012917. doi: 10.1161/CIRCEP.124.012917
51. Kim D, Yu HT, Shim J, Park J, Baek YS, Park SW, Kim DK, Park YA, Kim TH, Uhm JS, et al. Cryoballoon pulmonary vein isolation with versus without additional right atrial linear ablation for persistent atrial fibrillation: the CRALAL randomized clinical trial. *Circ Arrhythm Electrophysiol*. 2025:**18**:e013408. doi: 10.1161/CIRCEP.124.013408

5

The Left Atrium

As is the case for the right, the left atrium is made up of a body, an appendage, a venous component, and a vestibule. It is separated from the right atrium by the components of the atrial septum. The developmental parts are well seen at the beginning of the fetal period of development (Figure 5.1). Postnatally, the boundaries between the components are not as easy to identify in the left as in the right atrium. This is because most of the walls of the chamber are smooth, with the pectinate muscles confined within the tubular appendage (Figure 5.2).[1] Unlike the arrangement in the right atrium, where the pectinate muscles of the appendage almost completely surround the atrioventricular junction, there is no direct boundary in the left atrium between the body and vestibule. This feature of the smooth postero-inferior wall serves to distinguish the right and left atriums should the heart be congenitally malformed.

Anteriorly and medially, the vestibule is directly adjacent to the aortic root (Figure 5.3). The supero-anterior wall cranial to the vestibule, including the anterior interatrial groove, is part of the body. When traced laterally, the vestibular component separates the narrow neck of the appendage from the hinge of the aortic leaflet of the mitral valve. This area is the ***vestibular isthmus*** of the left atrium (Figure 5.4). When then traced further posteriorly, the vestibule forms the inferior part of the lateral wall of the left atrium. There are no obvious boundaries on the smooth endocardial surface of the lateral wall between the vestibular component, the body

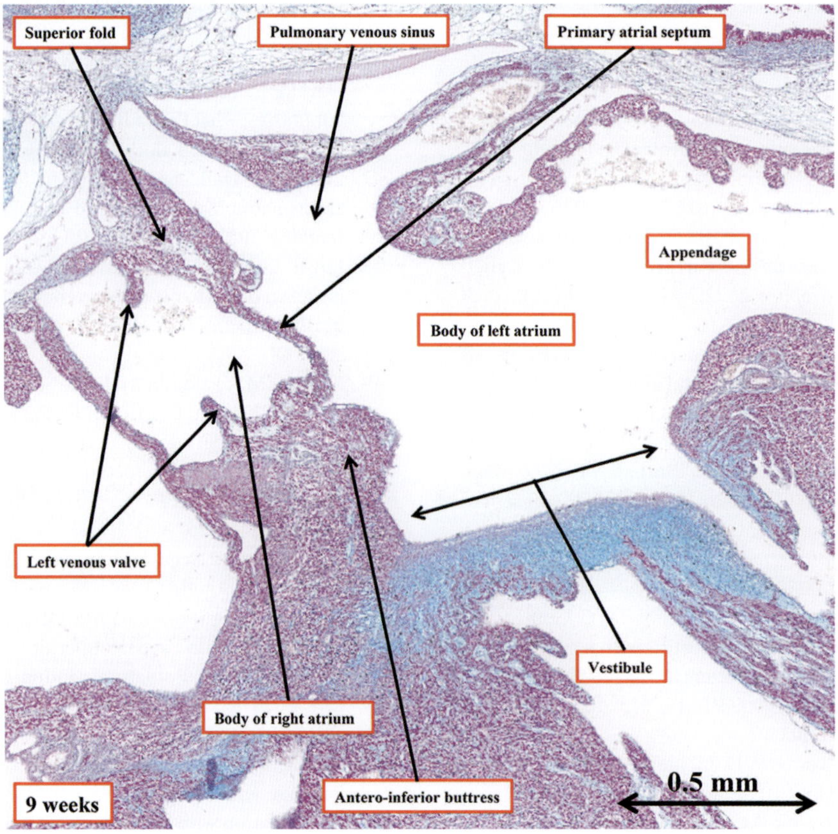

Figure 5.1. The image is from a human foetus sectioned in the frontal plane at 9 weeks gestation. It shows the developmental components of the left atrium. Note that the primary atrial septum is positioned to place the majority of the initial atrial component of the primary heart tube into the left atrium as its body. The part committed to the right atrium is the space between the primary septum and the left venous valve.

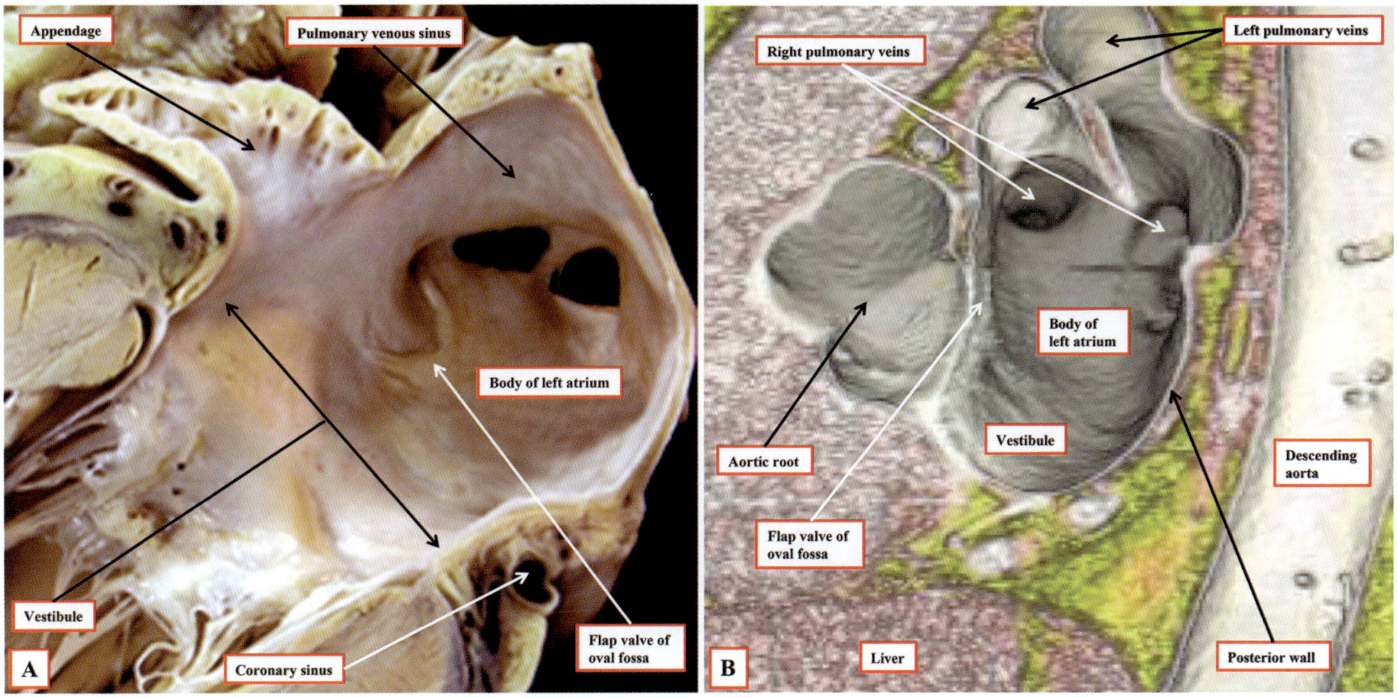

Figure 5.2. In panel A, the cavity of the left atrium is shown as seen in a heart sectioned along the long axis of its left side. As is the case for the right atrium, it is made up of a body, an appendage, a vestibule, and a venous component. In the left atrium, the pectinate muscles are confined within the tubular appendage, meaning that all the remaining walls are smooth. The chamber is separated from the right atrium by the septum, which is seen in the left side as the flap valve of the oval fossa. Note the location of the coronary sinus, with its own discrete walls, in the left atrioventricular groove. Panel B is a virtual section from a computed tomographic dataset. It can be seen that the body and vestibule provide the posterior wall of the left atrium, with the pulmonary veins connecting to the atrial roof to produce the pulmonary venous confluence. Courtesy of Dr Shumpei Mori.

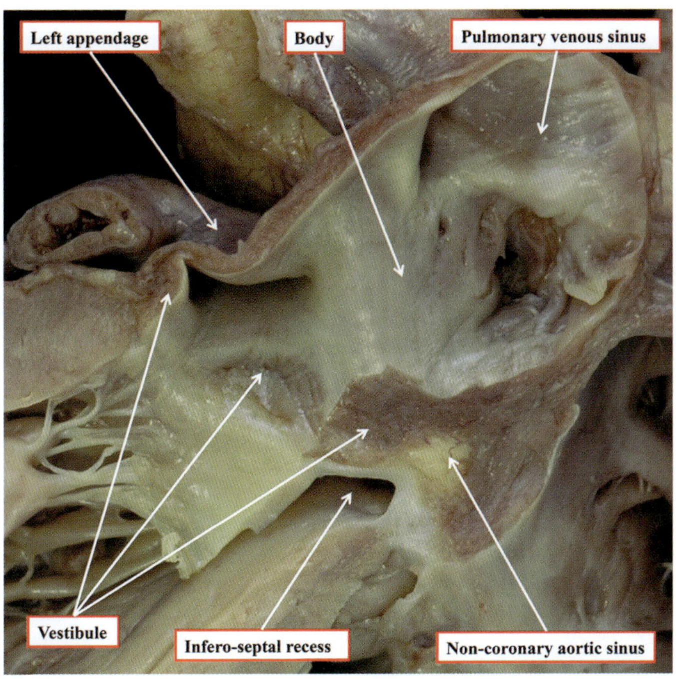

Figure 5.3. The heart has been sectioned in the frontal plane and the cavity of the left atrium is viewed from behind. The image shows how the vestibule, medially, is directly adjacent to the non-coronary sinus of the aortic root. When traced laterally, it interposes between the narrow neck of the appendage and the hinge of the aortic leaflet of the mitral valve. Note that the remainder of the anterior atrial wall is made up of the smooth walls of the body and the pulmonary venous sinus.

of the left atrium, and the cranial pulmonary venous sinus (Figure 5.4). The combined components derived from the vestibule and the body produce a second isthmus. This second area is much more extensive than the vestibular isthmus. It separates the orifice of the left inferior pulmonary vein from the hinge of the mural leaflet of the mitral valve and is described as the ***mitral isthmus***.[2] Ablation of the mitral isthmus may be needed for the elimination of macro-re-entrant atrial arrhythmias,[3] or as an adjunct to isolation of the pulmonary veins in patients with persistent atrial fibrillation.[4,5] The evidence regarding the efficacy of extensive linear ablation, when aimed at the septal, and especially at the posterior, walls has been controversial.[6-10]

An additional feature of clinical significance is found in the lateral wall. This is the ***left lateral ridge***. Also known as the ***Coumadin ridge***, it was identified initially as a "***taenia terminalis***". It is no more than a fold between the left inferior pulmonary vein and the left appendage (Figure 5.4). The structure is known to echocardiographers as the ***Q-tip sign***. It can be misinterpreted to represent a thrombus or atrial mass.[11] The vestibule can then be traced still further posteriorly, where it forms the atrial component of the left atrioventricular junction. Throughout its lateral and posterior parts, the vestibule supports the hinge of the mural leaflet of the mitral valve.

On the epicardial surface of the posterior part of the vestibule is found the ***coronary sinus*** (Figure 5.5). Although opening into the right atrium, the sinus is an integral component of the left atrioventricular groove. It is still frequently stated that the pulmonary venous component forms the posterior wall of the left atrium.[11] As shown in Figure 5.2 panel B and as was emphasized in Chapter 1,

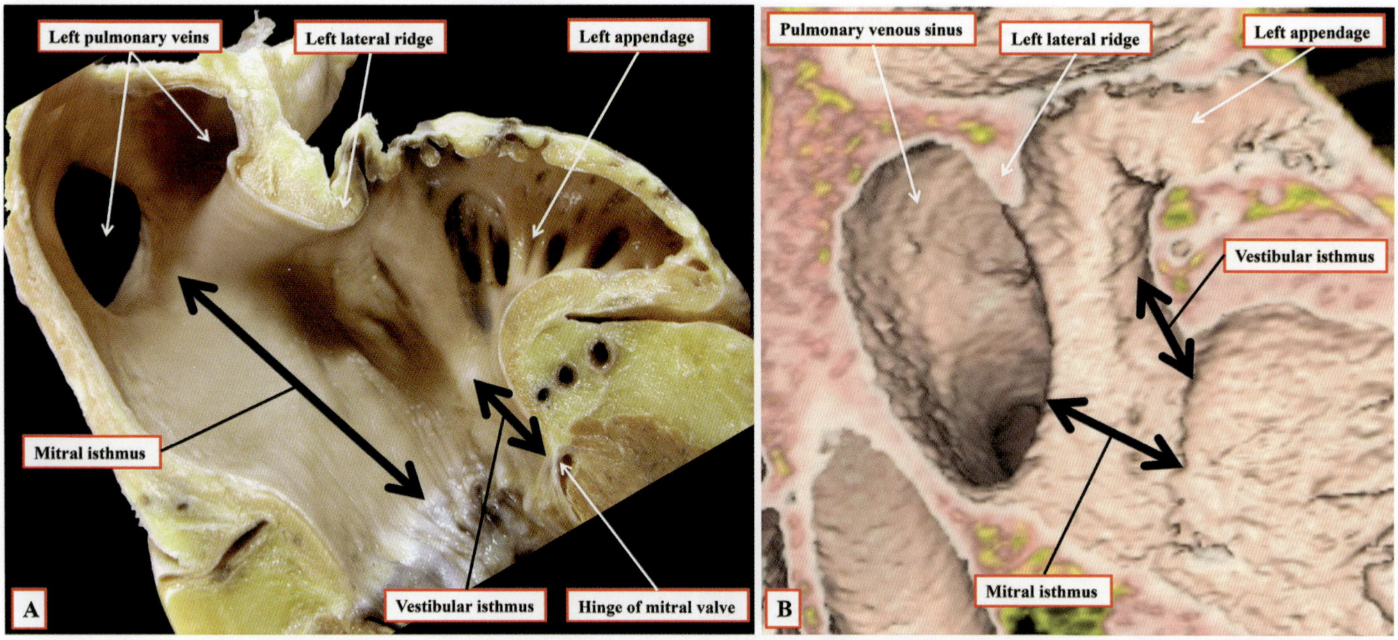

Figure 5.4. In panel A, the heart has been sectioned along the long axis of the left-sided chambers, but with the parietal part viewed from the septal aspect. The section shows the location of the anterior vestibular isthmus between the mouth of the left atrial appendage and the hinge of the leaflet of the mitral valve. There is then a second larger isthmus, the mitral isthmus, between the orifice of the left pulmonary vein and the hinge of the mural leaflet. The left lateral ridge is also seen between the neck of the appendage and the left superior pulmonary vein. Panel B shows how the isthmuses can now be identified using a virtual dissection of a computed tomographic dataset.

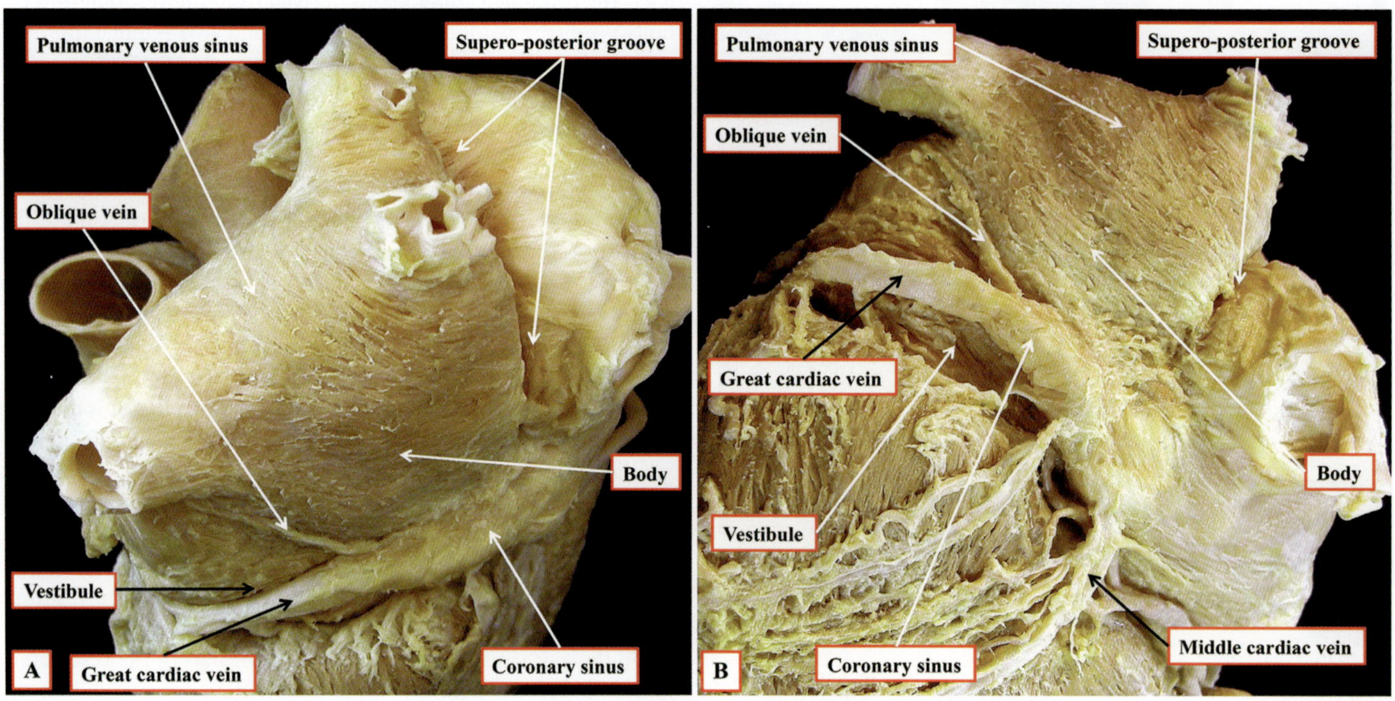

Figure 5.5. The posterior aspect of the left atrioventricular junction is viewed from the left side and above in panel A and from beneath in panel B. The images show the location of the coronary sinus in the groove, overlying the vestibular myocardium. Note the location of the oblique vein, which joins with the great cardiac vein to form the coronary sinus. The vestibular wall posteriorly is continuous with the wall of the body and the inferior part of the pulmonary venous sinus. Note the deep groove which separates the left atrium postero-superiorly from the cavity of the right atrium.

when viewed with the heart in an attitudinally appropriate position, it is the body that contributes the greater part of the posterior wall, with the vestibular component forming the most inferior part adjacent to the coronary sinus.[1]

Arising anteriorly from the left atrial body as a flattened tubular extension is its ***appendage*** (Figure 5.6 panel A). It varies significantly in terms of its shape and size, with the recognition of *cauliflower* (Figure 5.6 panel B), *chicken wing*, *cactus*, and *windsock* variants.[12] The distal end of the appendage is adjacent to the origin of the pulmonary trunk, with its cavity overlying the so-called ***left ventricular summit***, which contains the initial branches of the left coronary artery and the great cardiac vein.[13] The fine coral-like pectinate muscles are largely confined within the body of the appendage (Figure 5.7).

A few muscles can extend into the atrial body, with depressions or pits between them thinning the atrial wall. This means that care is needed when manipulating catheters or sheaths in this region so as to minimize the risk of atrial perforation. The left atrial appendage is the most frequent site for formation of thrombus. Almost half of the thrombuses complicating atrial fibrillation of valvar origin and nine-tenths of those found in non-valvar atrial fibrillation are localized in the appendage.[14] The narrow neck of the appendage provides the landing site for devices placed to block its cavity from the remainder of the left atrial chamber (Figure 5.8).[12,13] Such closure of the appendage is now used as a mechanical alternative to anticoagulation in patients at high risk of bleeding, or as an adjunct to ablative therapy.[15] Devices are also inserted to isolate the appendage in patients with atrial fibrillation having a relative or absolute contraindication to anticoagulation in the context of increased risk stratification scores.[15–18] The left atrial appendage has also been identified as a potential site of atrial arrhythmias and the locus for initiation of atrial fibrillation.[19,20] Recent data, however, do not support an empirical strategy of isolation of the appendage for patients with recurrent atrial fibrillation after previous ablation.[21]

The atrial body provides the scaffold anteriorly supporting the ***atrial septum***, with the septal components forming the greater part of the anterior wall of the chamber (Figure 5.2). The larger part of the septum itself is formed by the flap valve of the oval fossa. The horns of the valve are seen when the septum is viewed from the left atrial aspect. They overlap the superior interatrial fold as it turns anteriorly (Figure 5.2). As was discussed in Chapter 4, although the horns of the flap valve overlap the rims of the ***oval fossa*** in normal individuals, the two components are not fused together in up to one-third of normal individuals.[22] Such persistent probe-patency of the oval foramen is well appreciated from the left atrial aspect when a catheter is placed across the space between the flap valve and the rims (Figure 5.9). The flap valve is supported inferiorly by the buttress of the atrial septum, which forms the septal component of the vestibule.

The ***pulmonary veins*** enter the cavity of the left atrium cranially, with the wall between the right- and left-sided veins forming the atrial dome (Figure 5.10). In most individuals, veins enter the pulmonary venous sinus superiorly and inferiorly from both the right and left sides. This produces the arrangement in which the four orifices occupy the corners of the dome (Figure 5.10).

Variations in the manner of connection, however, are frequent (Figures 5.11).[23] The veins from one side can drain through a common orifice, most frequently on the right side, but shown on the left side in Figure 5.11. An additional vein can open directly into the dome itself, producing the so-called ***roof vein***.[24–26] The most frequent example of an extra vein is found when a separate vein drains

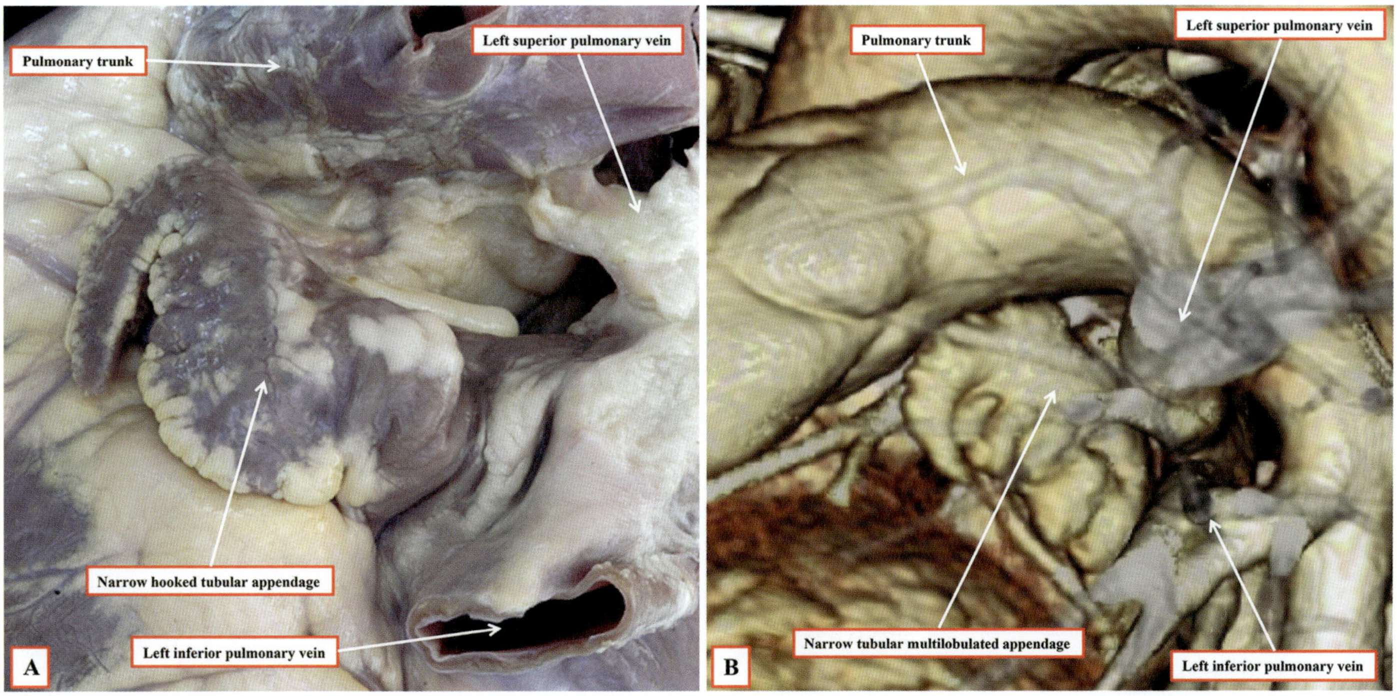

Figure 5.6. Panel A shows a lateral view of the left atrioventricular junction. The left atrial appendage extends forwards from the body of the atrium, overlapping the so-called summit of the left ventricle. Panel B is a reconstruction of a computed tomogram showing the same view of the appendage. The multilobulated arrangement produces the so-called cauliflower variant.

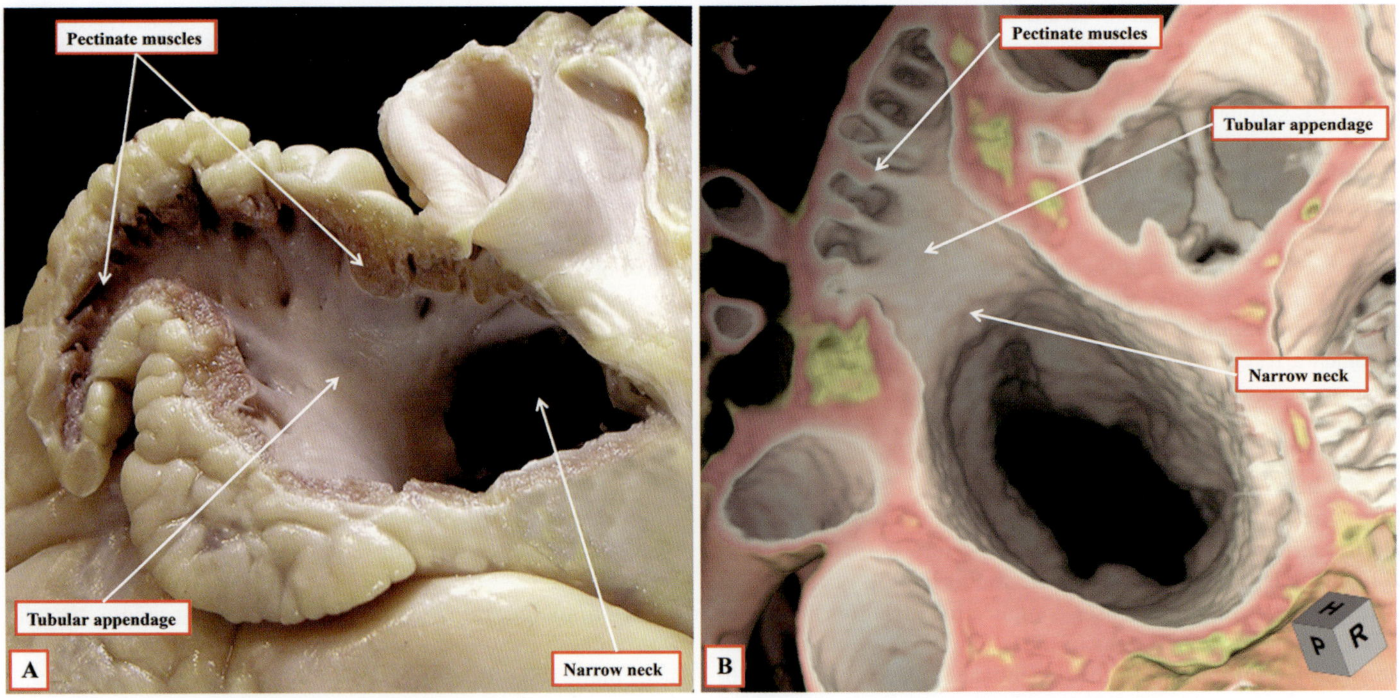

Figure 5.7. In panel A, the parietal wall of the left appendage, viewed in the same orientation as shown in Figure 5.6, has been removed to illustrate how the pectinate muscles are confined within its middle and distal parts, leaving a narrow smooth-walled neck with the atrial body. This arrangement is well seen in the virtual dissection, shown in the short axis, from a computed tomographic dataset.

the middle lobe of the right lung, with this variant reported in one study in one-quarter of patients (Figures 5.11 panel B, 5.12).[26] When found, the diameter of such a right middle vein is smaller than those of the other veins (Figure 5.11 panel B). It is usually the case that the myocardial sleeves extending along the superior veins are both larger and longer (Figure 5.13), with some being as long as 2 cm.

The myocardial architecture is complex at the ***venoatrial junctions***.[25] The myocardial sleeves are thickest and circumferential at these junctions, but become thinner and more irregular when traced towards the lung hilums (Figure 5.13). As described in Chapter 2, the pulmonary venous sinus is derived from mediastinal myocardium and has a different lineage from the systemic venous myocardium.[27]

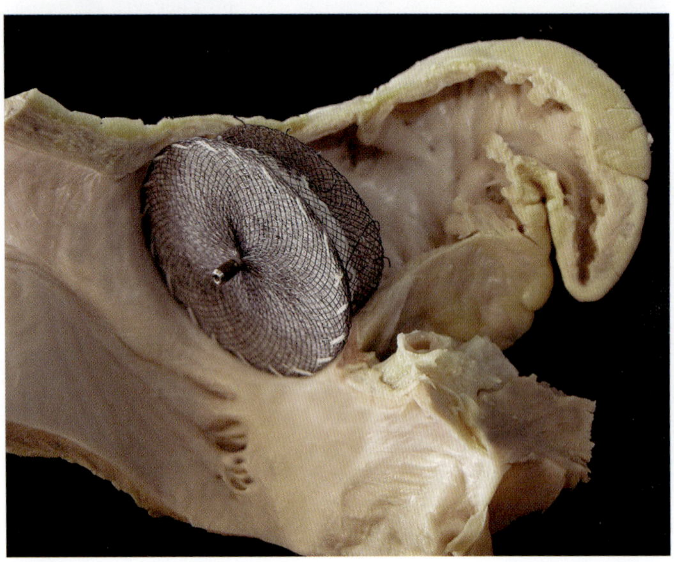

Figure 5.8. A device has been placed in the neck of the appendage to isolate its cavity from the remainder of the cavity of the left atrium. Note the pits in the atrial wall.

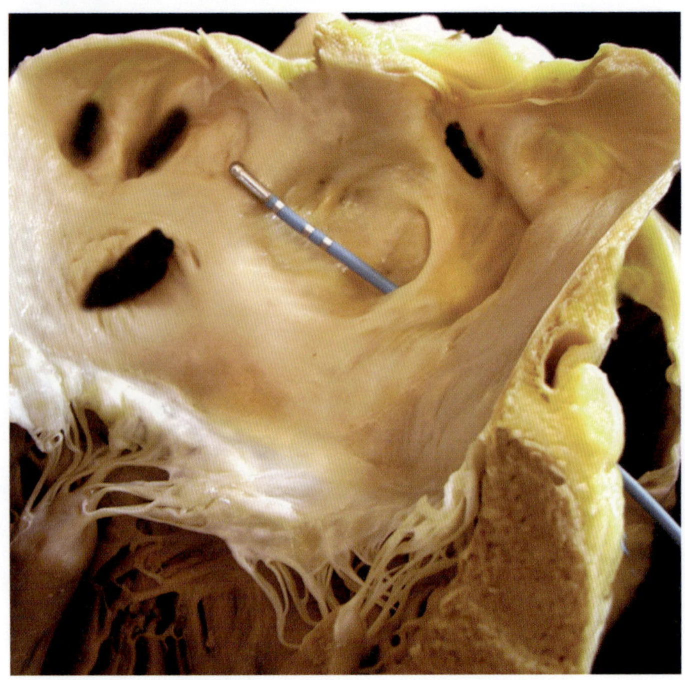

Figure 5.9. A catheter has been placed from the inferior caval vein across a persistently patent oval foramen, with the heart photographed from the left side. It separates the horns of the flap valve from the rims of the oval fossa.

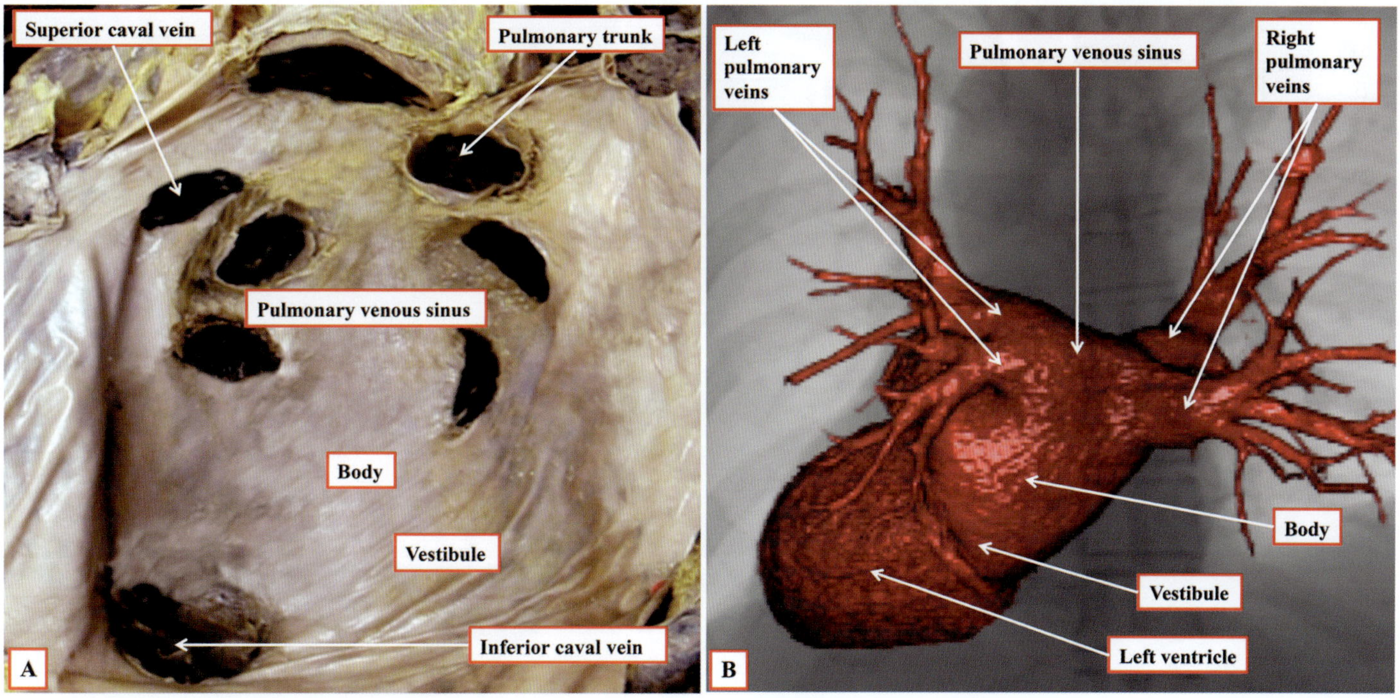

Figure 5.10. Panel A shows the posterior wall of the pericardial cavity, having removed the heart. The four pulmonary veins open superiorly into the cavity, as shown in panel B, which is a reconstruction of the heart viewed from behind made from a computed tomogram. The posterior wall of the atrium is made up of the vestibule and body, with the pulmonary venous sinus forming the atrial dome. Each of the pulmonary veins enters a corner of the pulmonary venous sinus.

The manner of aggregation of the cardiomyocytes within the sleeves is also complex. Within the thickness of the walls, some of the cardiomyocytes are aggregated in circumferential fashion, but these are interconnected with other aggregates having a longitudinal orientation (Figure 5.13).[26]

Such an arrangement may theoretically lead to anisotropic conduction between the bundles, which can act in itself as a focal trigger or a substrate for micro re-entry. The orifices of the veins have been considered the main source of the arrhythmias that initiate *atrial fibrillation*. Pulmonary venous isolation, therefore, has been the cornerstone of ablative procedures for both the paroxysmal and permanent types of fibrillation.[28–33] The role of the veins as substrates for fibrillation is supported by the fractal and mesh-based attributes of the myocardial architecture. It is further supported by genome-wide association studies. They have shown that the main locuses indicating a risk for development of atrial fibrillation are housed on chromosome 4q25 and are close to the gene *PITX2*. This is a transcription factor highly expressed in the left atrium during development, and one known to be involved in the formation of the pulmonary veins.[34,35] Variations in connexin genes have also been associated with fibrillation, which has been prevented in animal studies by connexin gene transfer.[36] Animal studies have also demonstrated the propensity of the pulmonary veins to exhibit automatic activity. Due to shorter refractory periods, as well as abrupt changes in orientation of the cardiomyocytes, the pulmonary veins at their junctions with the left atrium have a stronger potential to initiate and perpetuate atrial tachyarrhythmias.[37]

Data on the human heart are less conclusive in this respect. Several years ago, Perez-Lugones and colleagues claimed to have identified so-called "P cells" within the sleeves.[38] They provided no evidence, however, to show that these entities were any more than swollen working cardiomyocytes.[24] Other studies have reported the presence of Cajal-like cells and melanocyte-like cells that are potentially arrhythmogenic, but a causal relationship between these structures and clinical arrhythmias has not been proven.[26] What can be stated with certainty is that the overall mural architecture remains one of a three-dimensional intermingling of aggregated individual cardiomyocytes.[25,39] This suggests that other factors, such as the development of fibrosis or adiposis in the walls, herald the development of atrial fibrillation. Fibrillation, furthermore, can recur subsequent to isolation of the pulmonary veins.[40] Thus, although patients with atrial fibrillation have a higher number of pathological alterations of the pulmonary veins, the anatomical findings are similar.[26] The presence of fibrosis of the myocardial sleeves has been correlated with atrial fibrillation, but not with age. The nature of the fibrosis, furthermore, was different from the postnecrotic myocardial scars found in the setting of ischaemic heart disease.[26]

It is reasonable to suggest, therefore, that structural remodelling or stretch of the atrial chambers due to heart disease, genetic causes, or other non-identified mechanisms combine to produce electrical dissociation between the aggregated cardiomyocytes. Local heterogeneities in conduction are then able to facilitate the initiation and perpetuation of fibrillation.[41,42] The fibrotic and inflammatory changes have also been identified by biopsy and by late gadolinium contrast-enhanced cardiac magnetic resonance in patients with lone fibrillation.[43–46] Also of significance is the knowledge that the veins and their venoatrial junctions are highly innervated by nerves originating from the cardiac ganglionated neural plexuses.[47] Evidence now exists to show a neural role in the initiation and sustenance of

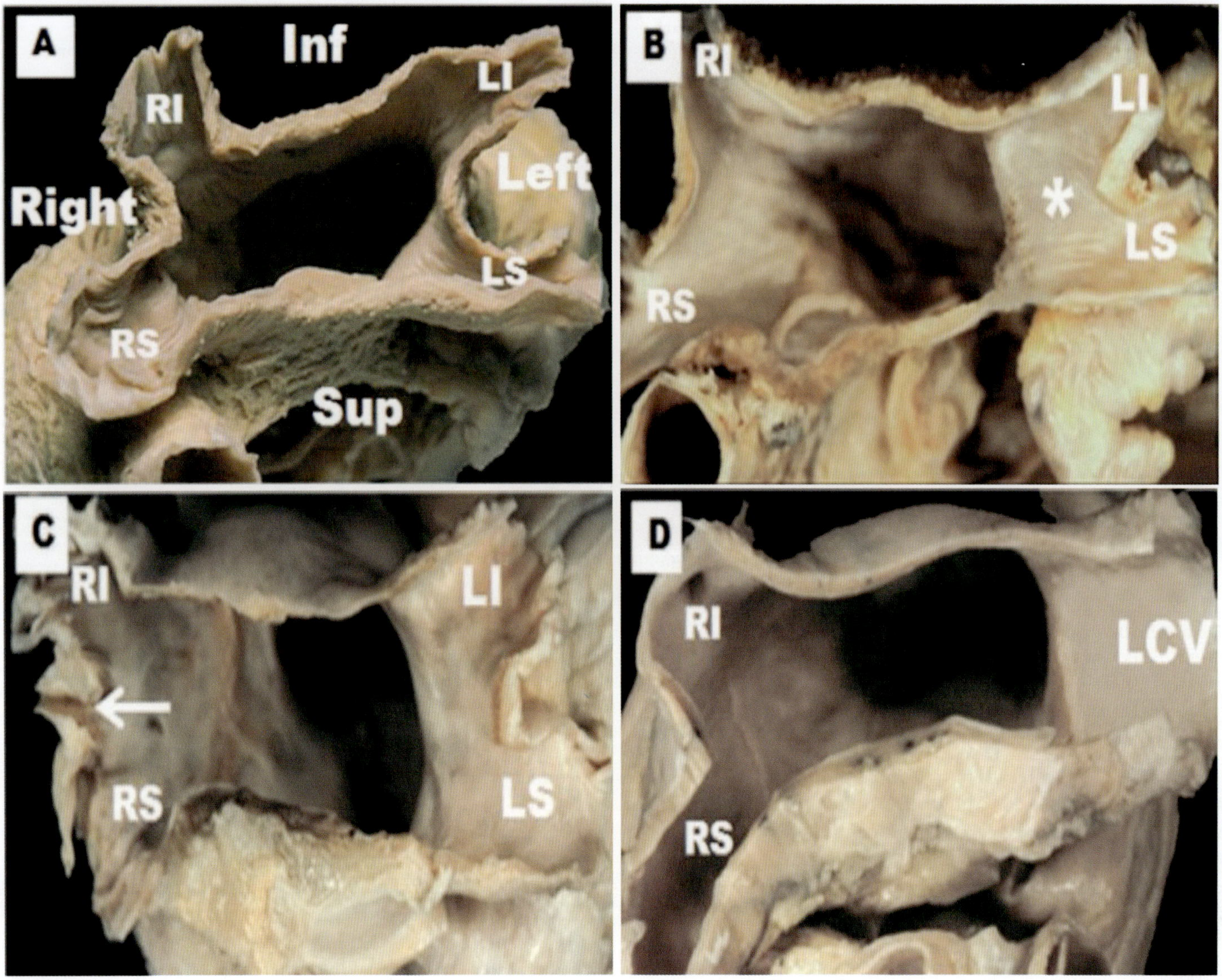

Figure 5.11. Four specimens are shown with the roof of the left atrium removed and the observer looking towards the mitral orifice. They illustrate some of the variability regarding the connections of the pulmonary veins to the pulmonary venous sinus. Panel A shows the anticipated arrangement, with a vein entering each corner of the venous sinus. In panel B, the left (L) veins enter the venous sinus through a common vestibule (asterisk). In panel C, three veins enter the sinus on the right (R) side (arrow), whereas in the variant shown in panel D there is a solitary left-sided vein (LCV). Additional abbreviations: I, Inf, inferior; S, Sup, superior.

atrial arrhythmias.[48,49] Thus, the cause of atrial fibrillation is multifactorial and complex.[50]

When functioning normally, the left atrial walls are activated from the sinus node. In this regard, although there is muscular continuity with the walls of the right atrium through the rims of the oval fossa and the strands that join the walls of the vestibule with the coronary sinus, the major pathway between the atrial chambers is ***Bachmann's bundle***. As was described in Chapter 4, the bundle is a direct continuation of the precaval component of the terminal crest of the right atrium. Having passed in front of the orifice of the superior caval vein, the precaval band continues into the roof and anterior wall of the left atrium through the cranial part of the interatrial groove. A major feature of the bundle is the parallel aggregation of its contained cardiomyocytes, thus favouring preferential conduction along its long axis (Figure 5.14). Changes in orientation and thickness at the boundary of these bundles, nonetheless, may lead to conduction block during the propagation of sinus rhythm, or provide the substrate for atrial arrhythmias.[51]

Although separated from the atrial walls by the fibrous pericardium, the relationship of the nerves tracking through the mediastinum is of clinical significance, as is the location of the oesophagus. The ***phrenic nerves*** track along the lateral parts of the fibrous pericardium. The right phrenic nerve has a close relationship with the superior caval vein and the anterior border of the orifice of the right superior pulmonary vein (Figure 5.15 panel A). On the left side, the phrenic nerve passes over the left appendage as it courses to supply the left diaphragm (Figure 5.15 panel B).[52] It is at risk of being damaged during cryoablation, although the risk is low, estimated at no more than 4%, and is usually reversible.[53,54]

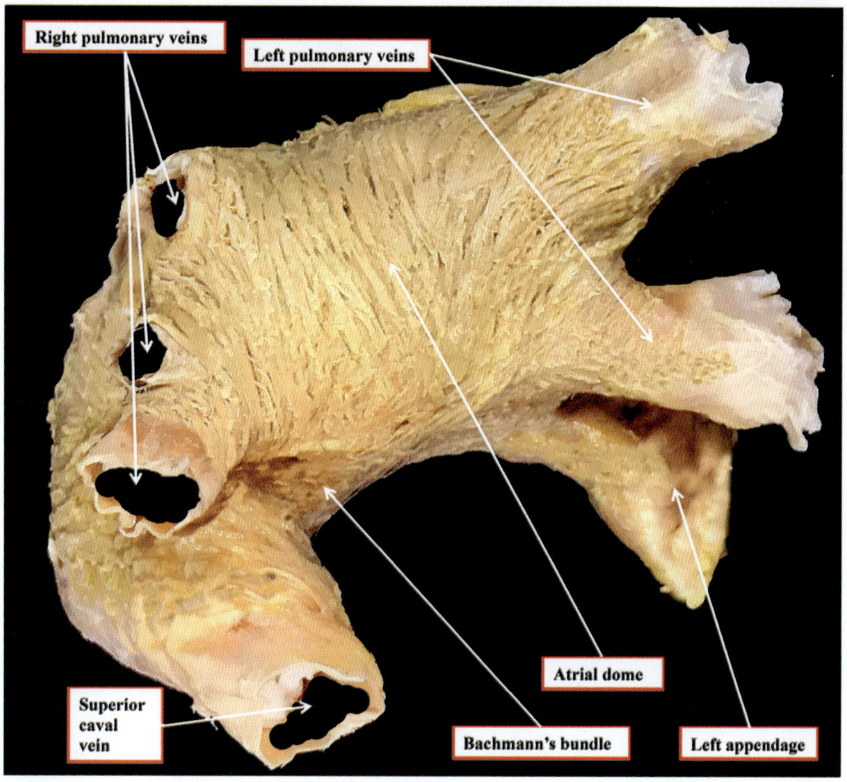

Figure 5.12. In this heart, viewed in comparable fashion to the specimens shown in Figure 5.11, but without removing the atrial dome, there are again three pulmonary veins entering the atrial roof on the right side. In this heart, the epicardial surface of the chambers has been removed to show the "grain" produced by the aggregation of the working cardiomyocytes making up the walls. The walls extend as sleeves for varying distances along the pulmonary veins.

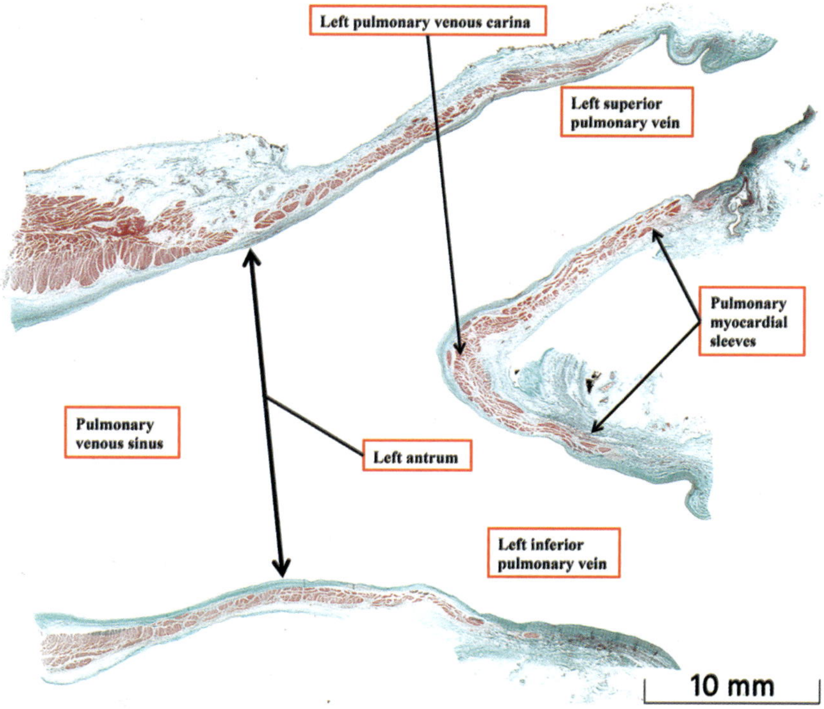

Figure 5.13. The histological section, stained using the trichrome technique, is through the left venoatrial junction. It shows the carina separating the superior and inferior veins, which themselves open to the venous sinus through the antrum. Note that the pulmonary venous sleeves are longer along the superior and the inferior veins. The walls are made up of aggregated working cardiomyocytes, but with a complex and variable architecture between the veins.

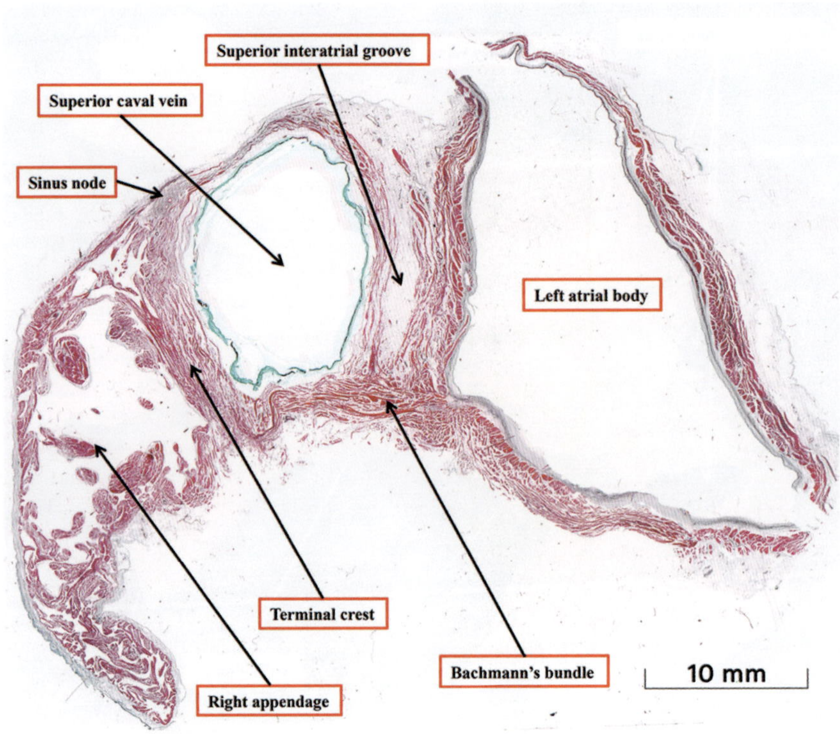

Figure 5.14. The histological section, stained using the trichrome technique and cut along the short axis of the atrial chambers, shows that the walls of the body of the left atrium are thicker than those of the right atrium, although the terminal crest of the right atrium is also thick. Note the parallel alignment of the cardiomyocytes in the terminal crest, which continue their parallel alignment into the walls of the left atrium. This is Bachmann's bundle.

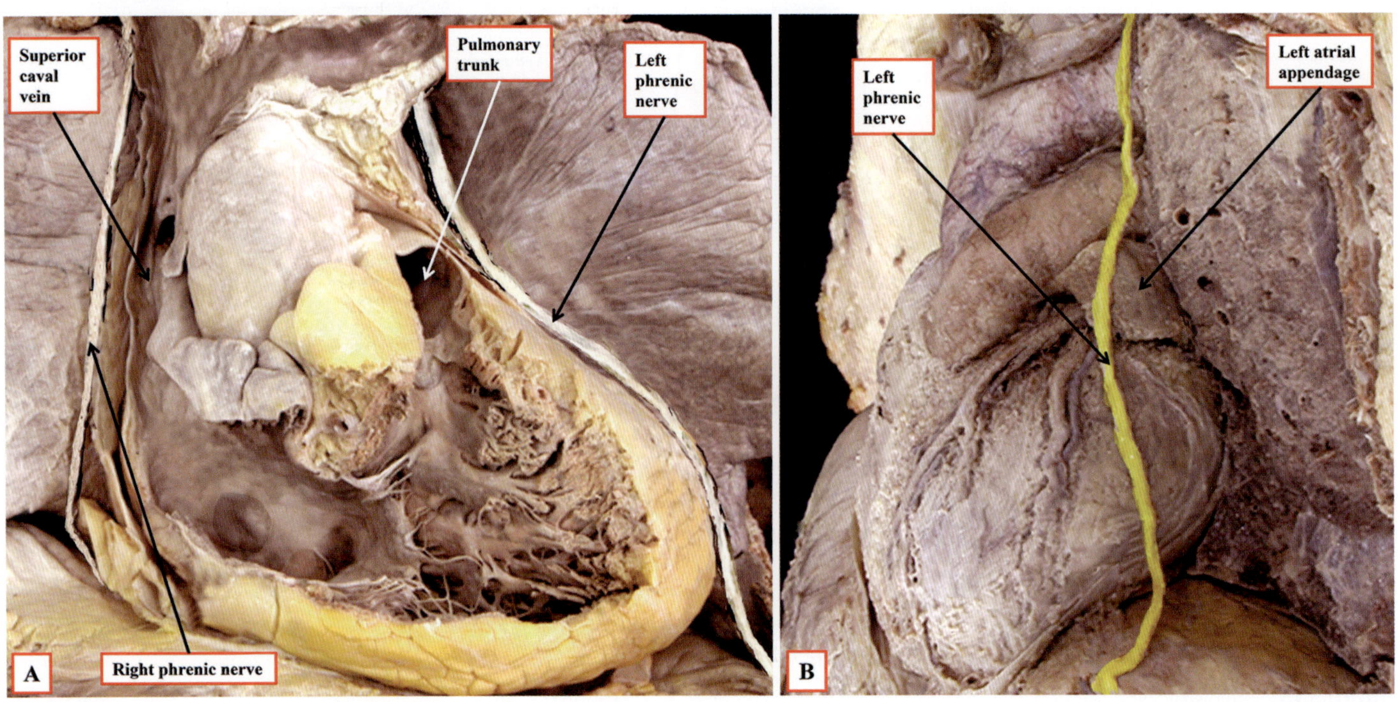

Figure 5.15. In panel A, the anterior walls of the pericardium have been removed to show the relationships of the right and left phrenic nerves to the cardiac chambers. In panel B, the entirety of the fibrous pericardium has been removed and the left phrenic nerve, coloured yellow, has been repositioned to show its relationship to the left atrial appendage.

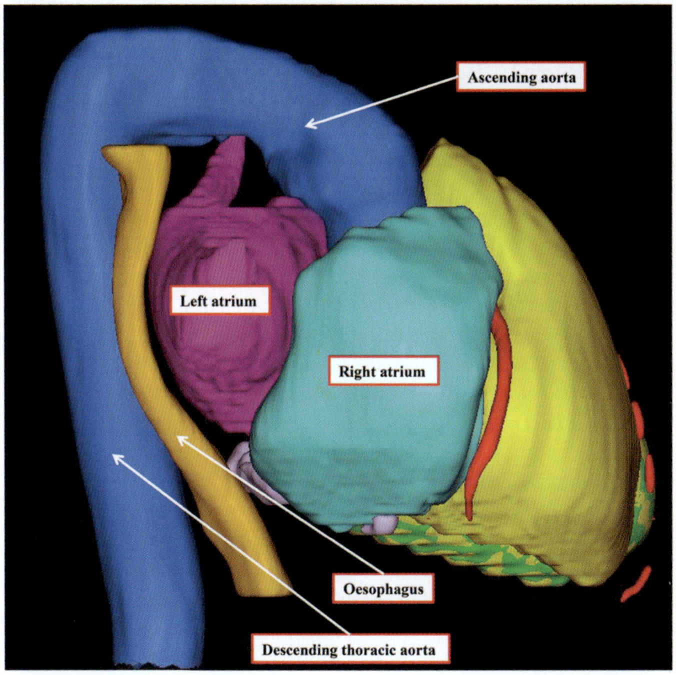

Figure 5.16. The images show a Carto map viewed from behind to show the relationship between the oesophagus and the descending aorta to the posterior wall of the left atrium. Courtesy of Dr Jose Angel Cabrera.

The ***oesophagus*** is located in close proximity to the posterior wall of the left atrium (Figure 5.16), with the vagal plexus descending on its anterior surface.[24] Damage to the oesophagus may occur in up to two-fifths of patients subjected to radiofrequency ablation for atrial fibrillation, especially when lines are made in the posterior wall. Creation of fistulous communications with the atrial cavity, however, is rare, occurring in approximately 0.04% of all patients with radiofrequency ablation. The risk is less with cryoablation, found in no more than 0.001%, whereas pulsed field ablation appears to avoid oesophageal damage. Should fistulas form, nonetheless, they are a significant problem. Depending on the availability of immediate surgical intervention, death has been reported to occur in two-thirds of such instances.[55–57]

REFERENCES

1. Elbatran AI, Anderson RH, Mori S, Saba MM. The rationale for isolation of the left atrial pulmonary venous component to control atrial fibrillation: a review article. *Heart Rhythm*. 2019;**16**:1392–1398. doi: 10.1016/j.hrthm.2019.03.012
2. Dudkiewicz D, Słodowska K, Jasińska KA, Dobrzynski H, Hołda M. The clinical anatomy of the left atrial structures used as landmarks in ablation of arrhythmogenic substrates and cardiac invasive procedures. *Translat Res Anat*. 2021;**23**:100102.
3. Neira V, Hanson M, Tso M, Khakh P, Burak C, Alam M, Sanhueza E, Bakker D, Pardy J, Redfearn D, et al. Comparison of anterior mitral line and mitral isthmus line for ablation of mitral annular flutter. *J Cardiovasc Electrophysiol*. 2024;**35**:1480–1486. doi: 10.1111/jce.16325
4. Davong B, Adelino R, Delasnerie H, Albenque JP, Combes N, Cardin C, Voglimacci-Stephanopoli Q, Combes S, Boveda S. Pulsed-field ablation on mitral isthmus in persistent atrial fibrillation: preliminary data on efficacy and safety. *JACC Clin Electrophysiol*. 2023;**9**:1070–1081. doi: 10.1016/j.jacep.2023.03.021
5. Shah S, Barakat AF, Saliba WI, Abdur Rehman K, Tarakji KG, Rickard J, Bassiouny M, Baranowski B, Tchou P, Bhargava M, et al. Recurrent atrial fibrillation after initial long-term ablation success: electrophysiological findings and outcomes of repeat ablation procedures. *Circ Arrhythm Electrophysiol*. 2018;**11**:e005785. doi: 10.1161/CIRCEP.117.005785
6. Huo Y, Gaspar T, Schönbauer R, Wójcik M, Fiedler L, Roithinger FX, Martinek M, Pürerfellner H, Kirstein B, Richter U, et al. Low-voltage myocardium-guided ablation trial of persistent atrial fibrillation. *NEJM Evidence*. 2022;**1**:EVIDoa2200141. doi: 10.1056/EVIDoa2200141
7. Junarta J, Siddiqui MU, Riley JM, Dikdan SJ, Patel A, Frisch DR. Low-voltage area substrate modification for atrial fibrillation ablation: a systematic review and meta-analysis of clinical trials. *Europace*. 2022;**24**:1585–1598. doi: 10.1093/europace/euac089
8. Ahn J, Shin DG, Han SJ, Lim HE. Does isolation of the left atrial posterior wall using cryoballoon ablation improve clinical outcomes in patients with persistent atrial fibrillation? A prospective randomized controlled trial. *Europace*. 2022;**24**:1093–1101. doi: 10.1093/europace/euac005
9. Tamborero D, Mont L, Berruezo A, Matiello M, Benito B, Sitges M, Vidal B, de Caralt TM, Perea RJ, Vatasescu R, et al. Left atrial posterior wall isolation does not improve the outcome of circumferential pulmonary vein ablation for atrial fibrillation: a prospective randomized study. *Circ Arrhythm Electrophysiol*. 2009;**2**:35–40. doi: 10.1161/CIRCEP.108.797944
10. Kistler PM, Chieng D, Sugumar H, Ling LH, Segan L, Azzopardi S, Al-Kaisey A, Parameswaran R, Anderson RD, Hawson J, et al. Effect of catheter ablation using pulmonary vein isolation with vs without posterior left atrial wall isolation on atrial arrhythmia recurrence in patients with persistent atrial fibrillation: the CAPLA randomized clinical trial. *JAMA*. 2023;**329**:127–135. doi: 10.1001/jama.2022.23722
11. Ho SY, Cabrera JA, Sanchez-Quintana D. Left atrial anatomy revisited. *Circ Arrhythm Electrophysiol*. 2012;**5**:220–228. doi: 10.1161/CIRCEP.111.962720
12. Wang Y, Di Biase L, Horton RP, Nguyen T, Morhanty P, Natale A. Left atrial appendage studied by computed tomography to help planning for appendage closure device placement. *J Cardiovasc Electrophysiol*. 2010;**21**:973–982. doi: 10.1111/j.1540-8167.2010.01814.x
13. Su P, McCarthy KP, Ho SY. Occluding the left atrial appendage: anatomical considerations. *Heart*. 2008;**94**:1166–1170. doi: 10.1136/hrt.2006.111989
14. Liu R, Li Y. Morphology and function assessment of left atrial appendage in patients with atrial fibrillation. *Echocardiography*. 2024;**41**:e70013. doi: 10.1111/echo.70013
15. Wazni OM, Saliba WI, Nair DG, Marijon E, Schmidt B, Hounshell T, Ebelt H, Skurk C, Oza S, Patel C, et al. Left atrial appendage closure after ablation for atrial fibrillation. *N Engl J Med*. 2025;**392**:1277–1287. doi: 10.1056/NEJMoa2408308
16. Galea R, De Marco F, Meneveau N, Aminian A, Anselme F, Grani C, Huber AT, Teiger E, Iriart X, Babongo Bosombo F, et al. Amulet or watchman device for percutaneous left atrial appendage closure: primary results of the SWISS-APERO randomized clinical trial. *Circulation*. 2022;**145**:724–738. doi: 10.1161/CIRCULATIONAHA.121.057859

17. Glikson M, Wolff R, Hindricks G, Mandrola J, Camm AJ, Lip GYH, Fauchier L, Betts TR, Lewalter T, Saw J, et al. EHRA/EAPCI expert consensus statement on catheter-based left atrial appendage occlusion—an update. *Europace*. 2020;**22**:184. doi: 10.1093/europace/euz258
18. Chew DS, Zhou K, Pokorney SD, Matchar DB, Vemulapalli S, Allen LA, Jackson KP, Samad Z, Patel MR, Freeman JV, et al. Left atrial appendage occlusion versus oral anticoagulation in atrial fibrillation: a decision analysis. *Ann Intern Med*. 2022;**175**:1230–1239. doi: 10.7326/M21-4653
19. Di Biase L, Burkhardt JD, Mohanty P, Mohanty S, Sanchez JE, Trivedi C, Gunes M, Gokoglan Y, Gianni C, Horton RP, et al. Left atrial appendage isolation in patients with longstanding persistent AF undergoing catheter ablation: BELIEF trial. *J Am Coll Cardiol*. 2016;**68**:1929–1940. doi: 10.1016/j.jacc.2016.07.770
20. Naksuk N, Padmanabhan D, Yogeswaran V, Asirvatham SJ. Left atrial appendage: embryology, anatomy, physiology, arrhythmia and therapeutic intervention. *JACC Clin Electrophysiol*. 2016;**2**:403–412. doi: 10.1016/j.jacep.2016.06.006
21. Schmidt B, Bordignon S, Metzner A, Sommer P, Steven D, Dahme T, Busch M, Tilz RR, Schaack D, Rillig A, et al. Ablation strategies for repeat procedures in atrial fibrillation recurrences despite durable pulmonary vein isolation: the prospective randomized ASTRO AF multicenter trial. *Circulation*. 2024;**150**:2007–2018. doi: 10.1161/CIRCULATIONAHA.124.069993
22. Hagen PT, Scholz DG, Edwards WD. Incidence and size of patent foramen ovale during the first 10 decades of life: an autopsy study of 965 normal hearts. *Mayo Clin Proc*. 1984;**59**:17–20. doi: 10.1016/s0025-6196(12)60336-x
23. Bonczar M, Piatek-Koziej K, Wolska J, Tomala O, Stitou EA, Pekala J, Pekala P, Walocha J, Holda M, Koziej M. Variations in human pulmonary vein ostia morphology: a systematic review with meta-analysis. *Clin Anat*. 2022;**35**:906–926. doi: 10.1002/ca.23896
24. Ho SY, Cabrera JA, Sanchez-Quintana D. Left atrial anatomy revisited. *Circ Arrhythm Electrophysiol*. 2012;**5**:220–228. doi: 10.1161/circep.111.962720
25. Ho SY, Cabrera JA, Tran VH, Farre J, Anderson RH, Sanchez-Quintana D. Architecture of the pulmonary veins: relevance to radiofrequency ablation. *Heart*. 2001;**86**:265–270. doi: https://doi.org/10.1136/heart.86.3.265
26. Sanchez-Quintana D, Lopez-Minguez JR, Pizarro G, Murillo M, Cabrera JA. Triggers and anatomical substrates in the genesis and perpetuation of atrial fibrillation. *Curr Cardiol Rev*. 2012;**8**:310–326. doi: 10.2174/157340312803760721
27. Sizarov A, Anderson RH, Christoffels VM, Moorman AF. Three-dimensional and molecular analysis of the venous pole of the developing human heart. *Circulation*. 2010;**122**:798–807. doi: 10.1161/CIRCULATIONAHA.110.953844
28. Russo AM, Zeitler EP, Giczewska A, Silverstein AP, Al-Khalidi HR, Cha YM, Monahan KH, Bahnson TD, Mark DB, Packer DL, et al. Association between sex and treatment outcomes of atrial fibrillation ablation versus drug therapy: results from the CABANA trial. *Circulation*. 2021;**143**:661–672. doi: 10.1161/CIRCULATIONAHA.120.051558
29. Calkins H, Reynolds MR, Spector P, Sondhi M, Xu Y, Martin A, Williams CJ, Sledge I. Treatment of atrial fibrillation with antiarrhythmic drugs or radiofrequency ablation: two systematic literature reviews and meta-analyses. *Circ Arrhythm Electrophysiol*. 2009;**2**:349–361. doi: 10.1161/CIRCEP.108.824789 CIRCEP.108.824789 [pii]
30. Nielsen JC, Johannessen A, Raatikainen P, Hindricks G, Walfridsson H, Pehrson SM, Englund A, Hartikainen J, Mortensen LS, Hansen PS, et al. Long-term efficacy of catheter ablation as first-line therapy for paroxysmal atrial fibrillation: 5-year outcome in a randomised clinical trial. *Heart*. 2017;**103**:368–376. doi: 10.1136/heartjnl-2016-309781
31. Mont L, Bisbal F, Hernandez-Madrid A, Perez-Castellano N, Vinolas X, Arenal A, Arribas F, Fernandez-Lozano I, Bodegas A, Cobos A, et al. Catheter ablation vs. antiarrhythmic drug treatment of persistent atrial fibrillation: a multicentre, randomized, controlled trial (SARA study). *Eur Heart J*. 2014;**35**:501–507. doi: 10.1093/eurheartj/eht457
32. Packer DL, Mark DB, Robb RA, Monahan KH, Bahnson TD, Poole JE, Noseworthy PA, Rosenberg YD, Jeffries N, Mitchell LB, et al. Effect of catheter ablation vs antiarrhythmic drug therapy on mortality, stroke, bleeding, and cardiac arrest among patients with atrial fibrillation: the CABANA randomized clinical trial. *JAMA*. 2019;**321**:1261–1274. doi: 10.1001/jama.2019.0693
33. Camm AJ. Left atrial ablation for management of atrial fibrillation: CABANA vs. real-world data. Apples and oranges? *Eur Heart J*. 2019;**40**:1265–1267. doi: 10.1093/eurheartj/ehz168
34. Mommersteeg MT, Brown NA, Prall OW, de Gier-de Vries C, Harvey RP, Moorman AF, Christoffels VM. Pitx2c and Nkx2-5 are required for the formation and identity of the pulmonary myocardium. *Circ Res*. 2007;**101**:902–909. doi: 10.1161/CIRCRESAHA.107.161182
35. Olesen MS, Holst AG, Jabbari J, Nielsen JB, Christophersen IE, Sajadieh A, Haunso S, Svendsen JH. Genetic loci on chromosomes 4q25, 7p31, and 12p12 are associated with onset of lone atrial fibrillation before the age of 40 years. *Can J Cardiol*. 2012;**28**:191–195. doi: 10.1016/j.cjca.2011.11.016
36. Kato T, Iwasaki YK, Nattel S. Connexins and atrial fibrillation: filling in the gaps. *Circulation*. 2012;**125**:203–206. doi: 10.1161/CIRCULATIONAHA.111.075432 CIRCULATIONAHA.111.075432 [pii]
37. Kumagai K, Ogawa M, Noguchi H, Yasuda T, Nakashima H, Saku K. Electrophysiologic properties of pulmonary veins assessed using a multielectrode basket catheter. *J Am Coll Cardiol*. 2004;**43**:2281–2289. doi: 10.1016/j.jacc.2004.01.051 S0735109704006825 [pii]
38. Perez-Lugones A, McMahon JT, Ratliff NB, Saliba WI, Schweikert RA, Marrouche NF, Saad EB, Navia JL, McCarthy PM, Tchou P, et al. Evidence of specialized conduction cells in human pulmonary veins of patients with atrial fibrillation. *J Cardiovasc Electrophysiol*. 2003;**14**:803–809. doi: 10.1046/j.1540-8167.2003.03075.x
39. Anderson RH. Subepicardial and endocardial myocardial layers within the roof of the left atrium. *Heart Rhythm*. 2021;**18**:358–359. doi: 10.1016/j.hrthm.2020.11.014
40. Asaeikheybari G, El-Harasis M, Gupta A, Shoemaker MB, Barnard J, Hunter J, Passman RS, Sun H, Kim HS, Schilling T, et al. Artificial intelligence-based feature analysis of pulmonary vein morphology on computed tomography scans and risk of atrial fibrillation recurrence after catheter ablation: a multi-site study. *Circ Arrhythm Electrophysiol*. 2024;**17**:e012679. doi: 10.1161/CIRCEP.123.012679
41. Lau DH, Schotten U, Mahajan R, Antic NA, Hatem SN, Pathak RK, Hendriks JM, Kalman JM, Sanders P. Novel mechanisms in the pathogenesis of atrial fibrillation: practical applications. *Eur Heart J*. 2016;**37**:1573–1581. doi: 10.1093/eurheartj/ehv375

42. Allessie M, Ausma J, Schotten U. Electrical, contractile and structural remodeling during atrial fibrillation. *Cardiovasc Res.* 2002;**54**:230–246. doi: S0008636302002584 [pii]
43. Gal P, Marrouche NF. Magnetic resonance imaging of atrial fibrosis: redefining atrial fibrillation to a syndrome. *Eur Heart J.* 2017;**38**:14–19. doi: 10.1093/eurheartj/ehv514
44. Haemers P, Hamdi H, Guedj K, Suffee N, Farahmand P, Popovic N, Claus P, LePrince P, Nicoletti A, Jalife J, et al. Atrial fibrillation is associated with the fibrotic remodelling of adipose tissue in the subepicardium of human and sheep atria. *Eur Heart J.* 2017;**38**:53–61. doi: 10.1093/eurheartj/ehv625
45. Delgado V, Di Biase L, Leung M, Romero J, Tops LF, Casadei B, Marrouche N, Bax JJ. Structure and function of the left atrium and left atrial appendage: AF and stroke implications. *J Am Coll Cardiol.* 2017;**70**:3157–3172. doi: https://doi.org/10.1016/j.jacc.2017.10.063
46. Gal P, Marrouche NF. Magnetic resonance imaging of atrial fibrosis: redefining atrial fibrillation to a syndrome. *Eur Heart J.* 2017;**38**:14–19. doi: 10.1093/eurheartj/ehv514
47. Chevalier P, Tabib A, Meyronnet D, Chalabreysse L, Restier L, Ludman V, Aliès A, Adeleine P, Thivolet F, Burri H, et al. Quantitative study of nerves of the human left atrium. *Heart Rhythm.* 2005;**2**:518–522. doi: https://doi.org/10.1016/j.hrthm.2005.01.022
48. Katritsis DG. Autonomic ablation and neuromodulation: novel concepts in search of novel technology. *Pacing Clin Electrophysiol.* 2016;**39**:405–406. doi: 10.1111/pace.12847
49. Katritsis GD, Katritsis DG. Cardiac autonomic denervation for ablation of atrial fibrillation. *Arrhythm Electrophysiol Rev.* 2014;**3**:113–115. doi: 10.15420/aer.2014.3.2.113
50. de Groot NMS, Kleber A, Narayan SM, Ciaccio EJ, Doessel O, Bernus O, Berenfeld O, Callans D, Fedorov V, Hummel J, et al. Atrial fibrillation nomenclature, definitions, and mechanisms: position paper from the International Working Group of the Signal Summit. *Heart Rhythm.* 2025;**22**:1480–1491. doi: 10.1016/j.hrthm.2024.11.012
51. Ariyarajah V, Spodick DH. The Bachmann bundle and interatrial conduction. *Cardiol Rev.* 2006;**14**:194–199. doi: 10.1097/01.crd.0000195221.26979.2b
52. Sanchez-Quintana D, Ho SY, Climent V, Murillo M, Cabrera JA. Anatomic evaluation of the left phrenic nerve relevant to epicardial and endocardial catheter ablation: implications for phrenic nerve injury. *Heart Rhythm.* 2009;**6**:764–768. doi: S1547-5271(09)00211-2 [pii] 10.1016/j.hrthm.2009.02.029 [doi]
53. Sorensen SK, Johannessen A, Worck R, Hansen ML, Hansen J. Radiofrequency versus cryoballoon catheter ablation for paroxysmal atrial fibrillation: durability of pulmonary vein isolation and effect on atrial fibrillation burden: the RACE-AF randomized controlled trial. *Circ Arrhythm Electrophysiol.* 2021;**14**:e009573. doi: 10.1161/CIRCEP.120.009573
54. Heeger CH, Sohns C, Pott A, Metzner A, Inaba O, Straube F, Kuniss M, Aryana A, Miyazaki S, Cay S, et al. Phrenic nerve injury during cryoballoon-based pulmonary vein isolation: results of the worldwide YETI Registry. *Circ Arrhythm Electrophysiol.* 2022;**15**:e010516. doi: 10.1161/CIRCEP.121.010516
55. Halbfass P, Pavlov B, Muller P, Nentwich K, Sonne K, Barth S, Hamm K, Fochler F, Mugge A, Lusebrink U, et al. Progression from esophageal thermal asymptomatic lesion to perforation complicating atrial fibrillation ablation: a single-center registry. *Circ Arrhythm Electrophysiol.* 2017;**10**:e005233. doi: 10.1161/CIRCEP.117.005233
56. Gandjbakhch E, Mandel F, Dagher Y, Hidden-Lucet F, Rollin A, Maury P. Incidence, epidemiology, diagnosis and prognosis of atrio-oesophageal fistula following percutaneous catheter ablation: a French nationwide survey. *Europace.* 2021;**23**:557–564. doi: 10.1093/europace/euaa278
57. Tilz RR, Schmidt V, Purerfellner H, Maury P, Chun K, Martinek M, Sohns C, Schmidt B, Mandel F, Gandjbakhch E, et al. A worldwide survey on incidence, management, and prognosis of oesophageal fistula formation following atrial fibrillation catheter ablation: the POTTER-AF study. *Eur Heart J.* 2023;**44**:2458–2469. doi: 10.1093/eurheartj/ehad250

6

The Atrioventricular and Ventriculo-Arterial Junctions

The extent of the ventricular septum and its components, remains controversial. It can be described simply as having muscular and membranous components. But part of the membranous septum is usually atrioventricular rather than being interventricular. And, relative to these septal components, the ventricular cavities and their valves spiral within the overall ventricular mass. These ventricular interrelationships become more significant when considering the junctions between the ventricular cavities with the cavities of their appropriate atrial partners, and with the intrapericardial arterial trunks. The junctions together occupy the base of the ventricular mass. They support the leaflets of both the atrioventricular and arterial valves, but not in comparable fashion.[1] This is because the atrioventricular junctions are unions, at the same time producing separation, between two myocardial components, namely the atrial and ventricular myocardial walls. The ventriculo-arterial junctions are more complex, since their larger parts are made up of a union between myocardial or fibrous ventricular walls and the arterial walls of the sinuses of the arterial roots. The semilunar hinging of the arterial valvar leaflets within the roots extends distally beyond the margins of the ventricular myocardial cone. There is, therefore, a fundamental difference found at the distal extent of the cone. On the one hand are the discrete myocardial–arterial junctions. On the other hand there are the lines that mark the distal extent of the ventricular cavities when the valves are closed. This complexity is not currently clarified by popular drawings, many of which show a fibrous "skeleton" within the junctions areas, which is presumed to provide the support for the leaflets of all the cardiac valves.[2] The skeleton thus depicted is often presumed also to provide anchorage for the myocardial ventricular walls.[3]

The concept of well-formed fibrous rings, or "annuluses", within the junctional areas is grossly exaggerated.[4] Simple dissection of the base of the ventricular mass points to the spurious nature of the drawings (Figure 6.1). Cardiac muscle, furthermore, cannot be compared to skeletal muscle.[5] The cardiomyocytes making up both the atrial and ventricular walls are attached to each other. They are aggregated together to produce a three-dimensional mesh within an overall supporting fibrous matrix. The valvar leaflets are then hinged in various ways from the crest of the ventricular cone, itself formed by aggregation of the individual cardiomyocytes. In the case of the pulmonary root, the leaflets are hinged within the free-standing infundibular myocardial sleeve. The atrioventricular junctions, furthermore, contain the major components of the cardiac vasculature, such as the major coronary arteries,[6] and the coronary sinus and its venous tributaries.[7] On occasion, they harbour the accessory myocardial connections which provide the substrate for the Wolff–Parkinson–White and Mahaim variants of ventricular pre-excitation.[8] This chapter will describe the specific features of all the junctions.

Atrioventricular Junctions

The anatomist tends to view the base of the ventricular cone from its atrial aspect (Figure 6.1). Such assessment reveals the central location of the aortic root, which is wedged between the right and left atrioventricular junctions. It also shows how the pulmonary root is lifted away from the base of the myocardial cone, placing the leaflets of the pulmonary valve in anterior and left-sided position, despite being supported by the right ventricle (Figures 6.1, 6.2 panel A). Assessment from the ventricular aspect (Figure 6.2 panel B) confirms the extent of the ***subpulmonary infundibulum***. It also reveals the presence of the significant ***infero-septal recess*** of the left ventricular outflow tract.[9] This space interposes between the inferior part of the muscular ventricular septum and the overall skirt of mitral valvar leaflet tissue. The view obtained by the anatomist is achieved by removing the walls of the atrial chambers and by separation of the arterial roots from the intrapericardial arterial trunks at their ***sinutubular junctions***. Attention to the trunks themselves, which will be expanded in Chapter 10, shows that, when traced distally from the sinutubular junctions, they spiral as they extend to the margins of the pericardial cavity (Figure 6.3).

Assessment from the ventricular aspect, as was emphasized in Chapter 1, demonstrates the importance of using the attitudinally appropriate approach when naming the leaflets of the atrioventricular valves. Even now, most clinicians continue to describe the valvar leaflets using the Valentine approach. When using this inappropriate approach, the leaflet of the ***tricuspid valve*** supported by the diaphragmatic component of the right atrioventricular junction is deemed to be "posterior".[10] Structures that are posterior, however, are those that are closest to the spine. As was shown in Chapter 1, the

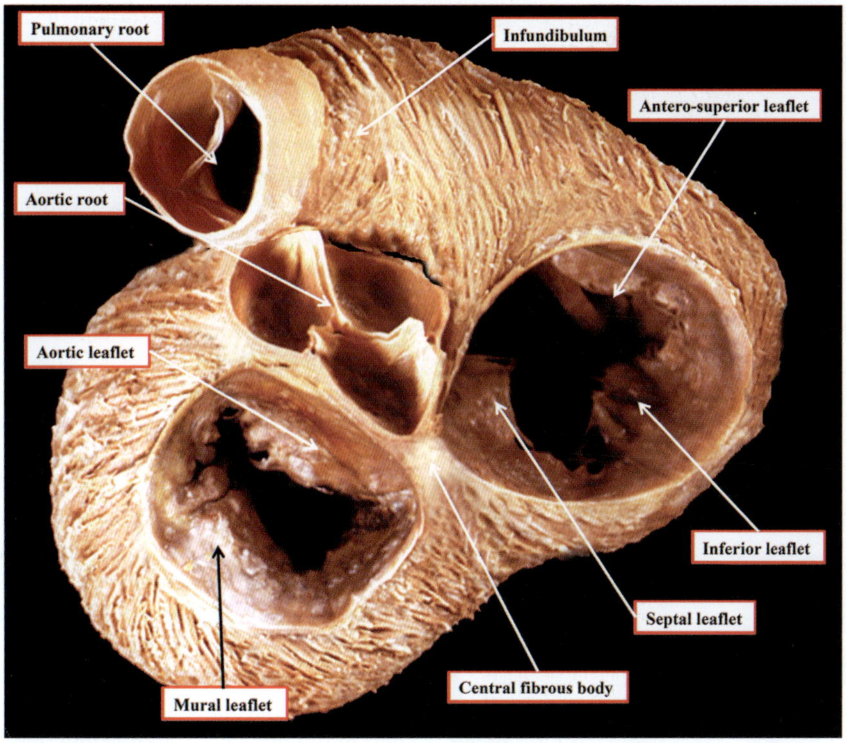

Figure 6.1. The heart has been dissected by removing the atrial walls and cutting back the arterial trunks to the level of the sinutubular junctions in the pulmonary root and the bases of the sinuses of the aortic root. There is no evidence of a so-called fibrous skeleton. The area best representing a "skeleton" is the region of fibrous continuity between the leaflets of the tricuspid and mitral valves called the central fibrous body.

images now available to clinicians directly reveal the relationship of the cardiac components not only to the sternum and the spine, but also to the diaphragm. Such assessment of the junctions, as for example when using computed tomography, reveals the septal leaflet of the tricuspid valve to be closest to the spine, and hence posterior. The leaflet supported by the diaphragmatic margin of the junction is inferiorly positioned. The third leaflet of the valve is then located antero-superiorly (Figure 6.2 panel B). Specific features of the valve, and its supporting tension apparatus, are provided in Chapter 7.

The leaflets of the ***mitral valve*** are conventionally described as being *anterior* and *posterior*.[11] This is reasonably accurate. The leaflet that is located towards the spine, however, wraps itself round the other leaflet (Figure 6.4). This feature, coupled with the obliquity of the valve relative to the bodily coordinates, offers the alternative approach of naming the leaflets as being ***aortic*** and ***mural***. Labelling in this fashion then emphasizes the significance of their support within the left atrioventricular junction. The aortic leaflet of the mitral valve is named in this fashion because of its continuity with the non-coronary and left coronary leaflets of the aortic valve (Figure 6.5).

The mural leaflet of the valve guards a much greater part of the circumference of the left atrioventricular junction (Figures 6.1, 6.6 panel A). The thickened rightward end of this area of continuity, described as the ***right fibrous trigone***, is part of the area within the junctions which is formed of fibrous tissues. Called the ***central fibrous body*** (Figures 6.5, 6.6), this area is frequently interpreted as being made up only by the right fibrous trigone and the membranous septum.[12] A significant contribution to the area is also provided by fibrous continuity between the leaflets of the mitral and tricuspid valves. This part of the central fibrous body provides the support for the ***antero-inferior buttress*** of the atrial septum (Figure 6.7).

The expansion of the atrioventricular junctions during the fetal period establishes the definitive arrangement of the area frequently described as the cardiac "***crux***" (Figure 6.8). During the process of cardiac septation, the primary atrial septum, which separates the atrial cavities, grows caudally towards the developing muscular ventricular septum. The two septal components come together at the level of the developing atrioventricular junctions. Relative to the plane provided by the atrioventricular cushions, they form an obvious cross, hence the naming of this part as the "***crux***". The crossing point of the septal components and the junctions becomes remodelled during the fetal period concomitant with inferior expansion of both the developing right and left atrioventricular junctions and the incorporation of the aortic root into the developing infero-septal recess of the left ventricular outflow tract (Figure 6.4). When seen in the four-chamber projection in the adult heart, there is then a marked off-setting of the planes of the atrial and ventricular septums (Figure 6.7). As part of the change produced by expansion of the atrioventricular junctions during fetal life, the atrial wall of the triangle of Koch similarly expands over the underlying ventricular walls to incorporate the fibrofatty epicardial tissues, thus producing the ***inferior pyramidal space*** (Figure 6.9). From the stance of the anatomist, it is the epicardial boundary of the space as seen on the diaphragmatic surface of the heart that represents the crux (Figure 6.8).

When viewed in this fashion, the site of the inferior component of the muscular ventricular septum is marked by the inferior interventricular artery and the middle cardiac vein. Electrophysiologists, however,

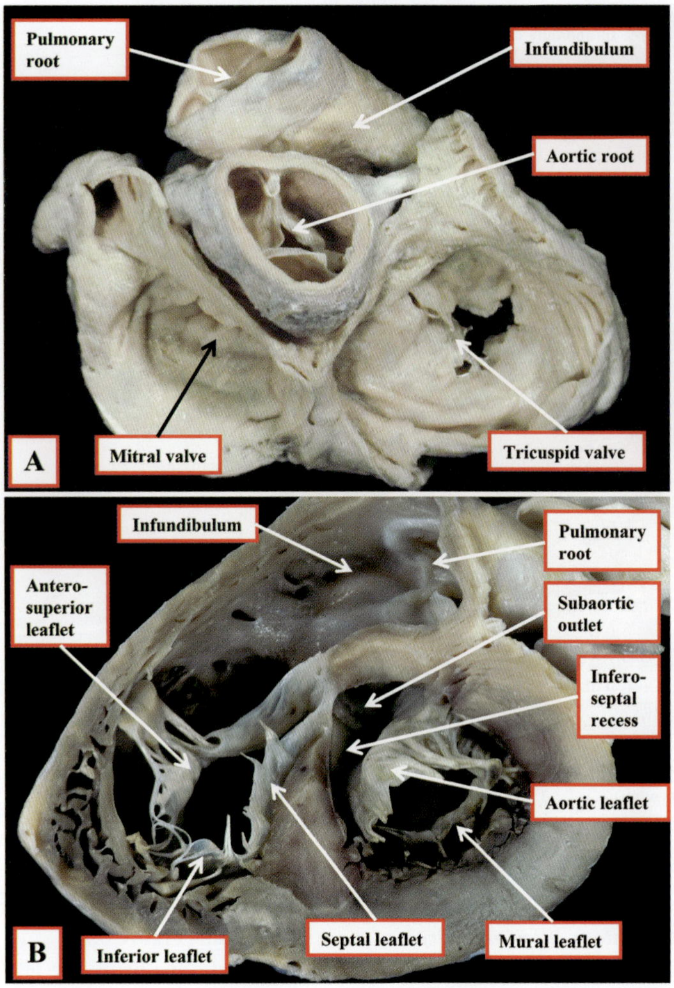

Figure 6.2. The images show the features of the base of the ventricular mass, which contains both the atrioventricular and ventriculo-arterial junction. Panel A shows the view from the atrial aspect, having cut back the atrial walls and removed the intrapericardial arterial trunks at the level of the sinutubular junctions. Panel B, from a different heart, shows the ventricular aspect, having sectioned the ventricular mass obliquely at the level of the mid-point of the subpulmonary infundibulum. In panel B, the labels show how the leaflets of the atrioventricular valves can be named in attitudinally appropriate fashion.

when assessing the focus of ventricular arrhythmias, now described the presence of "basal" and "apical" components of the crux, suggesting that these can be differentiated according to their relationship to the two vascular structures.[12–14] It is difficult to understand the logic of this categorization, the more so since the entirety of the ventricular border of the inferior pyramidal space is part of the basal surface of the ventricular cone. Forming the atrial walls of the pyramidal space, the vestibules diverge markedly when traced inferiorly from the central fibrous area. They can be removed to reveal the ventricular surface of the space (Figure 6.9 panel B). This ventricular component has usually been considered to be part of the septum. Some have labelled it as the "*posterior septal process*".[15] Sections taken across the base of the left ventricle, however, show that the ventricular myocardium in question is neither septal nor posterior. It is the diverging inferior wall of the left ventricle (Figure 6.10).

Because of the interposition of the fibroadipose epicardial tissues, ***accessory muscular atrioventricular connections*** found within the inferior pyramidal space are properly described as being ***paraseptal***, rather than ***septal***.[16] They have often been described as being located posteriorly. The pathways are located inferiorly when assessed in attitudinally appropriate fashion (Figure 6.11). In the same way, pathways frequently described as being "antero-septal" are located superiorly and in paraseptal location.[17] They are directly adjacent to the right coronary sinus of the aortic root (Figure 6.11 panel A). The only true septal component of the atrioventricular junctions is the atrioventricular component of the membranous septum, although this is often overlaid by atrial vestibular myocardium to produce a fibromuscular septum. This area often includes the atrioventricular conduction axis itself (Figure 6.11 panel B). It is unlikely that true septal accessory muscular connections could exist in this area. Hence, those previously labelled as being "***mid-septal***" are better considered to be ***mid-paraseptal*** (Figure 6.11 panel A).[18] It follows that appreciation of the make-up of the atrioventricular junctions provides the basis for understanding the arrangement of the various pathways producing the different forms of pre-excitation.

Neither the right nor the left junction contains a well-formed and continuous "***annulus***" supporting the hinges of the leaflets of the atrioventricular valves (Figure 6.12). Throughout the larger parts of the circumference of the right junction, for example, it is the epicardial fibroadipose tissues that separate the atrial vestibular myocardium from the underlying summit of the right ventricular walls. In areas within the circumference, however, it is possible, in the same heart, to find shelves of fibrous tissue separating the atrial and ventricular walls. Such "***disjunction***" is part of the normal arrangement (Figure 6.13).[19,20] A prominent "disjunction" between the atrial and ventricular components of the left atrioventricular junction has also been suggested to be associated with prolapse of the leaflets of the

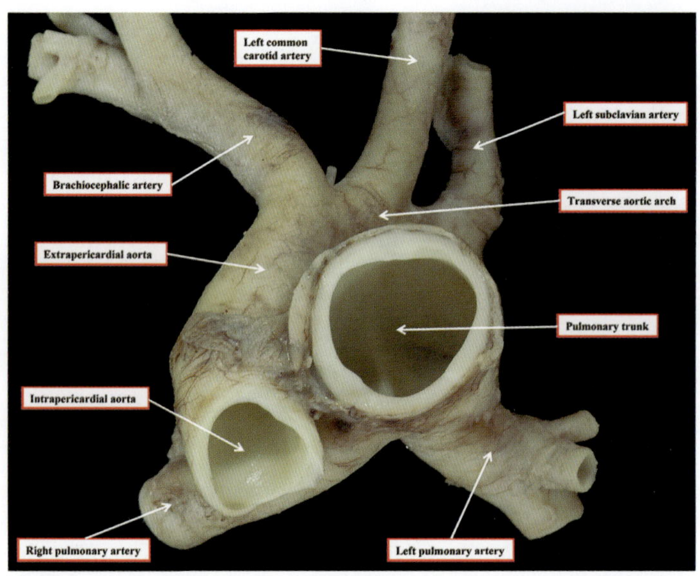

Figure 6.3. The intrapericardial arterial trunks have been removed from the heart at the level of the sinutubular junctions and photographed from the aspect of the base of the ventricular cone looking towards the margins of the pericardial cavity. The pericardium has then been removed to show their branching patterns. The trunks spiral as they extend to the margins of the pericardial cavity.

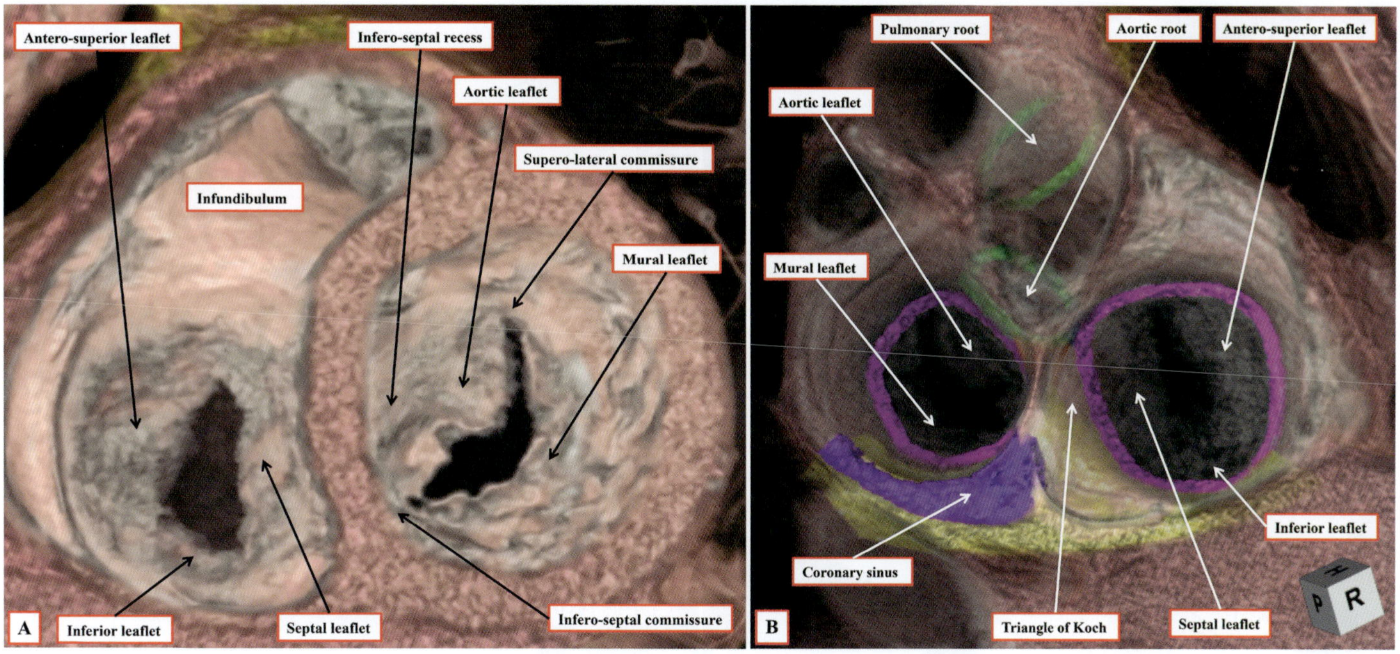

Figure 6.4. The image shown in panel A, taken from a computed tomographic dataset obtained from a living patient, shows the location of the leaflets of the atrioventricular valves as seen from the ventricular apex looking towards the base in left anterior oblique projection. The arrangement parallels the view obtained by the morphologist as shown in Figure 6.1B. In panel B, another computed tomographic dataset has been segmented to show the hinges of the leaflets within the atrioventricular junctions, coloured purple. In this figure, however, the junctions are viewed from the aspect of the atrial chambers looking towards the apex. The so-called annuluses of the arterial valves, as described by echocardiographers, have also been segmented and are shown in green. These rings are virtual entities, since the valvar leaflets are hinged in semilunar fashion within the arterial roots. The cavity of the coronary sinus has also been segmented, showing its location within the posterior part of the left atrioventricular junction. The "compass" box in the lower corner of the panel confirms that it is the septal leaflet of the tricuspid valve that is closest to the spine, and hence posterior.

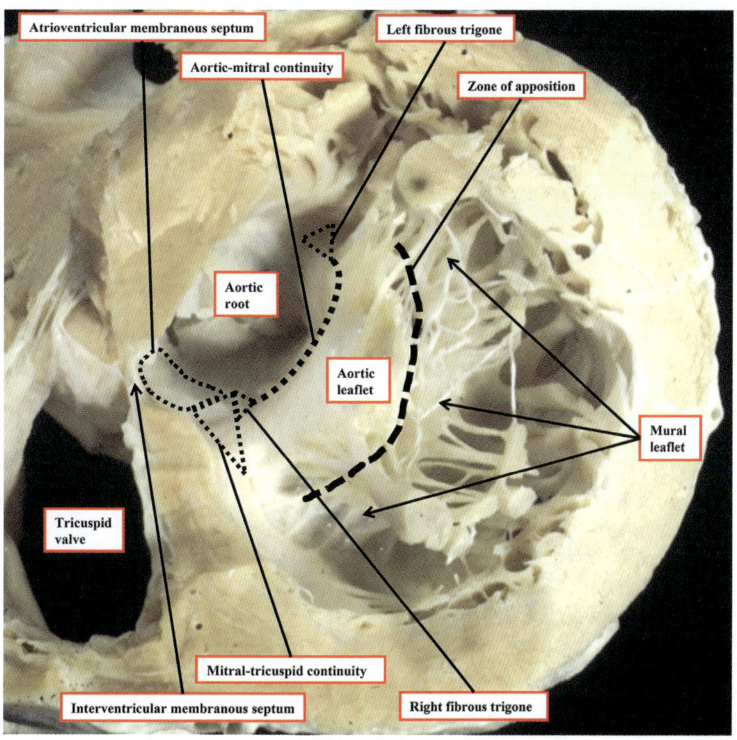

Figure 6.5. The image shows the structures making up the base of the left ventricle as viewed from the apex, with the heart positioned in attitudinally appropriate location. The mural leaflet of the mitral valve wraps itself around the aortic leaflet, the leaflets co-apting along a crescentic solitary zone of apposition. The aortic leaflet is in fibrous continuity, via the fibrous roof of the ventricle, with two of the leaflets of the aortic valve. The area of continuity is thickened at its rightward end to form the right fibrous trigone. The trigone then merges with the fibrous roof of the infero-septal recess, formed by an area of mitral-to-tricuspid valvar continuity, and also with the atrioventricular component of the membranous septum. These three fibrous areas together form the so-called central fibrous body.

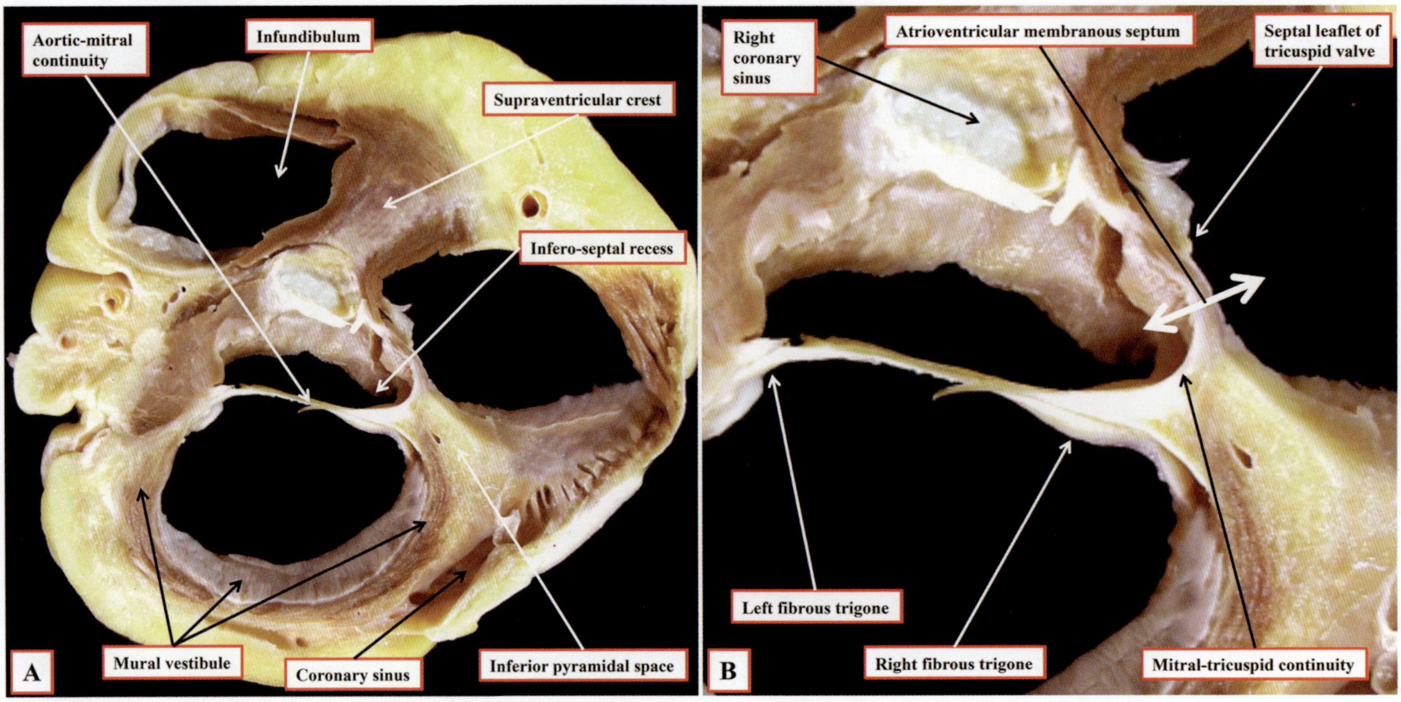

Figure 6.6. Panel A shows a section through the short axis of the atrioventricular junctions photographed from the atrial aspect. It shows the difference between the support provided to the aortic and mural leaflets of the mitral valve. The aortic leaflet is in fibrous continuity with the leaflets of the aortic valve. The larger part of the junction is contiguous with the mural vestibule of the left atrium. The section cuts through the curtain of aortic-to-mitral continuity. The area has been enlarged in panel B. The left end of the area of continuity is thickened to form the left fibrous trigone. The right end is also thickened to form the right fibrous trigone, but this area is continuous with a further area of fibrous continuity between the leaflets of the mitral and tricuspid valves. This area forms the roof of the infero-septal recess and is itself then continuous with the membranous septum. The section shows how the attachment of the septal leaflet of the tricuspid valve divided the membranous septum into atrioventricular and interventricular parts, although the interventricular part cannot be seen in this section. The right fibrous trigone, along with the roof of the infero-septal recess and the membranous septum, with its atrioventricular component shown by the double-headed white arrow, form the so-called central fibrous body.

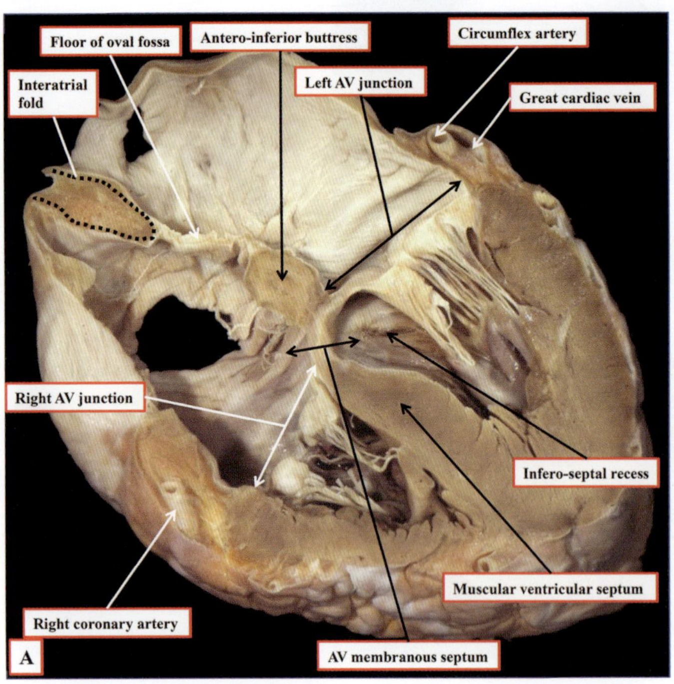

Figure 6.7. The heart has been sectioned along its long axis in the frontal plane. The section shows the off-setting of the right and left atrioventricular junctions, with the area of fibrous continuity between the leaflets of the tricuspid and mitral valves, also incorporating the atrioventricular (AV) component of the membranous septum, forming the roof of the infero-septal recess and supporting the antero-inferior buttress of the atrial septum.

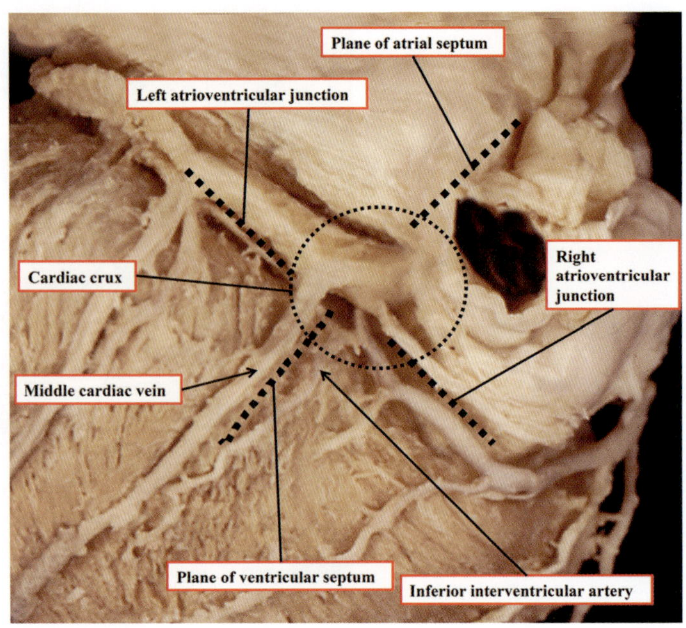

Figure 6.8. The diaphragmatic surface of the heart is viewed from beneath. The dashed lines show the planes, on the one hand, of the atrial and ventricular septums and, on the other hand, the right and left atrioventricular junctions. As is shown by the circle, when viewed from the diaphragmatic aspect, the planes cross to provide the area known to cardiologists as the "crux".

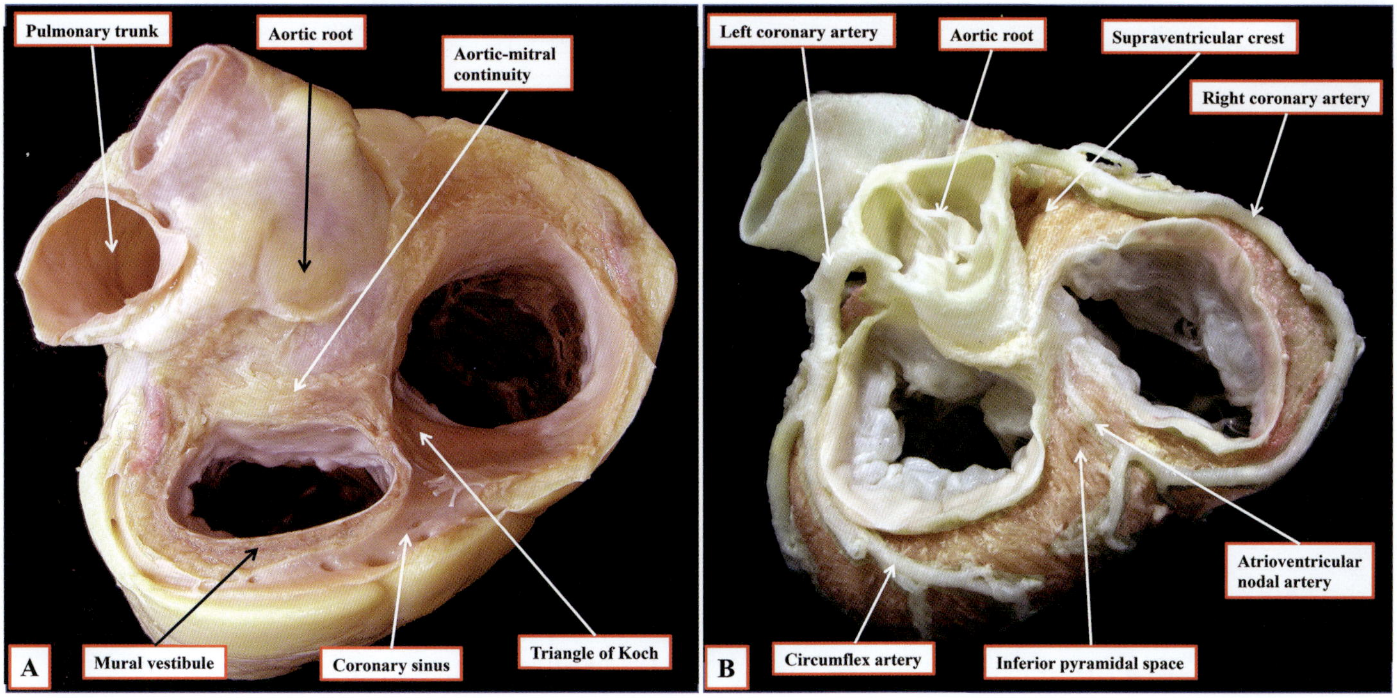

Figure 6.9. Two different hearts have been dissected to show the atrial view of the atrioventricular junctions. In panel A, the atrial vestibules have been left in place. Note again the difference between the mural part of the left atrioventricular junction and the area of continuity with the aortic root. In panel B, the vestibules have been removed, along with the coronary sinus and the cardiac veins, but leaving behind the coronary arteries. It can be seen that the floor of the triangle of Koch overlies diverging inferior margins of the right and left atrioventricular junctions. The area between the atrial wall and the underlying ventricular myocardium is the inferior pyramidal space.

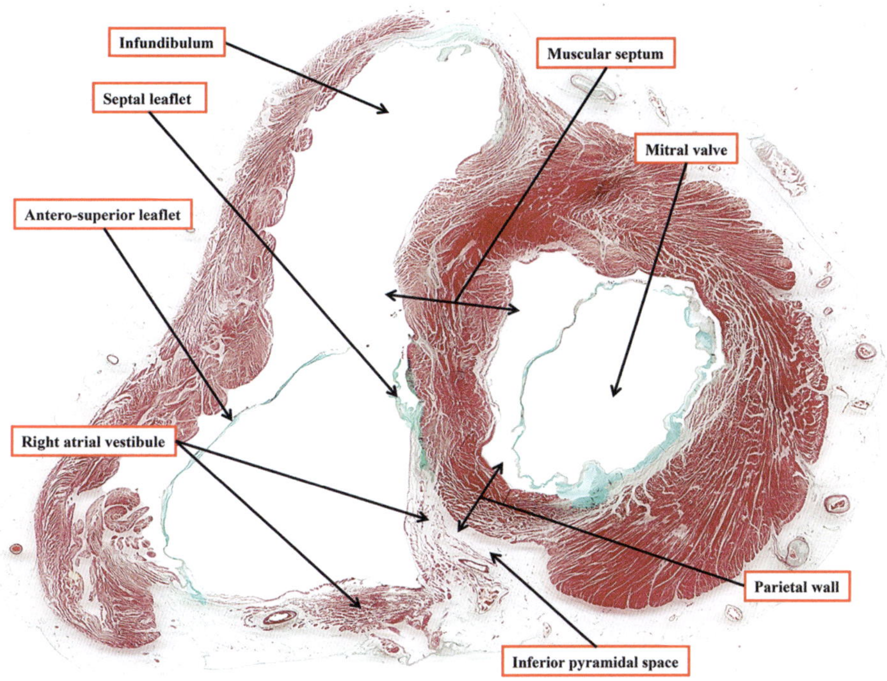

Figure 6.10. The image shows a section through the short axis of the ventricular mass that cuts through the vestibule of the right atrium supporting the inferior leaflet of the tricuspid valve. The section, which has been stained using the trichrome technique, is viewed from the apex looking towards the base. It shows that the ventricular surface of the inferior pyramidal space, marked by the double-headed arrow, is formed by a parietal component of the left ventricular wall. It does not represent a septal structure.

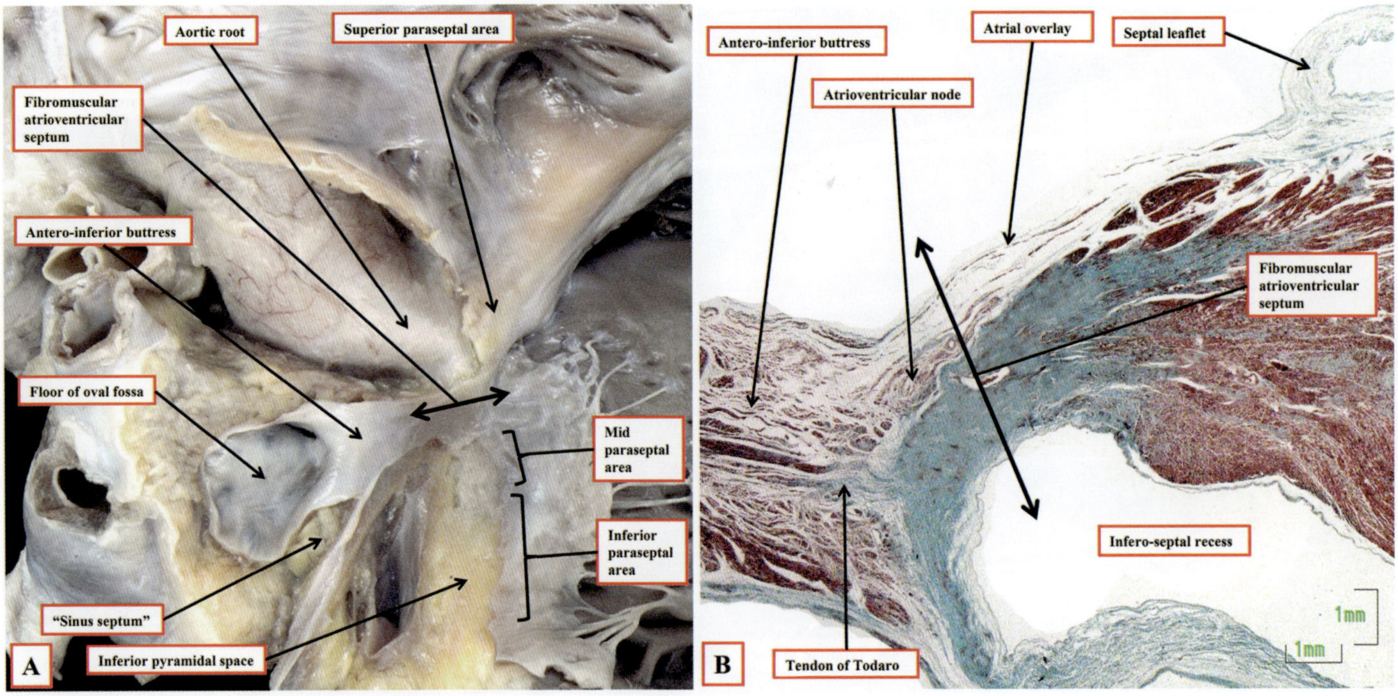

Figure 6.11. The dissection shown in panel A, viewed from the right side, has been prepared by removing the components of the atrial walls that are not septal. All that remains is the floor of the oval fossa and its antero-inferior buttress. The double-headed arrow then shows the location of the atrioventricular component of the membranous septum, which is the only septal part of the atrioventricular junctions. As is shown in panel B, however, which is a section across this area from a different heart, the fibrous component can be overlain by a layer of vestibular myocardium, producing a fibromuscular atrioventricular septum. In this heart, the septal area includes part of the atrioventricular conduction axis. The labels in panel A then show how the paraseptal areas can be divided into inferior, middle, and superior parts.

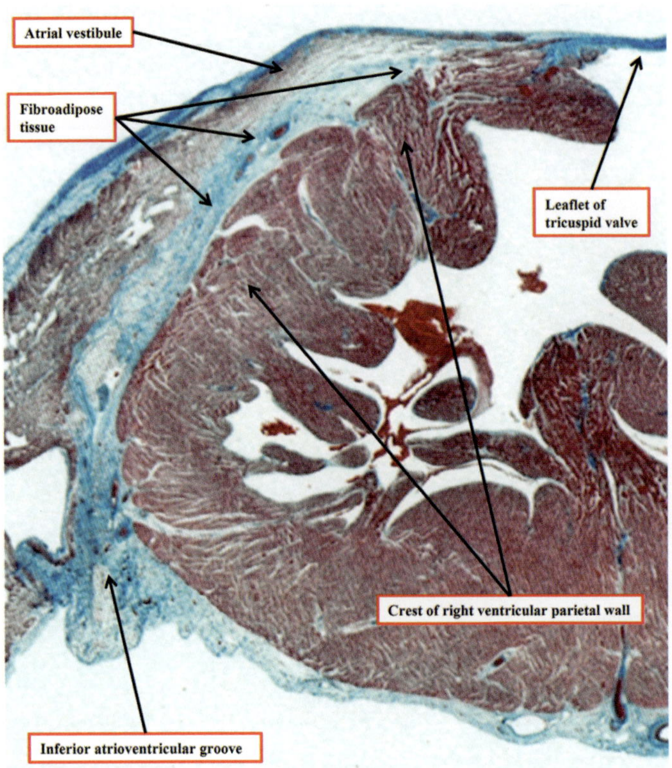

Figure 6.12. The histological section, stained using the trichrome technique, shows the typical arrangement of the support provided to the inferior and antero-septal leaflets of the tricuspid valve. It is the fibroadipose tissues of the junction that insulate the atrial myocardium from the underlying crest of the parietal right ventricular wall. There is no "annulus" as such supporting the hinge of the leaflet.

mitral valve and sudden cardiac death.[21] The finding of abnormal rhythms, particularly when severe, is known to be associated independently with long-term excess mortality and lower event-free survival.[18] These features are to be found irrespective of the presence or absence of mitral regurgitation and the severity of the so-called "disjunction", with the latter being a ubiquitous finding in the normal heart.[22] As yet, the distinction between the normal findings and their potential pathological significance remains to be proven.[20]

When found in the right atrioventricular junction, the ***accessory pathways*** responsible for ventricular pre-excitation traverse within the fibroadipose tissues on the epicardial aspect of the hinges of the valvar leaflets. With regard to pre-excitation, an additional feature of importance, to be found in the right atrioventricular junction, is the presence within the vestibular myocardium of remnants of the primary ring of conduction tissue found during embryonic development. With expansion of the atrioventricular junction, part of the ring is incorporated into the right atrial vestibule. It then encircles the parietal part of the orifice of the tricuspid valve. Most pathways for accessory conduction are made of working myocardium.[23] These pathways can traverse the epicardial tissues of the junction at any site from the hinge of the leaflet to the epicardial covering, and can be found anywhere within the parietal parts of the right junction. On occasion, however, the remnants of the primary ring can persist as the atrial origin of right-sided pathways (Figure 6.14 panel A). These are the so-called "***atriofascicular tracts***".[24] The ventricular parts of the tracts can insert into the right bundle branch. They are insulated as they join the ventricular walls, usually adjacent to the hinge of the antero-superior leaflet of the tricuspid valve at the acute margin

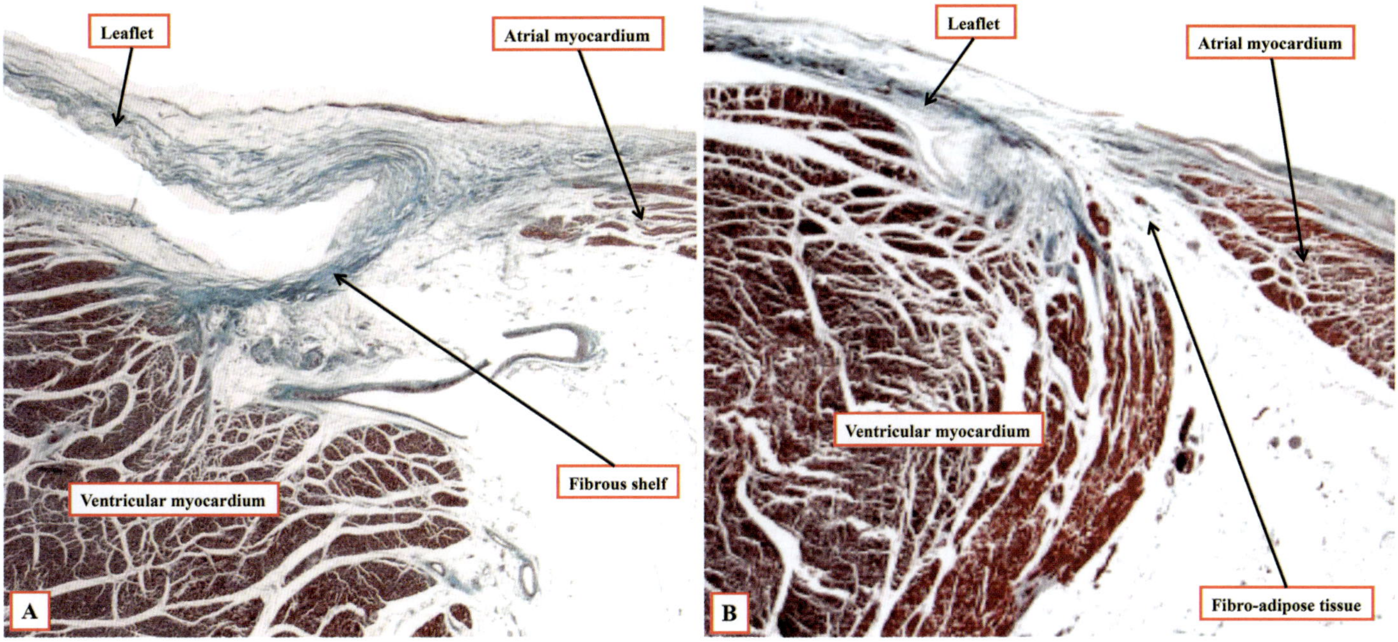

Figure 6.13. The panels show the variation, in the same heart, of the support offered to the mural leaflet of the mitral valve. The arrangement shown in panel A, described as "disjunction", is a normal finding.

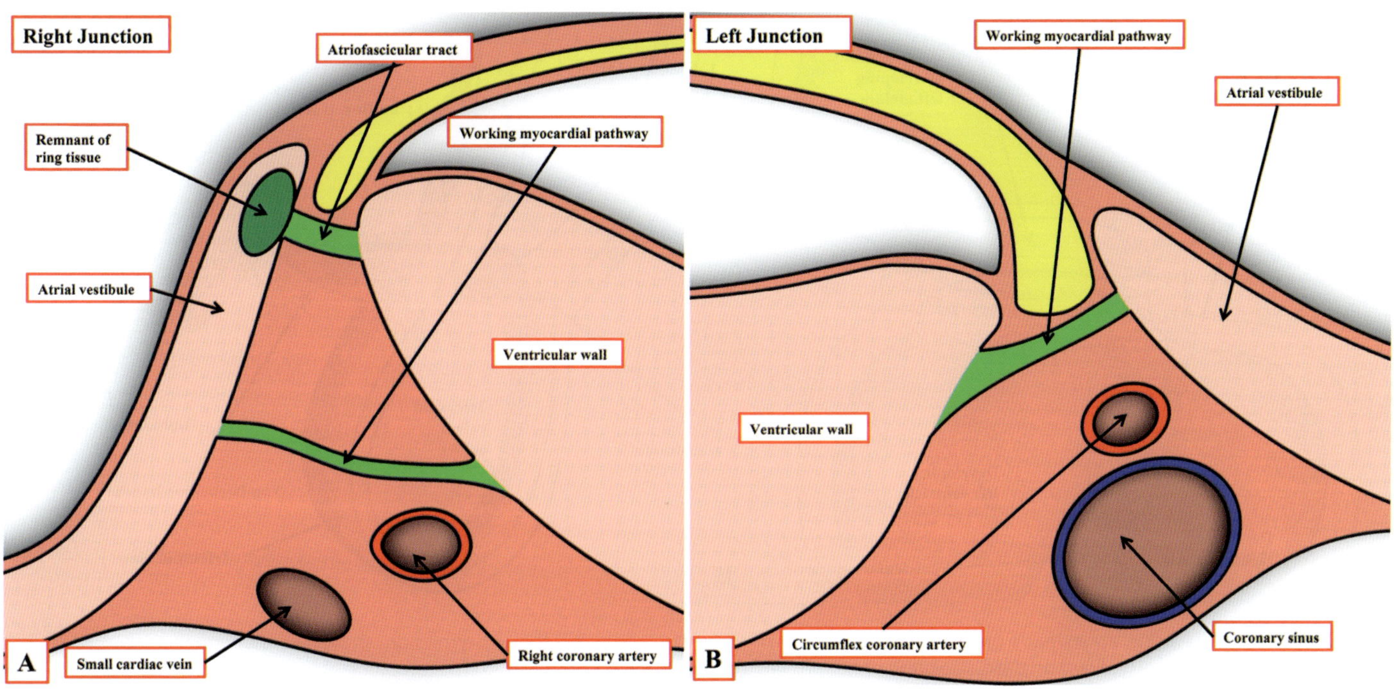

Figure 6.14. The drawings, originally made by Mrs Gemma Price and modified with her permission, contrast the make-up of the right (panel A) and left (panel B) parietal atrioventricular junctions in the context of the accessory muscular connections responsible for producing ventricular pre-excitation. Only the right junction contains the remnants of the ring of conduction tissue that surrounded the primary interventricular foramen. These remnants can persist as the atrial components of the so-called atriofascicular tracts. In both junctions the pathways of working myocardium, which are the anatomical substrates for regular Wolff–Parkinson–White pre-excitation, run on the epicardial aspect of the hinges of the leaflets of the tricuspid and mitral valves. Note that, in either junction, the pathways can be closely related to vascular branches.

of the right atrioventricular junction. The atriofascicular tracts conduct in decremental fashion. Such decrementally conducting tracts can also be found producing pre-excitation in the left atrioventricular junction.[25] Whatever is responsible for the decremental features of the left-sided pathways, it cannot be because they originate in remnants of the primary ring, which are found only in the right-sided vestibule. The vestibular myocardium of the left atrioventricular junction, nonetheless, is derived from the embryonic atrioventricular canal. As such, it does have the capacity to delay atrioventricular conduction. The primary ring, therefore, encircles only the right atrioventricular junction (Figure 6.15). During its development, it terminated in a second nodal remnant formed within the base of the atrial septum. This is the ***retro-aortic node***.[26] As yet, the function of the node during normal atrioventricular conduction has yet to be established. It is likely involved in some of the arrhythmias that are cured by ablation from the non-coronary sinus of the aortic root.[27]

The pathways for accessory conduction found within the left atrioventricular junction are mostly within its mural component. It was suggested for quite some time that the pathways passed through "gaps" in the fibrous annulus of the mitral valve.[28] This is not possible, since as with the right atrioventricular junction, there is no continuous "annulus" supporting the mural leaflet of the mitral valve. As in the right junction, the accessory myocardial pathways extend between the atrial and ventricular muscle masses by running within the fibroadipose tissues of the atrioventricular groove (Figure 6.16 panel B).[28]

The mural leaflet of the mitral valve, as was the case for the tricuspid valve, can in the same heart be hinged from a shelf of fibrous tissue, or directly from the crest of the ventricular wall. Irrespective of its make-up, the pathways producing pre-excitation within the left junction skirt the hinge of the mural leaflet of the mitral valve. As such, they can be closely related to the circumflex artery and the coronary sinus (Figure 6.17). The pathways would be particularly close to the circumflex artery when the artery itself is dominant, supplying the inferior interventricular artery and the artery to the atrioventricular node. Although the pathways are known to exist throughout the parietal left atrioventricular groove, on occasion pathways have been described in relation to the aortic leaflet of the mitral valve. Since, in almost all individuals, this leaflet is in fibrous continuity with two of the leaflets of the aortic valve, it is difficult to envisage how an accessory myocardial pathway could extend from the atrial to the ventricular myocardial masses in this area. The obvious explanation is that the pathways are found in that rare circumstance where the aortic root remains supported by the myocardium of the inner heart circumference. Such myocardium is present during the early stages of embryonic life, but attenuates during the initial stages of fetal development.[29] Should such myocardium

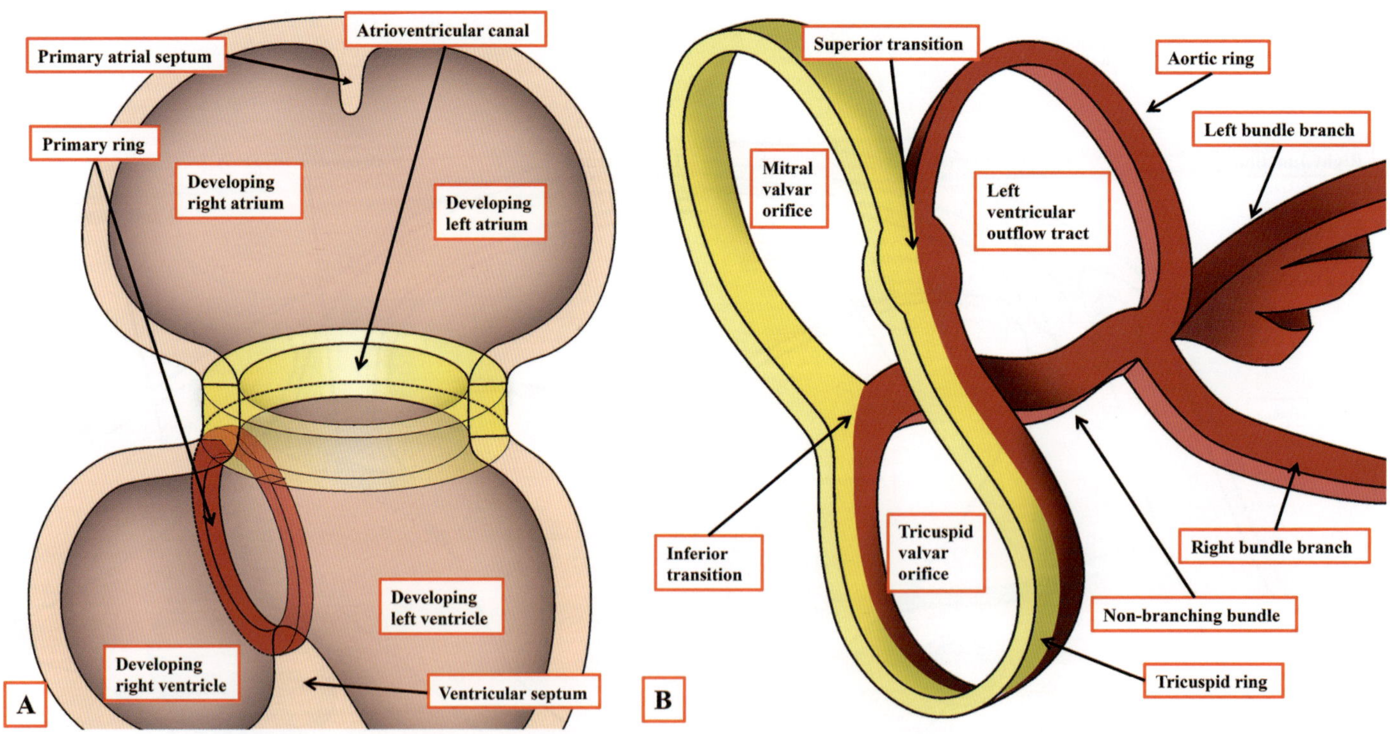

Figure 6.15. The drawings, again made originally by Mrs Gemma Price and relabelled with her permission, show the influence of expansion of the atrioventricular canal (yellow) on the disposition of the primary ring (red). With rightward expansion of the atrioventricular canal, the primary ring itself bends at a right angle, with the dorsal part then encircling the newly formed right atrioventricular junction as part of the right atrioventricular canal. The inferior transition forms the basis of the regular atrioventricular node. Remnants of the rightward part persist as ring tissues. The component encircling the left ventricular outflow tract also eventually attenuates, but the superior transition remains as the so-called retro-aortic node.

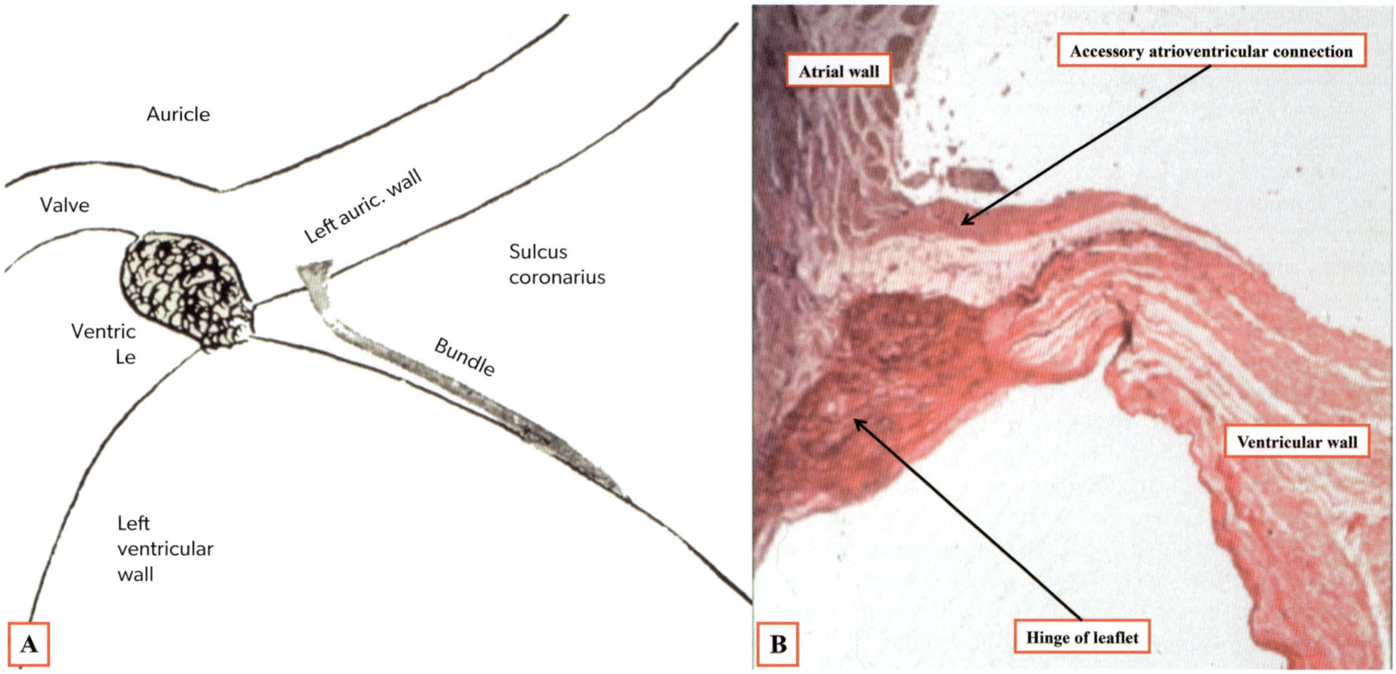

Figure 6.16. Panel A shows the drawing made by Öhnell when describing the first histological confirmation of the anatomic substrate for Wolff–Parkinson–White syndrome type A. Panel B shows a histological section from a patient known to have died with the arrhythmia. The similarity between the drawing and the histology is striking. Note that the pathway skirts the fibrous tissue supporting the hinge of the mural leaflet of the mitral valve.

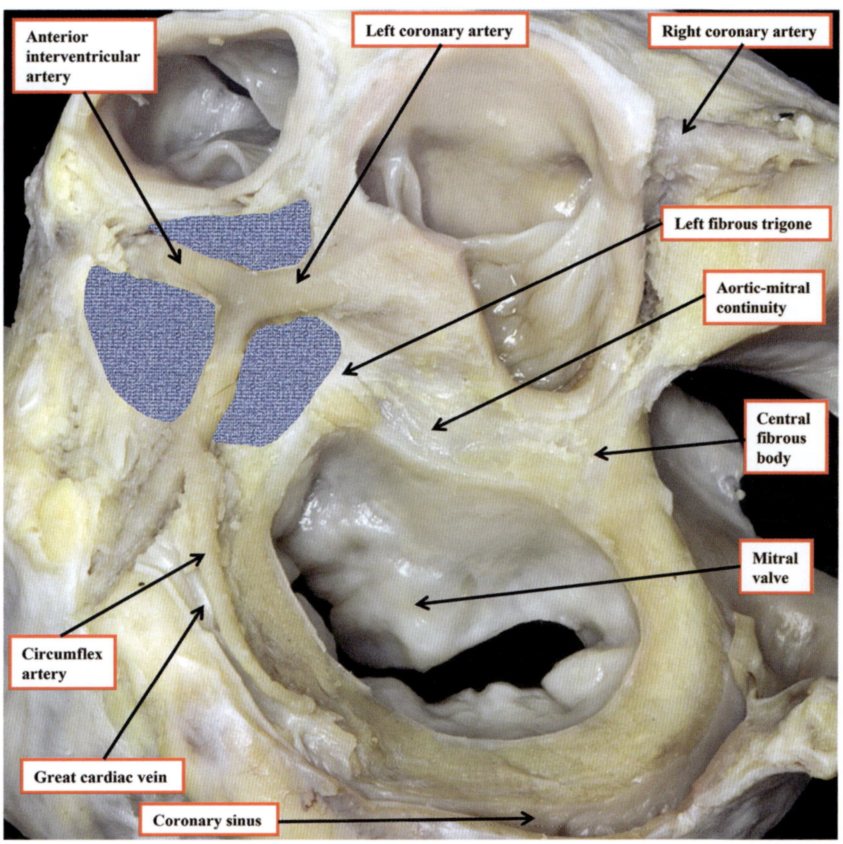

Figure 6.17. The base of the ventricular mass is shown from its atrial aspect, focusing on the left atrioventricular junction. The region known as the summit of the left ventricle is shown by the textured area. The left coronary artery divides into its anterior interventricular and circumflex branches within the area. The great cardiac vein also runs through the summit as it joins the oblique vein of the left atrium to become the coronary sinus.

persist postnatally,[30] then it would provide a potential myocardial substrate for an accessory atrioventricular pathway. It is also known that the accessory pathways can be associated with diverticulums of the coronary sinus.[31] Specific features of all the different accessory pathways are given greater consideration in Chapter 12, which is devoted to the conduction system.

Key components of both atrioventricular junctions are the vascular channels supplying and receiving blood from the walls of the cardiac chambers. The blood supply to the walls is provided by the right and left coronary arteries (Figure 6.18).[6] These major arteries emerge from the sinuses of the aortic root adjacent to the pulmonary trunk (Figure 6.18). The ***right coronary artery*** enters the right atrioventricular groove directly above the supraventricular crest of the right ventricle. It then encircles the parts of the junction hinging the antero-superior and -inferior leaflets of the tricuspid valve. In nine-tenths of individuals, the right coronary artery is dominant, supplying the inferior interventricular artery, along with the artery to the atrioventricular node, and then continuing into the left atrioventricular groove to supply blood to the diaphragmatic wall of the left ventricle. In around half of individuals, the ***first branch of the artery supplies the sinus node***. At the acute margin of the junction it gives rise to the ***acute marginal artery***. As it enters the inferior right atrioventricular junction it is accompanied by the ***small cardiac vein***, with the venous tributary then draining to the ***coronary sinus***.

The ***left coronary artery***, having exited from the aortic root as a solitary vessel, enters the space directly behind the subpulmonary infundibulum, with the tubular left atrial appendage forming the roof of the space. This area of the ventricular base was named the ***left ventricular summit*** (Figure 6.17). It received this name because, when viewed attitudinally, it is the most superior part of the myocardium making up the ventricular cone.[32] The crest of the left ventricular wall extending inferiorly and posteriorly from the area of the summit is the mural component of the left atrioventricular junction. As the left coronary artery enters the area now described as the summit, it branches into the ***anterior*** interventricular and ***circumflex*** arteries, often giving off a third ***intermediate*** branch (Figure 6.19). A detailed discussion of the coronary arteries will be found in Chapter 11, specifically devoted to the coronary circulation. Also entering the summit is the ***great cardiac vein***.[33] It ascends alongside the anterior interventricular artery to reach the summit, exiting to enter the inferior left atrioventricular groove, where it joins with the ***oblique vein*** of the left atrium to form the coronary sinus. The venous components of the summit have become important, since it has been observed that they can be catheterized so as to obtain access to the crest of the muscular ventricular septum. The septal part of the summit supports the left coronary leaflet of the aortic valve, with a varying extent of myocardium incorporated at the base of the left coronary sinus.[34] As already discussed, the coronary sinus itself is an integral part of the left junction, along with the circumflex artery in the one-tenth of the population in which it is dominant.

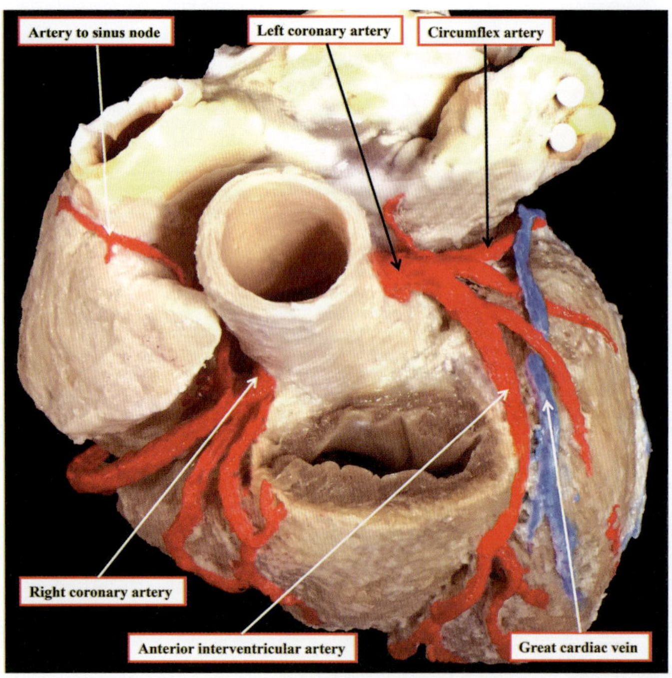

Figure 6.18. The heart is photographed from the front, having removed the subpulmonary infundibulum and reflected the tubular left atrial appendage. The right coronary artery is seen entering the right atrioventricular groove above the supraventricular crest of the right ventricle. The left coronary artery enters the area known as the left ventricular summit, where it is divided into the anterior interventricular and circumflex coronary arteries, with the circumflex artery joined by the great cardiac vein.

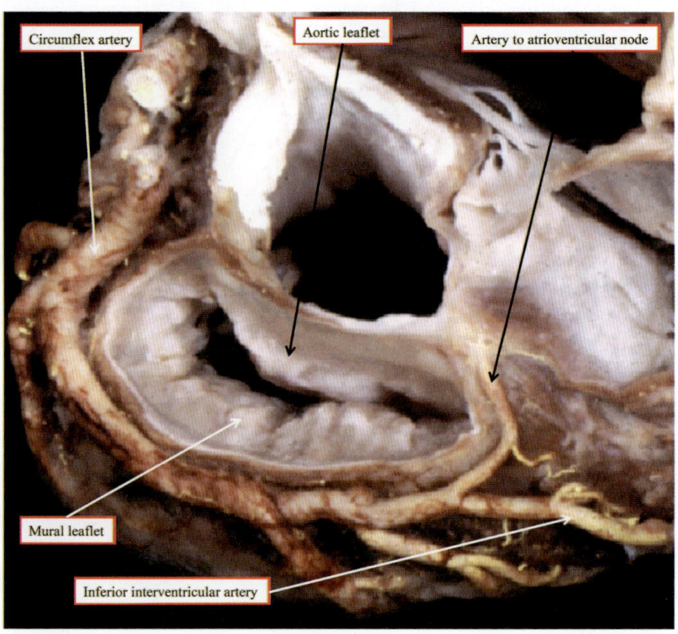

Figure 6.19. In this heart, the circumflex artery is dominant, supplying the inferior interventricular artery and the artery to the atrioventricular node. The heart has been dissected to show the adjacency of the artery to the entirety of the mural leaflet of the mitral valve. The artery would also be directly adjacent to any accessory atrioventricular connection in a patient with a dominant circumflex artery.

And, on occasion, diverticulums of the sinus can be the substrates for Wolff–Parkinson–White syndrome.[31]

Ventriculo-Arterial Junctions

The junctions of the ventricular mass with the arterial roots are more complex in terms of their anatomy than are the junctions between the atrial and ventricular myocardial components. This is because the leaflets of the atrioventricular valves, although not supported by a continuous fibrous "***annulus***", are hinged within their junctions in relatively circular fashion (Figure 6.20). This is not the case with the leaflets of the arterial valves. They are hinged within their supporting roots in semilunar fashion (Figure 6.20).

This arrangement creates significant problems when attempts are made to define an "annulus". Further problems with nomenclature arise when considering how to account for the moving flaps of tissue that come together to close both the atrioventricular and the ventriculo-arterial junctions. These entities traditionally were described as "***cusps***". A cusp, of course, is a point or elevation. The word is used by anatomists to describe the surfaces of the molar and premolar teeth. This shows why, when the closed arterial roots are viewed from their ventricular aspect, anatomists had thought it appropriate also to describe the valves as having "cusps" (Figure 6.21). Such usage has become compromised with the passage of time. Thus, some now suggest that it is only the leaflets of the arterial valves that should be nominated as representing "cusps", with "leaflets" reserved for description of the moving parts of the atrioventricular valves.[28] This is less than satisfactory since one of the atrioventricular valves is itself said to be tricuspid. Electrophysiologists seeking to cure outflow tract arrhythmias, furthermore, frequently describe their procedures as ablating the valvar cusps. It is hoped that they are ablating the myocardium at the bases of the valvar sinuses, rather than the valvar leaflets. And even those who favour making the distinction between leaflets and cusps have described the coronary arteries as arising from the "cusps" of the aortic root.[35] All of these potential problems can be avoided simply by avoiding totally the use of "cusp".[36] The moving parts can then be described as leaflets in both the atrioventricular and arterial valves. For the arterial valves, the ***leaflets*** are then supported by the ***valvar sinuses***.

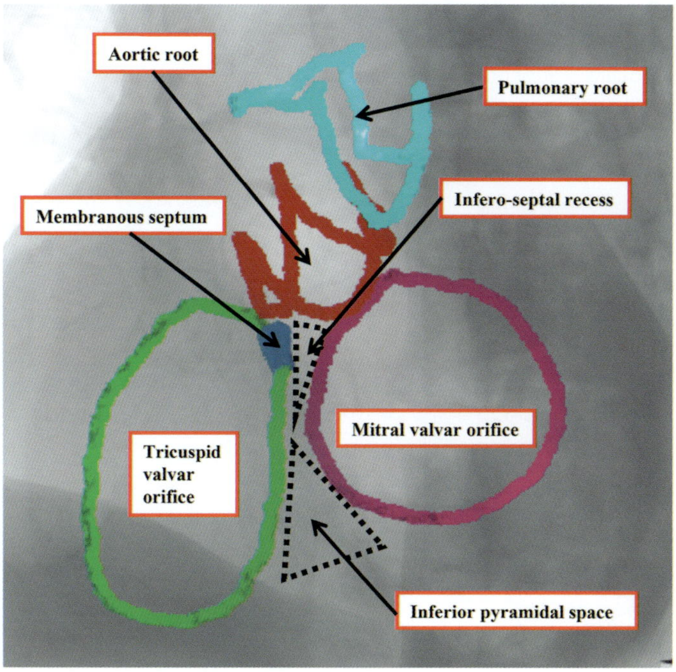

Figure 6.20. The image from a computed tomographic dataset in left anterior oblique projection has been segmented to show the hinges of the atrioventricular valvar leaflets within the right and left atrioventricular junctions, and the hinges of the aortic and pulmonary valves within the arterial roots. The membranous septum has also been segmented. The hinges of the leaflets of the atrioventricular valves are relatively circular. In contrast the leaflets within the arterial roots are hinged in semilunar fashion, producing a crown-like arrangement, with marked tilting of axes of the pulmonary root relative to the aortic root. The image has been marked to show the locations of the inferior pyramidal space and the infero-septal recess of the left ventricle.

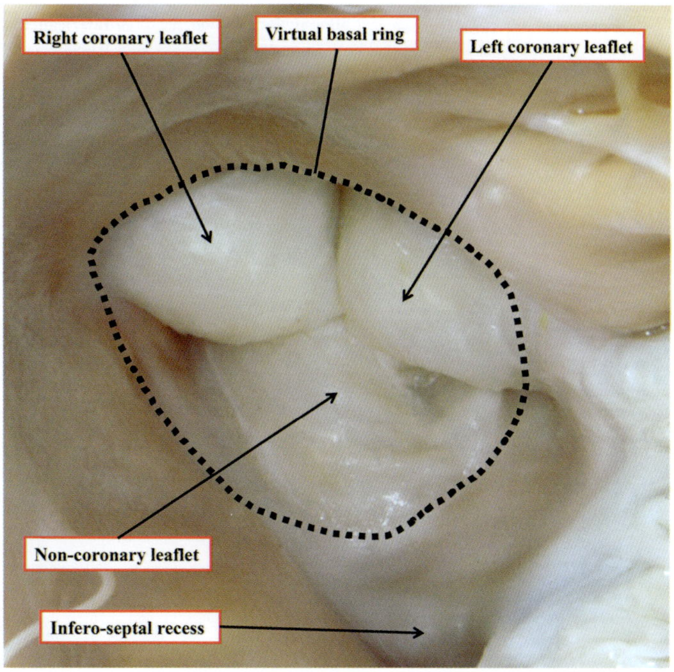

Figure 6.21. The image shows the aortic root viewed from the ventricular aspect with its leaflets in their closed position. The resemblance of the surfaces of the leaflets to the surfaces of the molar teeth offers an explanation as to why the leaflets were initially described as being "cusps", a similar arrangement being observed when the tricuspid valve is viewed in closed position from its atrial aspect. The photograph also shows the infero-septal recess, which is an extension of the left ventricular outflow tract but not part of the aortic root. The proximal boundary of the root is a virtual basal ring, constructed by joining together the nadirs of the semilunar valvar leaflets (black dashed ring). Note that extensions of the cavity of the outflow tract extend between the semilunar hinges towards the sinutubular junction. These extensions have fibrous walls and are the interleaflet triangles.

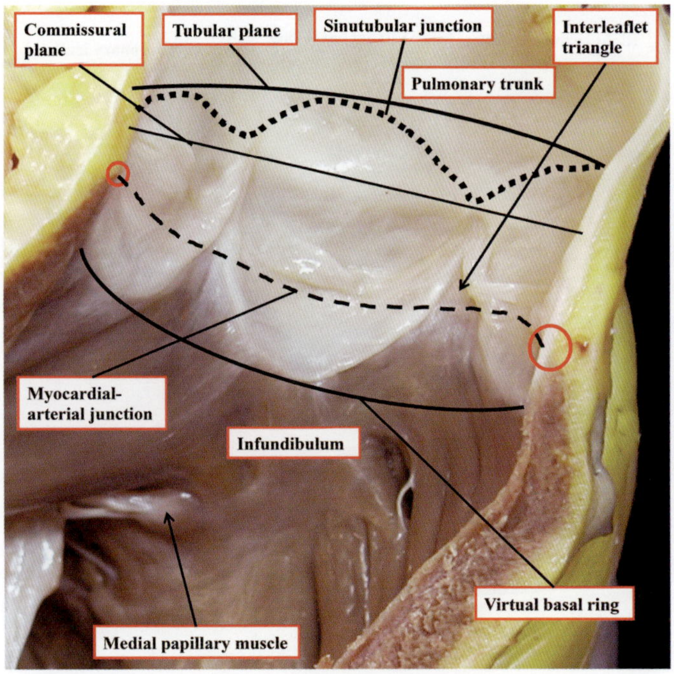

Figure 6.22. The subpulmonary infundibulum has been opened to show the complex anatomical arrangement of the pulmonary root, reflecting the semilunar hinging of the pulmonary valvar leaflets. The hinges of each leaflet cross the myocardial–arterial junction (red circles) so as to incorporate myocardium at the base of all three sinuses. Fibrous interleaflet triangles then extend between the hinges to the level of the sinutubular junction such that part of the distal wall of the ventricular cavity is arterial rather than myocardial. The semilunar hinges come together at the sinutubular junction to form the valvar commissures. Joining together the level of the commissures creates the commissural plane. Joining together the nadirs of the semilunar hinges creates the "annulus" defined by echocardiographers. It is a virtual anatomical entity. The sinusal walls, however, extend distally at their mid-portions relative to the plane that is created by joining together the levels of the valvar commissures. The zeniths of the sinusal walls can then be joined to create the tubular plane, which is another virtual entity.

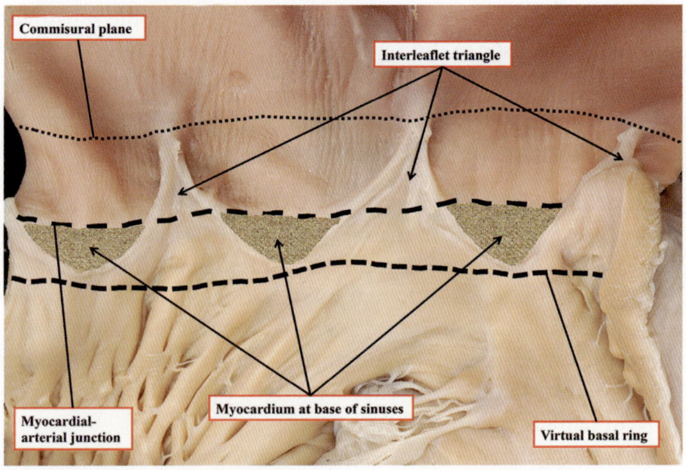

Figure 6.23. As with the heart shown in Figure 6.21, the pulmonary root has been opened and spread to show its component parts. In this heart, however, the valvar leaflets have been removed, leaving only their semilunar hinges. This makes it easier to recognize the myocardial–arterial junction. When the root is closed, it forms an obvious circle. Joining together the levels of the commissures creates another circle, but, as shown in Figure 6.21, the sinutubular junction extends distally relative to the commissural plane at the mid-points of each sinus. Joining together the zeniths of the sinuses creates the virtual tubular plane. The proximal boundary of the root, again circular, is anatomically another virtual entity. It is constructed by joining together the nadirs of the valvar hinges. It is this virtual basal ring that is recognized by echocardiographers as the valvar annulus.

Opening the ***pulmonary root*** then illustrates the anatomical complexity of a seemingly simple structure. The semilunar hinges of the leaflets, which come together distally at the ***sinutubular junction***, cross the anatomical junction between the distal extent of the myocardial right ventricular infundibulum and the arterial walls of the valvar sinuses (Figure 6.22). Removing the leaflets reveals the myocardial–arterial junction formed within the root to be an obvious ring. The sinutubular junction forms the distal extent of the root (Figure 6.23). It is not a planar junction. When assessed in three dimensions, the walls of the sinuses at their mid-points extend further distally than do the points at which the semilunar hinges join together at the sinutubular junction. The points of peripheral junction are described as the valvar ***commissures***. Another virtual ring, described as the ***tubular ring***, can be created by joining together the distal margins of the sinuses themselves.[32] This means that the tubular ring, along with the part of the root recognized by echocardiographers as the valvar annulus, with an annulus itself being a little ring, have no anatomic counterparts (Figure 6.22). They are virtual entities, yet the proximal virtual ring is still nominated by echocardiographers as an annulus. The myocardial–arterial junction, in

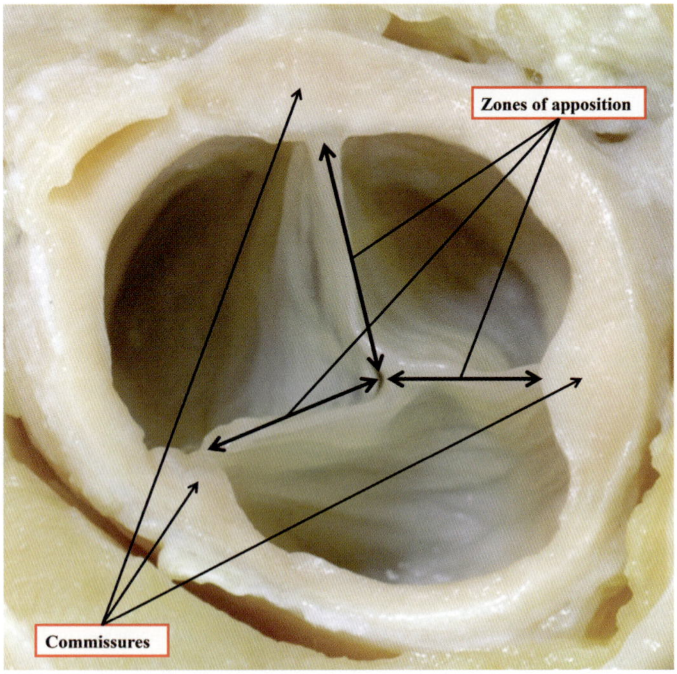

Figure 6.24. The closed aortic valve is photographed from above, showing how the leaflets come together when the valve is in its closed position. The attachments of the adjacent leaflets at the sinutubular junction constitute the valvar commissures. They are the distal ends of the zones of apposition between the leaflets, which extend from the commissures to the centroid of the valvar orifice. The centroid, present only when the valve is closed, is well below the level of the sinutubular junction.

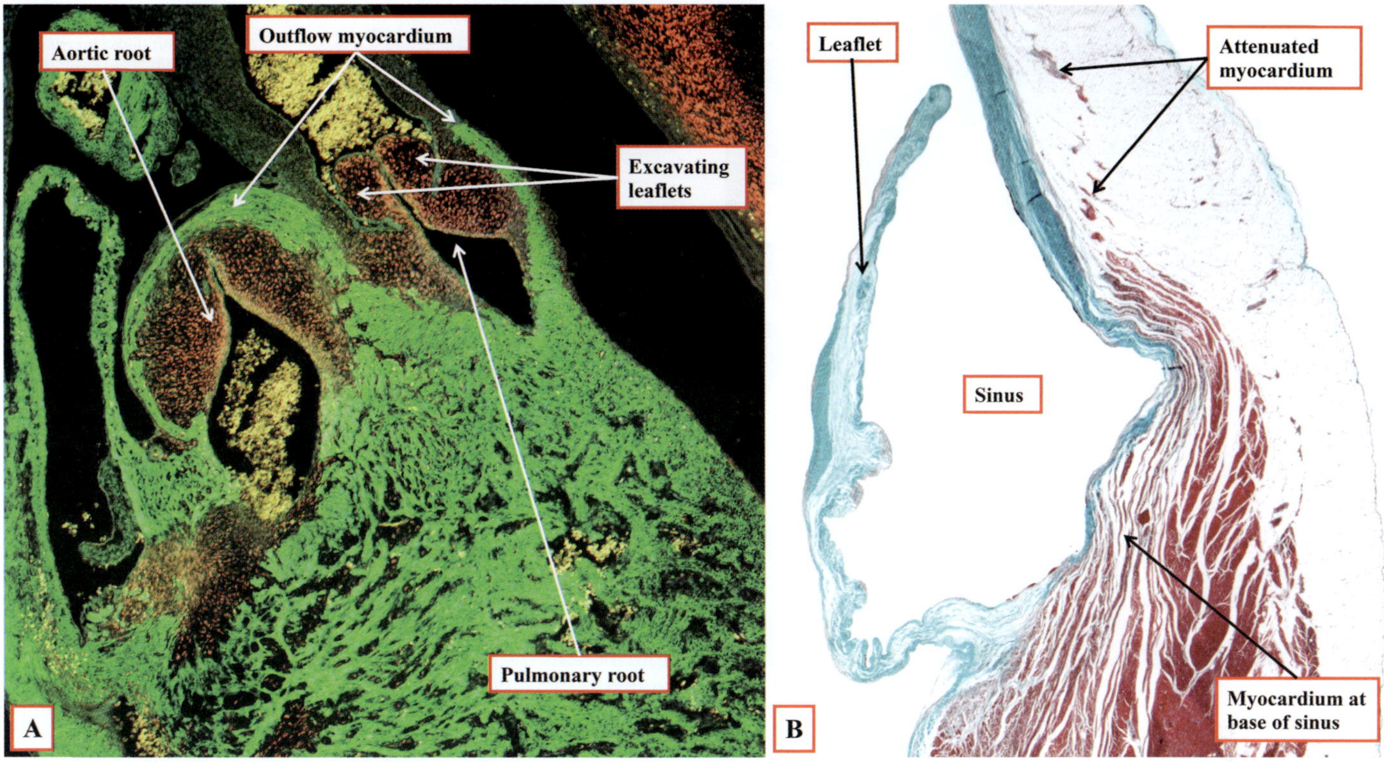

Figure 6.25. The panels show the evolution of the outflow tract myocardium that supports the arterial roots during their development. Panel A shows the arrangement at Carnegie stage 20 when the human embryo has progressed through around 7 weeks of development. The myocardium, stained in green, supports both arterial roots. At this stage, it extends distally to reach the level that will become the sinutubular junction. In the pulmonary root, it is possible to recognize the excavation of the outflow cushions and the intercalated valvar swelling that will form the leaflets of the definitive valve. Panel B shows a section through the non-adjacent sinus of the adult pulmonary root. The myocardium has now regressed to a level much closer to the virtual basal ring, leaving myocardium forming the base of the sinus. Remnants of the myocardium that initially extended to the sinutubular junction can still be observed on the epicardial aspect of the distal wall of the valvar sinus.

contrast, which is a true anatomical ring, is not currently described as being an "annulus", and nor is the sinutubular junction, another obvious anatomical ring. Still further confusion is created when it is appreciated that many surgeons define the semilunar hinges of the leaflets themselves as the "annuluses" of both arterial valves. Indeed, the anatomical study which emphasized the significance of the tubular ring also suggested that the semilunar hinges should be considered as the "true" annulus of the pulmonary root.[32] Irrespective of these linguistic niceties, there are no morphological entities that correspond with the planes created by joining together the nadirs of the semilunar leaflets or the zeniths marking the distal extent of the sinusal walls (Figure 6.22). They are best described, therefore, as the ***virtual basal ring***[33] and the ***tubular ring***.[32]

As indicated, the semilunar hinges of the valvar leaflets come together at the sinutubular junction as the valvar ***commissures*** (Figure 6.24). The use of this word then creates yet another problem for the anatomist. This is because anatomists usually define commissures as the zones of apposition between adjacent structures, such as the commissures between the lips or the eyelids. In the setting of arterial valvar function, therefore, since clinicians define the commissures for only the distal ends of the zones of apposition, it is necessary to provide a name for the apposing surfaces of the leaflets. They are the ***zones of apposition***. The leaflets come together in a snug fashion along the zones of apposition in each arterial root when the leaflets are closed, meeting together at the valvar centroid (Figure 6.24).

Assessment of Figures 6.22, 6.23 also shows that, at the base of each of the sinuses supporting a leaflet of the pulmonary valve, there is a myocardial crescent. These myocardial crescents are the remnants of the outflow myocardium that, during development, supported the entirety of the developing arterial roots (Figure 6.25 panel A).[29] During cardiac development, such myocardium initially extends to the margins of the pericardial cavity. With the formation of the intrapericardial arterial trunks, the level of myocardium regresses to what will become the sinutubular junction.[37] During ongoing embryonic, and later fetal, life there is then continuing attenuation and regression of the myocardium supporting the epicardial aspect of the developing arterial valvar sinuses. Remnants of this epicardial myocardium can still be recognized postnatally in the pulmonary root (Figure 6.25 panel B).

The myocardium found uniformly at the bases of all three pulmonary valvar sinuses (Figures 6.22, 6.23) shows that the regression of the outflow myocardium does not reach the level of the virtual basal ring. It is the myocardium remaining at the bases of the sinuses

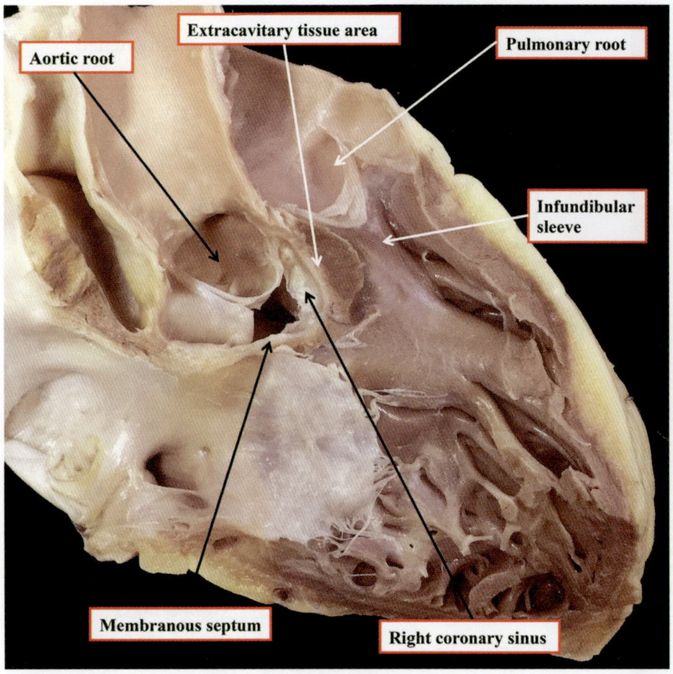

Figure 6.26. The heart has been dissected to show the relationship between the aortic and pulmonary roots. The leaflets of the pulmonary valve are lifted away from the ventricular base by the free-standing infundibular sleeve. An extracavitary area containing fibroadipose tissue separates the infundibulum from the sinuses of the aortic root that give rise to the coronary arteries.

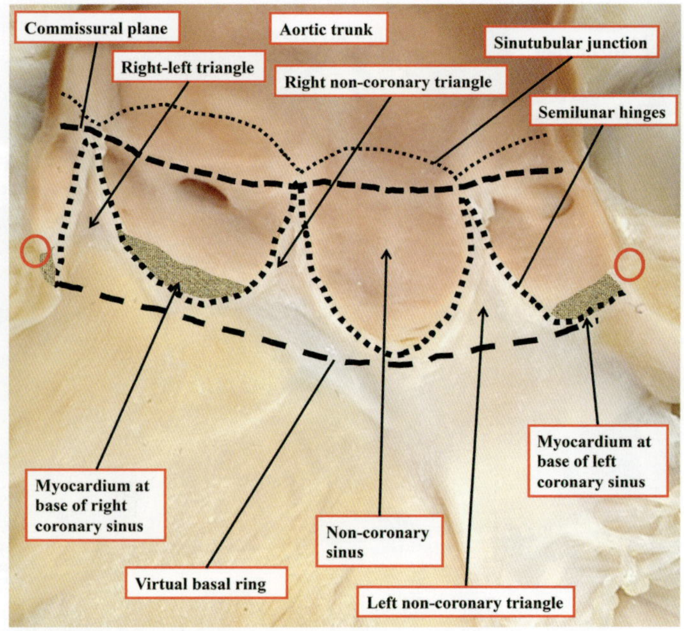

Figure 6.27. The aortic root has been opened by making a cut through the left coronary aortic sinus, with the root then spread to produce an image comparable to those shown for the pulmonary root in Figures 6.22 and 6.23. Unlike the arrangement in the pulmonary root, however, myocardium in the aortic root is found only at the bases of the two sinuses that give rise to the coronary arteries (brown textured areas). The two red circles show the level of the myocardial–arterial junction at the site of the incision through the left coronary aortic sinus used to open the root. As in the pulmonary root, it remains possible to recognize the sinutubular junction, with its zeniths marking the tubular plane. The commissural plane and the virtual basal ring have also been marked. The leaflets of the aortic valve have been removed in this heart to show the semilunar nature of their hinges. This reveals the presence of the interleaflet fibrous triangles. Separating the valvar sinuses, these fibrous components of the left ventricular outflow tract extend to the level of the commissural plane.

that is a target of electrophysiologists as they seek to ablate outflow tract arrhythmias.[38,39] Whether the myocardium remaining within the epicardial tissues could also serve as a substrate for the arrhythmias remains to be determined.[40] The finding of the myocardium incorporated at the bases of all three sinuses of the pulmonary root reflects the fact that, in the postnatal heart, the root itself is lifted away from the base of the ventricular cone by the free-standing infundibular sleeve of the right ventricle. This means that, in the postnatal heart, there is no "*outlet septum*". The sinuses of the pulmonary root adjacent to the aortic root are separated from the aortic valvar sinuses by extracavitary fibroadipose tissue (Figure 6.26).

The uniform inclusion of myocardium within the bases of the pulmonary valvar sinuses is not the case for the ***aortic root***. Only the bases of the two aortic valvar sinuses that give rise to the coronary arteries contain myocardium (Figure 6.27). A significant part of the base of the root is supported by the fibrous continuity that exists between the non-coronary and right coronary leaflets of the aortic valve and one of the leaflets of the mitral valve. It is this feature that permits the involved leaflet of the mitral valve to be described as being ***aortic*** (Figure 6.5). On occasions, the aortic root may be supported by a complete muscular infundibulum, but this is rare.[30] It is presumably for this reason that it is even rarer to find accessory myocardial pathways in relation to the aortic leaflet of the mitral valve. It is of note, nonetheless, that patients with hypertrophic cardiomyopathy have been observed to retain myocardium in the inner heart curvature, separating the hinges of the leaflets of the aortic and mitral valves.[41] The fibrous parts of the root adjacent to the septum are important since they constitute the so-called ***central fibrous body***. In most instances, part of this fibrous area is produced by continuity between the leaflets of the mitral and tricuspid valves. This area forms the roof of the ***infero-septal recess*** of the left ventricular outflow tract.[42] It is not an integral part of the aortic root. Another part of the fibrous support is then provided by the membranous septum.

As with the pulmonary root, the proximal boundary of the aortic root is the virtual basal plane that can be constructed by joining together the nadirs of the semilunar hinges of the aortic valvar leaflets (Figure 6.21). In keeping with the arrangement found in the pulmonary root, the sinutubular junction forms its distal boundary. But again, as in the pulmonary root, the junction is not a planar entity. A tubular ring can also be identified in the aortic root by joining together the zeniths of the walls of the valvar sinuses (Figure 6.28).[38] When the aortic root is assessed in its opened state in the autopsy

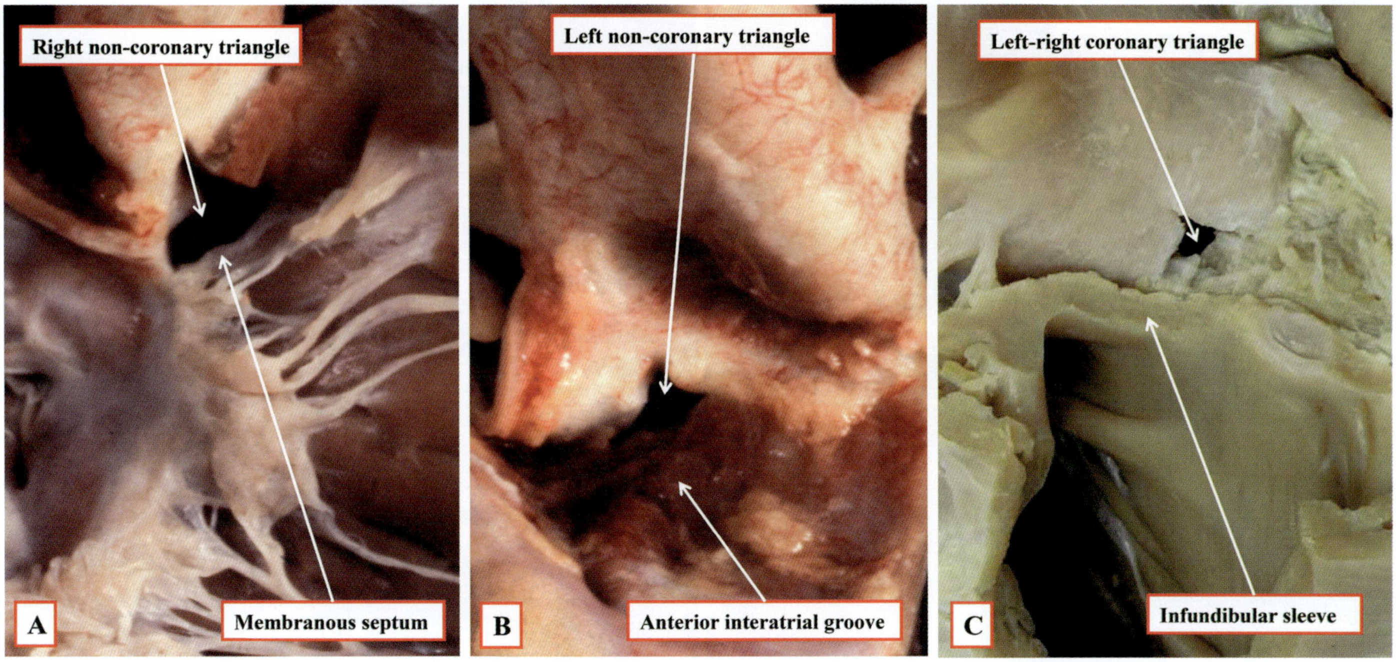

Figure 6.28. In these images, hearts have been dissected to show the sites of opening of the three interleaflet triangles demonstrated in Figure 6.27. In each panel, the fibrous wall of the interleaflet triangle has been removed and the heart photographed from outside the root. As shown in panel A, the triangle between the right coronary and non-coronary sinuses opens with its apex within the rightward extent of the transverse pericardial sinus. Its base is supported by the interventricular component of the membranous septum. Panel B shows that the apex of the triangle between the non-coronary and left coronary sinuses opens into the mid-portion of the transverse pericardial sinus, with the sinus bordered posteriorly by the anterior walls of the atrial chambers. So as to reveal the opening of the triangle between the right and left coronary aortic sinuses, as shown in panel C, it was first necessary to remove the pulmonary root and the distal part of the subpulmonary infundibulum. This shows how the tip of the triangle opens into the fibroadipose extracavitary tissue area that separates the aortic root from the subpulmonary infundibulum.

room, fibrous interleaflet triangles are much more obvious when compared to the triangles seen in the pulmonary root (compare Figures 6.22, 6.27).[43] During development, the epicardial surfaces of all the triangles include the outflow tract myocardium. Removal of the fibrous walls of the triangles reveals that, subsequent to regression of the myocardium, a potential communication is produced between the left ventricular outflow tract and extracavitary spaces (Figure 6.28). The triangles between the non-coronary sinus and its neighbours both open potentially to the transverse sinus of the pericardium (Figure 6.28, panels A and B). The triangle between the two sinuses giving rise to the coronary arteries, in contrast, would communicate if opened with the extracavitary area of tissue separating the free-standing infundibular sleeve from the aortic root (Figures 6.27, 6.28 panel C). As was the case with the pulmonary valve, the semilunar hinging of the leaflets within the valvar sinuses of the aortic root permits them to come together snugly under the pressure of the column of arterial blood that ensures valvar closure during ventricular diastole (Figure 6.23). When closed, the centroid of the valvar skirt is well below the level of the sinutubular junction (Figure 6.29).

The ability to measure the dimensions of the leaflets, along with the ability to correlate this information with their coaptation, and understand their relationship to the overall arrangement of the aortic root (Figure 6.30) has now revolutionized the approach to surgical repair of the aortic valve.[44,45] Such multimodality imaging is similarly critical for those contemplating transcatheter replacement of the aortic valve. It permits insertion of the correct device and guides the most appropriate route for access.[46,47]

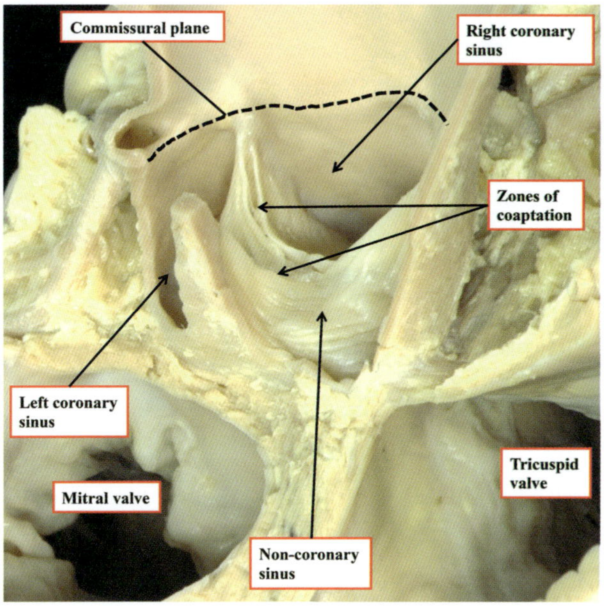

Figure 6.29. The aortic root has been dissected by removing the fibrous walls of the non-coronary and left coronary valvar sinuses with the leaflets in closed position. In this heart, the left coronary artery arose from the root distal to the sinutubular junction. The leaflets close together such that the centroid of the closed orifice is midway between the levels of the virtual basal ring and the commissural plane. Extensions of the cavity of the root extend to the level of the sinutubular junction at the commissures, walled by the fibrous interleaflet triangles, as shown by the post separating the cavities of the left and non-coronary sinuses. The opening of this triangle to the transverse pericardial sinus, when excised in a different heart, was shown in panel B of Figure 6.28.

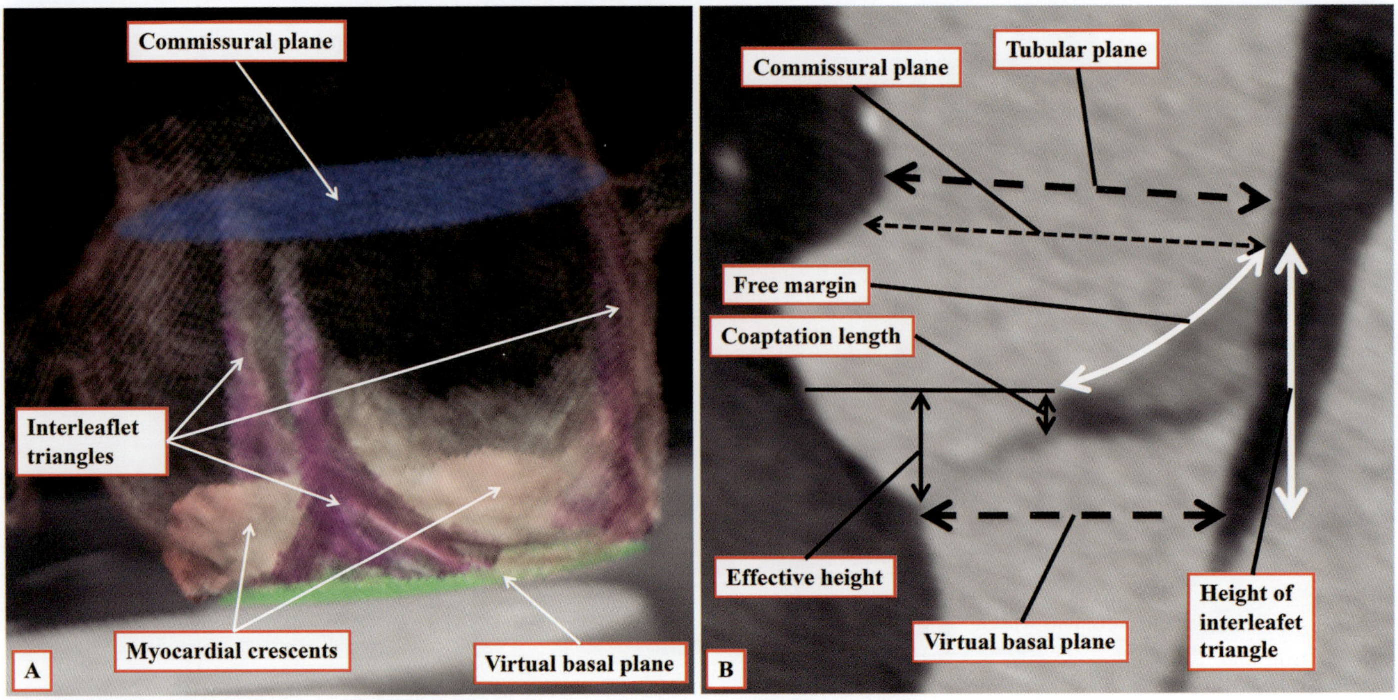

Figure 6.30. The images are prepared from computed tomographic datasets obtained from living patients. Panel A shows how it is now possible to demonstrate all features of the aortic root, with the myocardium incorporated in the sinuses giving rise to the coronary arteries segmented in pink. Panel B shows the measurements that can now be made to optimize surgical repair of diseased or congenitally malformed valves. Note that the tubular plane, made by joining together the zeniths of the sinuses at the sinutubular junction, is distal to the commissural plane, which is created by joining together the levels of the commissures.

REFERENCES

1. Spicer DE, Bridgeman JM, Brown NA, Mohun TJ, Anderson RH. The anatomy and development of the cardiac valves. *Cardiol Young*. 2014;**24**:1008–1022. doi: 10.1017/S1047951114001942
2. Buratto E, Konstantinov IE. Atrioventricular valve surgery: restoration of the fibrous skeleton of the heart. *J Thorac Cardiovasc Surg*. 2021;**162**:360–365. doi: 10.1016/j.jtcvs.2021.03.128
3. Zimmerman J, Bailey CP. The surgical significance of the fibrous skeleton of the heart. . *J Thorac Cardiovasc Surg*. 1962;**44**:701–712.
4. Saremi F, Sanchez-Quintana D, Mori S, Muresian H, Spicer DE, Hassani C, Anderson RH. Fibrous skeleton of the heart: anatomic overview and evaluation of pathologic conditions with CT and MR imaging. *Radiographics*. 2017;**37**:1330–1351. doi: 10.1148/rg.2017170004
5. Anderson RH, Smerup M, Sanchez-Quintana D, Loukas M, Lunkenheimer PP. The three-dimensional arrangement of the myocytes in the ventricular walls. *Clin Anat*. 2009;**22**:64–76. doi: 10.1002/ca.20645
6. Loukas M, Groat C, Khangura R, Owens DG, Anderson RH. The normal and abnormal anatomy of the coronary arteries. *Clin Anat*. 2009;**22**:114–128. doi: 10.1002/ca.20761
7. Ortale JR, Gabriel EA, Iost C, Marquez CQ. The anatomy of the coronary sinus and its tributaries. *Surg Radiol Anat*. 2001;**23**:15–21. doi: 10.1007/s00276-001-0015-0
8. Anderson RH, Ho SY. Anatomy of the atrioventricular junctions with regard to ventricular preexcitation. *Pacing Clin Electrophysiol*. 1997;**20**:2072–2076. doi: 10.1111/j.1540-8159.1997.tb03631.x
9. Li A, Zuberi Z, Bradfield JS, Zarif JK, Ward DE, Anderson RH, Shivkumar K, Saba MM. Endocardial ablation of ventricular ectopic beats arising from the basal inferoseptal process of the left ventricle. *Heart Rhythm*. 2018;**15**:1356–1362. doi: 10.1016/j.hrthm.2018.04.029
10. Hahn RT, Weckbach LT, Noack T, Hamid N, Kitamura M, Bae R, Lurz P, Kodali SK, Sorajja P, Hausleiter J, et al. Proposal for a standard echocardiographic tricuspid valve nomenclature. *JACC Cardiovasc Imaging*. 2021;**14**:1299–1305. doi: 10.1016/j.jcmg.2021.01.012
11. Ranganathan N, Lam JH, Wigle ED, Silver MD. Morphology of the human mitral valve. II. The value leaflets. *Circulation*. 1970;**41**:459–467. doi: 10.1161/01.cir.41.3.459
12. Kawamura M, Gerstenfeld EP, Vedantham V, Rodrigues DM, Burkhardt JD, Kobayashi Y, Hsia HH, Marcus GM, Marchlinski FE, Scheinman MM, et al. Idiopathic ventricular arrhythmia originating from the cardiac crux or inferior septum: epicardial idiopathic ventricular arrhythmia. *Circ Arrhythm Electrophysiol*. 2014;**7**:1152–1158. doi: 10.1161/CIRCEP.114.001704
13. Larroussi L, Badhwar N. Ventricular tachycardia arising from cardiac crux: electrocardiogram recognition and site of ablation. *Card Electrophysiol Clin*. 2016;**8**:109–113. doi: 10.1016/j.ccep.2015.10.010
14. Yoneda ZT, Stevenson WG. Idiopathic annular ventricular arrhythmias. *Arrhythm Electrophysiol Rev*. 2024;**13**:e21. doi: 10.15420/aer.2024.40
15. McAlpine WA. The left ventricle—general considerations. In: *Heart and Coronary Arteries: An Anatomical Atlas for Clinical*

Diagnosis, Radiological Investigation, and Surgical Treatment, pp. 27–38. New York: Springer; 1975.
16. Farre J, Anderson RH, Rubio JM, Tretter JT, Sanchez-Quintana D, Garcia-Talavera C, Bansal R, Lokhandwala YY, Cabrera JA, Wellens HJJ, et al. Miniseries 2—Septal and paraseptal accessory pathways—Part IV: Inferior paraseptal accessory pathways—lessons from surgical and catheter ablation. *Europace*. 2022;**24**:676–690. doi: 10.1093/europace/euab295
17. Farre J, Anderson RH, Sanchez-Quintana D, Mori S, Rubio JM, Garcia-Talavera C, Bansal R, Lokhandwala Y, Cabrera JA, Wellens HJJ, et al. Miniseries 2—Septal and paraseptal accessory pathways—Part II: Para-Hisian accessory pathways—so-called anteroseptal pathways revisited. *Europace*. 2022;**24**:650–661. doi: 10.1093/europace/euab293
18. Farre J, Anderson RH, Rubio JM, Garcia-Talavera C, Sanchez-Quintana D, Bansal R, Lokhandwala Y, Cabrera JA, Wellens HJJ, Back Sternick E. Miniseries 2—Septal and paraseptal accessory pathways—Part III: Mid-paraseptal accessory pathways—revisiting bypass tracts crossing the pyramidal space. *Europace*. 2022;**24**:662–675. doi: 10.1093/europace/euab294
19. Toh H, Mori S, Izawa Y, Toba T, Nishii T, Hirata KI. Revival of mitral and tricuspid annular disjunctions: are these really abnormal findings? *JACC Cardiovasc Imaging*. 2021;**14**:1682–1684. doi: 10.1016/j.jcmg.2021.05.026
20. Anderson RH, Garbi M, Zugwitz D, Petersen SE, Nijveldt R. Anatomy of the mitral valve relative to controversies concerning the so-called annular disjunction. *Heart*. 2023;**109**:734–739. doi: 10.1136/heartjnl-2022-322043
21. Dejgaard LA, Skjolsvik ET, Lie OH, Ribe M, Stokke MK, Hegbom F, Scheirlynck ES, Gjertsen E, Andresen K, Helle-Valle TM, et al. The mitral annulus disjunction arrhythmic syndrome. *J Am Coll Cardiol*. 2018;**72**:1600–1609. doi: 10.1016/j.jacc.2018.07.070
22. Essayagh B, Sabbag A, Antoine C, Benfari G, Yang LT, Maalouf J, Asirvatham S, Michelena H, Enriquez-Sarano M. Presentation and outcome of arrhythmic mitral valve prolapse. *J Am Coll Cardiol*. 2020;**76**:637–649. doi: 10.1016/j.jacc.2020.06.029
23. Becker AE, Anderson RH, Durrer D, Wellens HJ. The anatomical substrates of Wolff–Parkinson–White syndrome. A clinicopathologic correlation in seven patients. *Circulation*. 1978;**57**:870–879. doi: 10.1161/01.cir.57.5.870
24. Anderson RH, Sanchez-Quintana D, Mori S, Lokhandwala Y, Correa FS, Wellens HJ, Sternick EB. Unusual variants of pre-excitation: from anatomy to ablation: Part I—Understanding the anatomy of the variants of ventricular pre-excitation. *J Cardiovasc Electrophysiol*. 2019;**30**:2170–2180. doi: 10.1111/jce.14106
25. Katritsis DG, Wellens HJ, Josephson ME. Mahaim accessory pathways. *Arrhythm Electrophysiol Rev*. 2017;**6**:29–32. doi: 10.15420/aer.2016:35:1
26. Yanni J, Boyett MR, Anderson RH, Dobrzynski H. The extent of the specialized atrioventricular ring tissues. *Heart Rhythm*. 2009;**6**:672–680. doi: 10.1016/j.hrthm.2009.01.021
27. Bohora S, Lokhandwala Y, Sternick EB, Anderson RH, Wellens HJJ. Reappraisal and new observations on atrial tachycardia ablated from the non-coronary aortic sinus of Valsalva. *Europace*. 2018;**20**:124–133. doi: 10.1093/europace/euw324
28. Lunel AA. Significance of annulus fibrosus of heart in relation to AV conduction and ventricular activation in cases of Wolff–Parkinson–White syndrome. *Br Heart J*. 1972;**34**:1263–1271. doi: 10.1136/hrt.34.12.1263
29. Anderson RH, Lamers WH, Hikspoors J, Mohun TJ, Bamforth SD, Chaudhry B, Eley L, Kerwin J, Crosier M, Henderson DJ. Development of the arterial roots and ventricular outflow tracts. *J Anat*. 2024;**244**:497–513. doi: 10.1111/joa.13973
30. Rosenquist GC, Clark EB, Sweeney LJ, McAllister HA. The normal spectrum of mitral and aortic valve discontinuity. *Circulation*. 1976;**54**:298–301. doi: 10.1161/01.cir.54.2.298
31. Guiraudon GM, Guiraudon CM, Klein GJ, Sharma AD, Yee R. The coronary sinus diverticulum: a pathologic entity associated with the Wolff–Parkinson–White syndrome. *Am J Cardiol*. 1988;**62**:733–735. doi: 10.1016/0002-9149(88)91212-x
32. McAlpine WA. *Heart and Coronary Arteries: An Anatomical Atlas for Clinical Diagnosis, Radiological Investigation, and Surgical Treatment*. New York: Springer; 1975.
33. Mori S, Bradfield JS, Fukuzawa K, Shivkumar K. Comprehensive anatomy of the summit of the left ventricle. *JACC Clin Electrophysiol*. 2024;**10**:168–184. doi: 10.1016/j.jacep.2023.09.022
34. Toh H, Mori S, Tretter JT, Izawa Y, Shimoyama S, Suzuki M, Takahashi Y, Tsuda D, Toba T, Fujiwara S, et al. Living anatomy of the ventricular myocardial crescents supporting the coronary aortic sinuses. *Semin Thorac Cardiovasc Surg*. 2020;**32**:230–241. doi: 10.1053/j.semtcvs.2020.01.001
35. Michelena HI, Della Corte A, Evangelista A, Maleszewski JJ, Edwards WD, Roman MJ, Devereux RB, Fernandez B, Asch FM, Barker AJ, et al. International consensus statement on nomenclature and classification of the congenital bicuspid aortic valve and its aortopathy, for clinical, surgical, interventional and research purposes. *Eur J Cardio-thorac Surg*. 2021;**60**:448–476. doi: 10.1093/ejcts/ezab038
36. Anderson RH, Mori S. Nomenclature of the components of the aortic root. *Eur J Cardio-thorac Surg*. 2019;**55**:1020. doi: 10.1093/ejcts/ezy358
37. Anderson RH, Chaudhry B, Mohun TJ, Bamforth SD, Hoyland D, Phillips HM, Webb S, Moorman AF, Brown NA, Henderson DJ. Normal and abnormal development of the intrapericardial arterial trunks in humans and mice. *Cardiovasc Res*. 2012;**95**:108–115. doi: 10.1093/cvr/cvs147
38. Joshi S, Wilber DJ. Ablation of idiopathic right ventricular outflow tract tachycardia: current perspectives. *J Cardiovasc Electrophysiol*. 2005;**16** Suppl 1:S52–58. doi: 10.1111/j.1540-8167.2005.50163.x
39. Pathak RK, Ariyarathna N, Garcia FC, Sanders P, Marchlinski FE. Catheter ablation of idiopathic ventricular arrhythmias. *Heart Lung Circ*. 2019;**28**:102–109. doi: 10.1016/j.hlc.2018.10.012
40. Anderson RH, Mohun TJ, Sanchez-Quintana D, Mori S, Spicer DE, Cheung JW, Lerman BB. The anatomic substrates for outflow tract arrhythmias. *Heart Rhythm*. 2019;**16**:290–297. doi: 10.1016/j.hrthm.2018.08.014
41. Ferrazzi P, Spirito P, Binaco I, Zyrianov A, Poggio D, Vaccari G, Grillo M, Pezzoli L, Scatigno A, Dorobantu L, et al. Congenital muscular mitral-aortic discontinuity identified in patients with obstructive hypertrophic cardiomyopathy. *J Am Coll Cardiol*. 2020;**76**:2238–2247. doi: 10.1016/j.jacc.2020.09.534
42. Crucean A, Spicer DE, Tretter JT, Mohun TJ, Cook AC, Sanchez-Quintana D, Hikspoors J, Lamers WH, Anderson RH. Revisiting the anatomy of the left ventricle in the light of knowledge of its development. *J Anat*. 2024;**245**:201–216. doi: 10.1111/joa.14048
43. Sutton JP, 3rd, Ho SY, Anderson RH. The forgotten interleaflet triangles: a review of the surgical anatomy of the aortic valve. *Ann Thorac Surg*. 1995;**59**:419–427. doi: 10.1016/0003-4975(94)00893-c
44. Tretter JT, Burbano-Vera NH, Najm HK. Multi-modality imaging evaluation and pre-surgical planning for aortic valve-sparing operations in patients with aortic root aneurysm.

Ann Cardiothorac Surg. 2023;**12**:295–317. doi: 10.21037/acs-2023-avs2-0040
45. Tretter JT, Izawa Y, Spicer DE, Okada K, Anderson RH, Quintessenza JA, Mori S. Understanding the aortic root using computed tomographic assessment: a potential pathway to improved customized surgical repair. *Circ Cardiovasc Imaging*. 2021;**14**:e013134. doi: 10.1161/CIRCIMAGING.121.013134
46. Agricola E, Ancona F, Bartel T, Brochet E, Dweck M, Faletra F, Lancellotti P, Mahmoud-Elsayed H, Marsan NA, Maurovich-Hovart P, et al. Multimodality imaging for patient selection, procedural guidance, and follow-up of transcatheter interventions for structural heart disease: a consensus document of the EACVI Task Force on Interventional Cardiovascular Imaging: Part 1: Access routes, transcatheter aortic valve implantation, and transcatheter mitral valve interventions. *Eur Heart J Cardiovasc Imaging*. 2023;**24**:e209–e268. doi: 10.1093/ehjci/jead096
47. Reindl M, Lechner I, Holzknecht M, Tiller C, Fink P, Oberhollenzer F, von der Emde S, Pamminger M, Troger F, Kremser C, et al. Cardiac magnetic resonance imaging versus computed tomography to guide transcatheter aortic valve replacement: a randomized, open-label, noninferiority trial. *Circulation*. 2023;**148**:1220–1230. doi: 10.1161/CIRCULATIONAHA.123.066498

7

The Right Ventricle

As was shown in Chapter 1, although termed the "right", the ventricle to be described in this chapter is positioned, for the most part, anteriorly relative to its morphologically left partner (Figure 7.1).[1]

The first indication of its formation becomes evident with the ballooning of its apical component from the outlet of the developing ventricular part of the primary heart tube. At this initial stage, the developing right ventricle supports the entirety of the outlet component of the heart tube but lacks a direct inlet. The chamber obtains its inlet component subsequent to expansion of the atrioventricular canal but then cedes part of the outlet component to the left ventricle. Subsequent to these developmental processes, the myocardial components of the chamber extend from the atrioventricular junction to the base of the pulmonary root. The ventricular myocardium, however, does not extend distally to the level of the ***sinutubular junction***. Despite this subtlety, the definitive ventricle is well described as possessing functional ***inlet***, ***apical*** trabecular, and ***outlet*** components.[1] The cavity of the outlet part, when the pulmonary valvar leaflets are closed, is limited distally by the attachments of the adjacent leaflets at the sinutubular junction. There are, however, no discrete anatomical boundaries between the functional components (Figure 7.2).

As was described in Chapter 6, the ***right atrioventricular junction*** provides the proximal boundary of the ventricular cavity. It is formed throughout by fibroadipose tissues, which for the greater part of the junction separate the vestibular components of the atrial walls from the crest of the ventricular myocardial mass (Figure 7.3). No obvious "*annulus*" is found within the junction in the sense of a complete fibrous ring interposed between the atrial and ventricular myocardial masses. Instead, the leaflets of the tricuspid valve are mostly hinged from the ventricular walls and the septum at the level of the insulating plane provided by the fibroadipose tissues, although in places the myocardial masses can be separated by shelves of fibrous tissue, producing the feature described as "***disjunction***" when seen in the left atrioventricular junction.[2]

When traced distally, the ventricular cavity extends between the semilunar hinges of the adjacent leaflets of the pulmonary valve to reach their attachments at the ***sinutubular junction*** (Figure 7.4).[3] The myocardial walls, in contrast, stop short of the sinutubular junction.[4,5] There is a difference, therefore, between the distal extent of the right ventricular myocardium, which forms a discrete anatomical myocardial–arterial junction, and the haemodynamic ventriculo-arterial junction, which is formed by the leaflets of the pulmonary valve when they close during ventricular diastole.

The ***inlet*** component of the right ventricle surrounds and supports the tricuspid valve (Figure 7.5). It extends from the atrioventricular junction to the distal extent of the valvar tension apparatus, where the bases of the papillary muscles forming this distal boundary become continuous with the apical trabeculations (Figure 7.6).

Beyond the distal attachments, the coarsely trabeculated ***apical component*** occupies the outer curvature of the ventricular cavity (Figure 7.2). The ventricular walls then continue basally as a free-standing myocardial sleeve, which forms the ***subpulmonary infundibulum*** (Figure 7.7). The inlet and outlet ventricular components meet within the inner curvature of the ventricle at the site of the ***membranous septum*** (Figure 7.8).

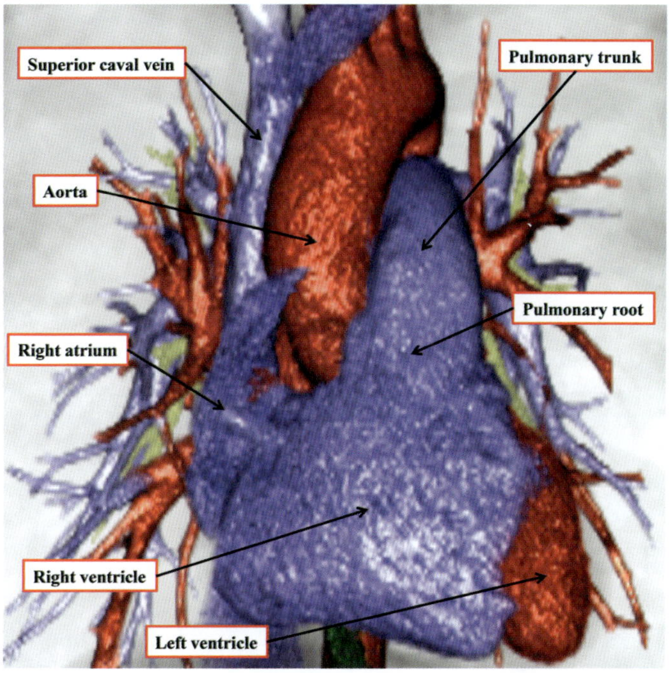

Figure 7.1. The image is from a segmented computerized tomographic dataset of a normal human heart viewed in frontal projection. The right ventricle, along with the right atrium and the pulmonary trunk, has been coloured blue. The left ventricle and the aorta are coloured red. As can be seen, although termed the "right" ventricle, the larger part of the chamber is situated in front of its left-sided counterpart. Its inferior margin lies on the diaphragm. Courtesy of Dr Shumpei Mori.

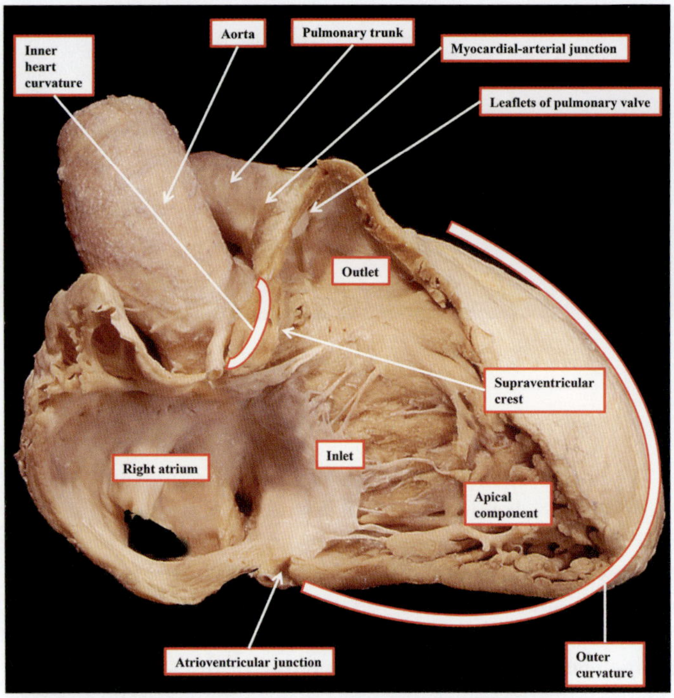

Figure 7.2. The image shows the extent and make-up of the myocardial walls of the right ventricle, with the ventricular cavity revealed by removal of its parietal wall. The septal leaflet of the tricuspid valve is seen, with the overall valve guarding the ventricular inlet. The distal boundary of the cavity is delineated by the undersurface of the leaflets of the pulmonary valve, which guard the ventricular outlet. As is shown in Figure 7.4, the cavity of the outlet extends beyond the distal myocardial–arterial junction. The ventricle wraps itself around the aortic root, having a trabeculated outer curvature, which encloses the apical ventricular component, and a smooth inner curvature, with the latter fold forming the supraventricular crest.

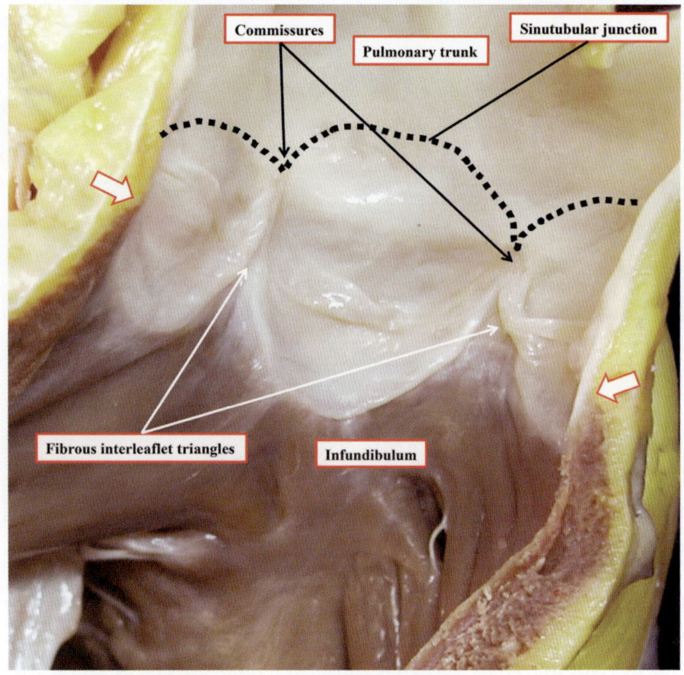

Figure 7.4. The pulmonary root has been opened to show the semilunar attachments of the leaflets of the pulmonary valve. The hinge lines of the adjacent leaflets come together distally at the sinutubular junction. When the leaflets are closed, it is the level of the sinutubular junction at these commissures that marks the distal extent of the ventricular cavity. This is distal to the junction between the ventricular myocardium and the fibro-elastic walls of the pulmonary valvar sinuses, shown by the white arrows with red borders. The space between the adjacent leaflets as they extend to attach at the sinutubular junction is filled by the fibrous interleaflet triangles, which themselves form the walls of the ventricular cavity distal to the myocardial–arterial junction.

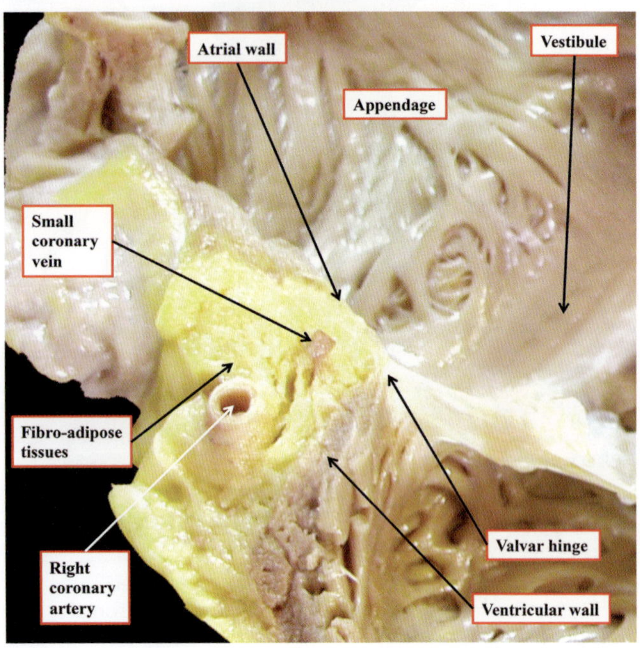

Figure 7.3. The cut across the inferior atrioventricular junction shows how the inferior leaflet of the tricuspid valve is hinged at the junction, which is between the vestibular component of the right atrium and the crest of the parietal ventricular wall. The junction itself is filled by fibro-adipose tissue, which encloses the right coronary artery and the small cardiac vein.

This small fibrous part of the septum is usually crossed by the septal leaflet of the tricuspid valve, separating it into atrioventricular and interventricular components, with the components well seen when the septum is transilluminated from the left side and viewed from the right ventricular aspect (Figure 7.9 panel A). When transilluminated from the right side and viewed from the cavity of the left ventricle, the membranous septum is seen usually to fill the base of the interleaflet triangle separating the non-coronary and right coronary sinuses of the aortic root (Figure 7.9 panel B).

The precise location of its interventricular component can vary depending on the rotation of the aortic root relative to the base of the ventricular mass.[6] The atrioventricular component, however, is more constant in its location. It forms the apex of the triangle of Koch. As such it provides an excellent landmark for predicting the location of the atrioventricular conduction axis (Figure 7.9). Segmentation of the conduction axis in hearts visualized using Synchrotron scanning now confirms the utility of these landmarks as guides to the likely location of the conduction axis (Figure 7.10).[7]

The much more extensive ***muscular septum*** interposes for its greater part between the apical components of the ventricles. Its inferior component separates the inlet of the right from the outlet of the left ventricle (Figure 7.11).[1] This apparent paradox reflects the presence, in the left ventricle, of the deep infero-septal recess, which lifts the mitral valvar leaflets away from the septum.[8] The roof of the recess is an area of fibrous continuity between the leaflets

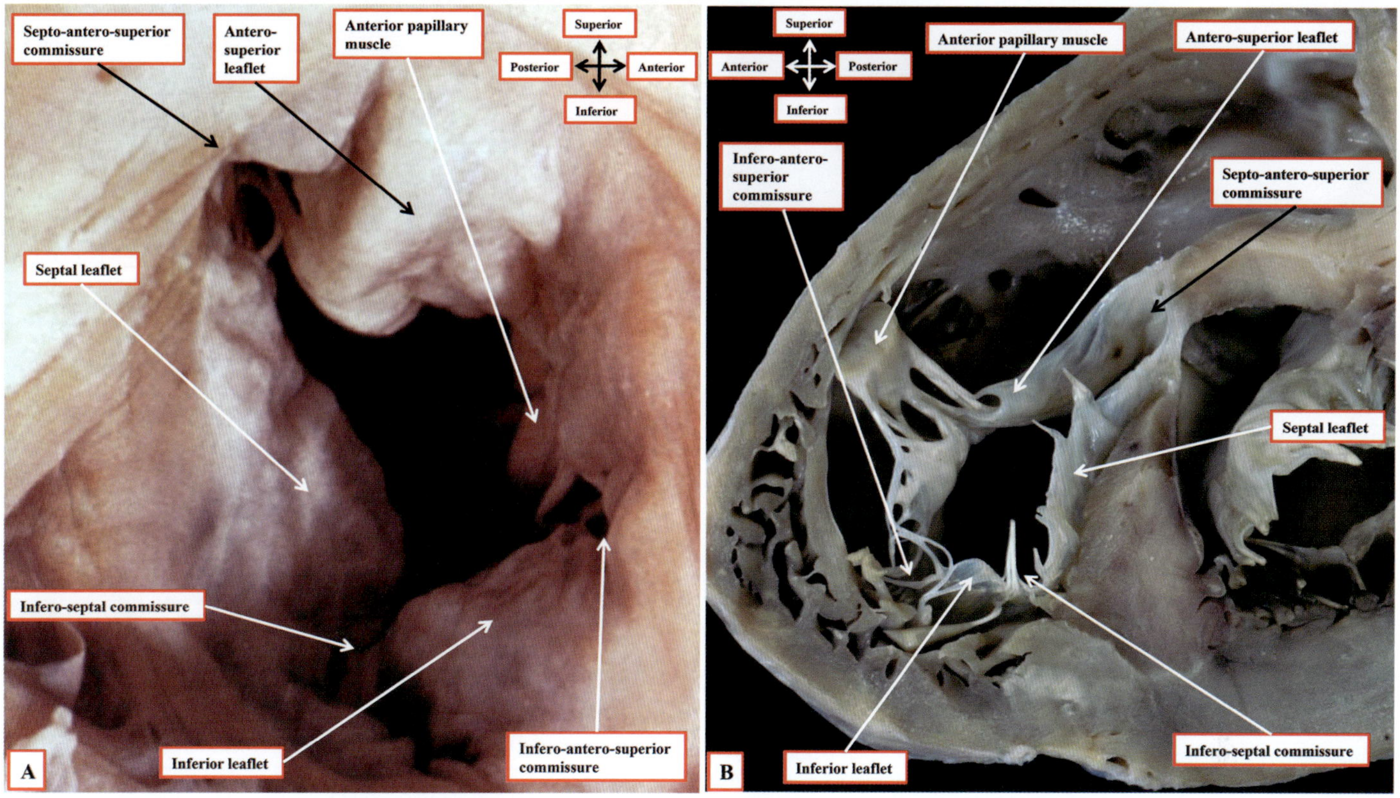

Figure 7.5. The images show how the leaflets of the tricuspid valve guard the inlet of the right ventricle. Panel A shows the view from the atrial aspect, and panel B shows the ventricular view, having removed the apical part of the ventricular cone. The valve closes in trifoliate fashion, with its leaflets positioned inferiorly, septally, and antero-superiorly.

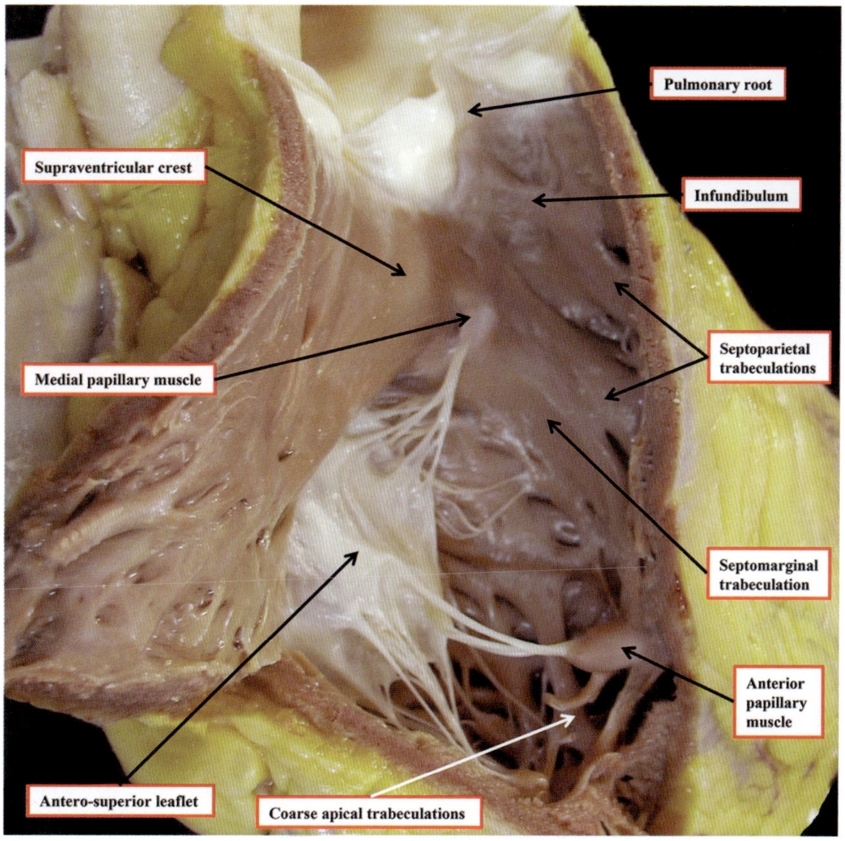

Figure 7.6. The parietal wall of the right ventricle has been opened by making a cut adjacent to the anterior interventricular artery, with the parietal wall then reflected to show the transition between the ventricular inlet and apical components at the insertion of the tension apparatus of the tricuspid valve into the apical trabeculations.

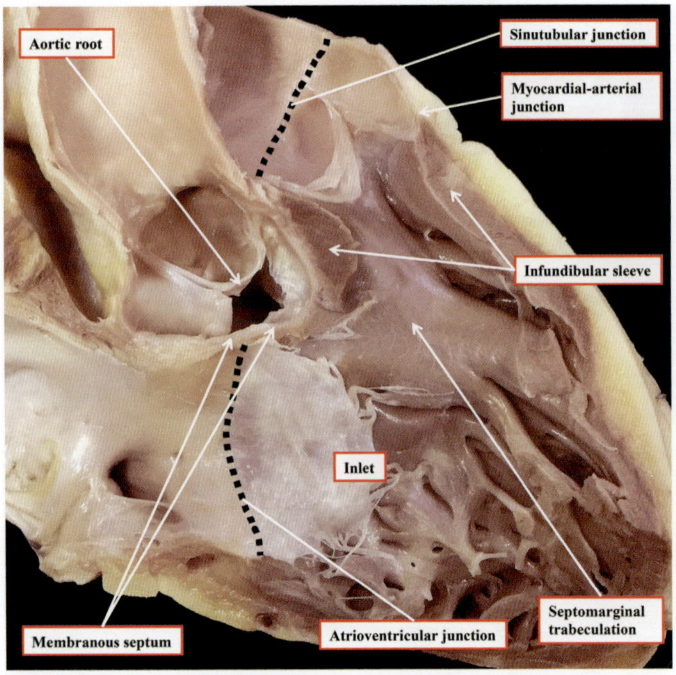

Figure 7.7. The parietal wall of the right ventricle, as in Figure 7.2, has been removed to show the inlet, apical, and outlet ventricular components. In this dissection, the right coronary sinus of the aortic root has also been removed, showing how the membranous septum occupies the inner curvature, being crossed by the hinge of the septal leaflet, which marks the atrioventricular junction, to divide it into its atrioventricular and interventricular components (see Figure 7.8). The removal of the right coronary sinus also reveals the free-standing nature of the subpulmonary infundibular sleeve, which lifts the leaflets of the pulmonary valve away from the base of the ventricular mass. Note again that the myocardial-arterial junction does not extend distally to reach the level of the sinutubular junction.

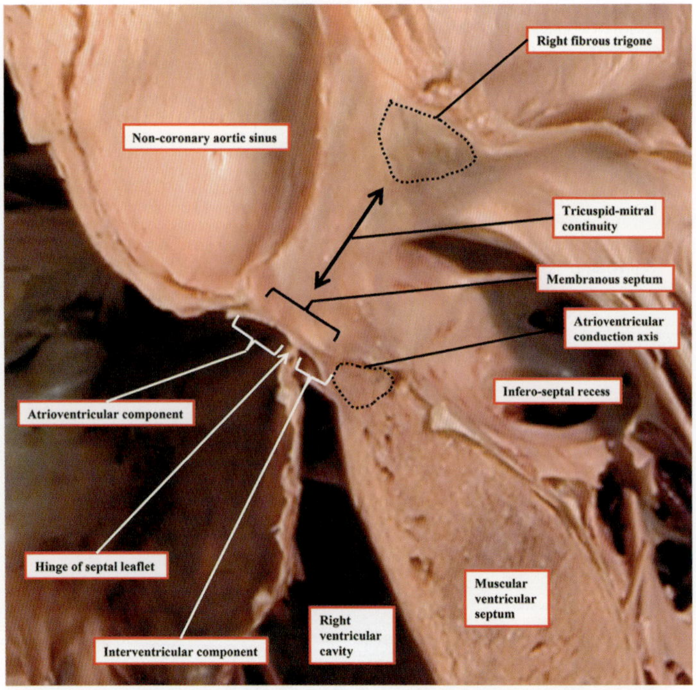

Figure 7.8. The image shows a close-up view of a frontal section made through the membranous part of the ventricular septum. It shows how the hinge of the septal leaflet of the tricuspid valve separates the fibrous membranous septum into atrioventricular and interventricular parts. In this heart, the ventricular component of the atrioventricular conduction axis can be seen to be wedged between the distal attachment of the interventricular part of the membranous septum and the crest of the muscular ventricular septum. The non-coronary leaflet of the aortic root has been removed. It is possible to recognize the components of the central fibrous body, which is made up of the atrioventricular component of the membranous septum, the area of tricuspid-to-mitral continuity which supports the base of the atrial septum, and the right fibrous trigone.

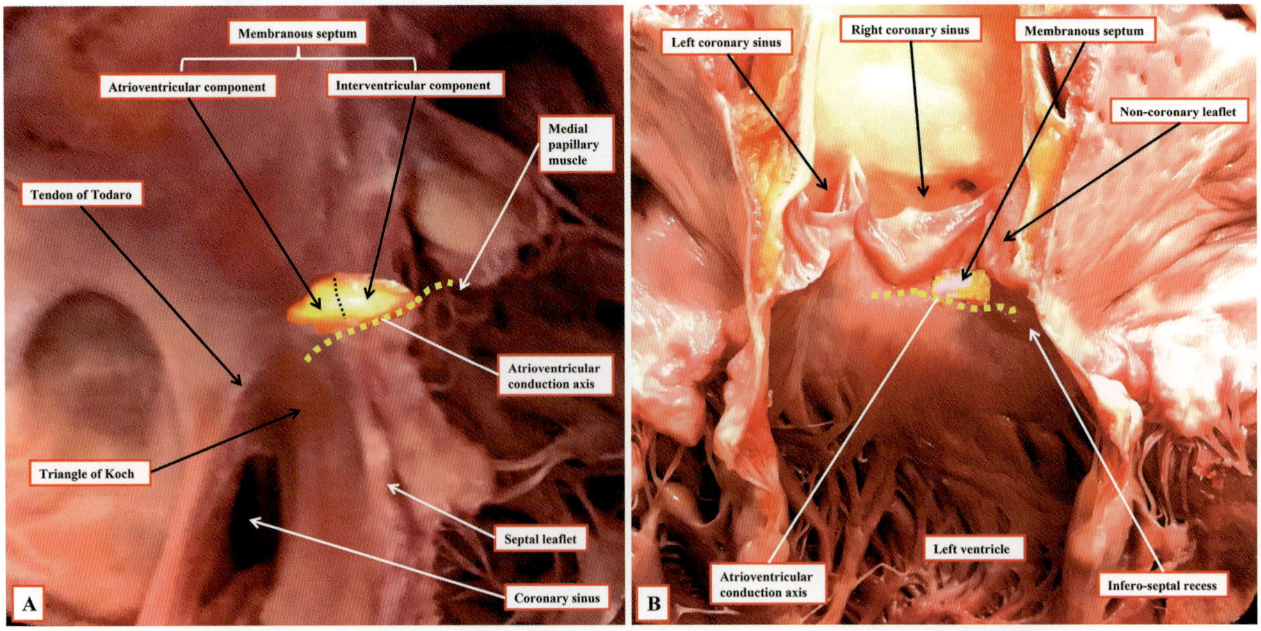

Figure 7.9. The heart has been transilluminated to show the location of the membranous septum. In panel A, the transillumination is from the left side. The base of the membranous septum provides the landmark for recognition of the location of the atrioventricular conduction axis, which passes from the apex of the triangle of Koch, re-emerging in the right ventricle in the region of the medial papillary muscle. The dotted black line shows how the hinge of the septal leaflet of the tricuspid valve separated the membranous septum into its atrioventricular and interventricular components. Panel B shows the comparable view after transillumination from the right side, having opened the aortic root by making an incision through the aortic leaflet of the mitral valve. The location of the conduction axis is again shown, in this heart being adjacent to the nadir of the hinge of the right coronary leaflet of the aortic valve. The membranous septum itself occupies the base of the triangle between the right and non-coronary sinuses of the aortic root.

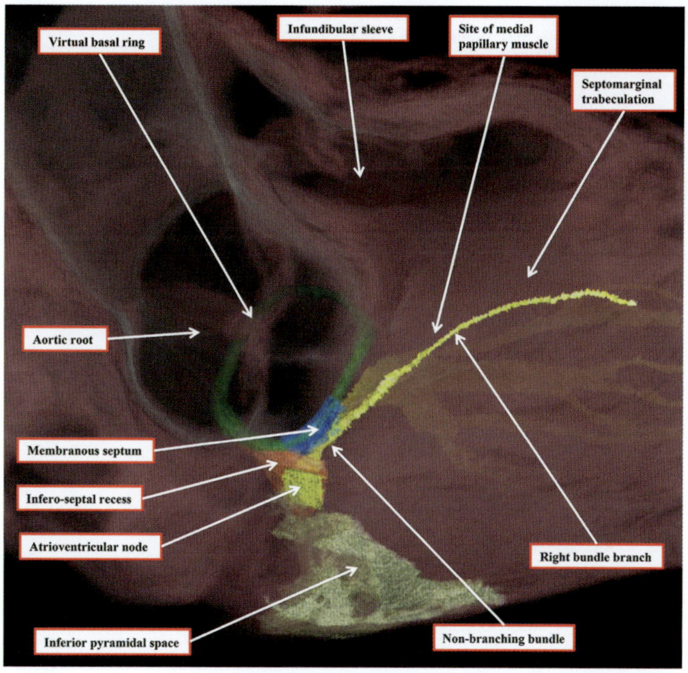

Figure 7.10. The image shows the reconstruction of an adult heart scanned using Synchrotron technology, with the location of the atrioventricular conduction axis established by segmentation of the individual sections from the three-dimensional dataset. The colours show the locations of the virtual basal ring of the aortic root (green), the roof of the infero-septal recess (orange), the membranous septum (blue), and the tissues occupying the inferior pyramidal space (pale yellow). All of these items were also segmented in the three-dimensional dataset. The image is shown in right anterior oblique orientation. The findings validate the landmarks to the conduction axis as shown in Figure 7.9.

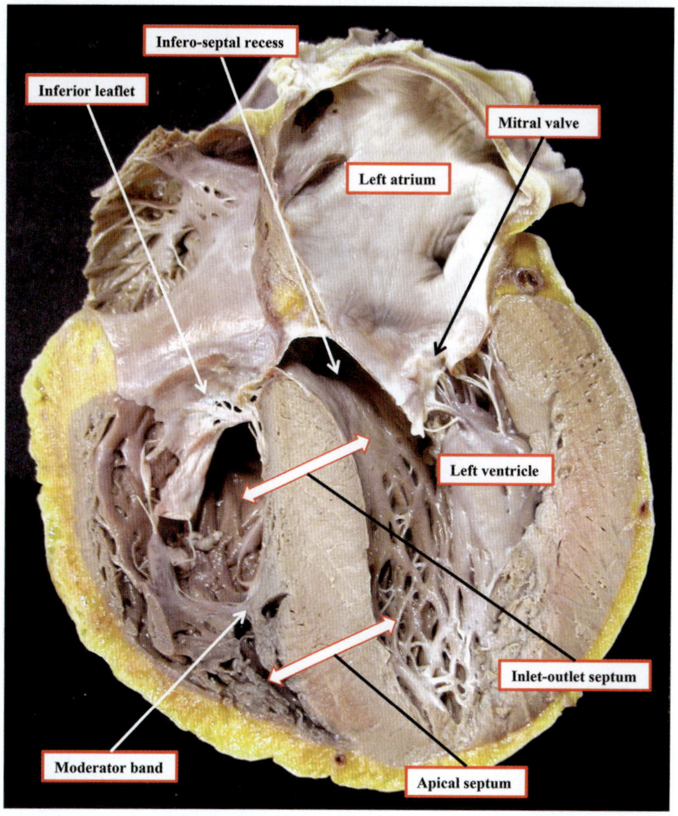

Figure 7.11. The four-chamber cut through the heart, viewed from the front, shows how the deep infero-septal recess of the left ventricle lifts the leaflets of the mitral valve away from the surface of the ventricular septum. This means that the inferior part of the muscular septum interposes between the inlet of the right ventricle and the infero-septal extension of the outlet of the left ventricle. Beyond the moderator band, the muscular septum separates the ventricular apical components. The section shows how the roof of the infero-septal recess is formed by an area of fibrous continuity between the leaflets of the mitral and tricuspid valves.

of the mitral and tricuspid valves.[9,10] This area, which is part of the so-called central fibrous body, provides the support for the antero-inferior buttress of the atrial septum. The distal part of the ventricular cavity is formed by the free-standing infundibular sleeve, which posteriorly separates the cavity of the infundibulum from the aortic root (Figures 7.12, 7.13). This means that there is no anatomically discrete conal, outlet, or infundibular septum to be found in the normal heart.[11]

The fibrous tissues forming the overall skirt of the ***tricuspid valve*** itself, as the name suggests, close in trifoliate fashion (Figure 7.5).[12] It has been suggested that the valve can have four leaflets[13] or be restricted to two leaflets.[14] These categorizations depend very much on whether the valve is assessed when opened or according to the manner of its closure. The very nature of the right atrioventricular junction dictates that, when seen during motion, the leaflets come together in trifoliate fashion. When assessed attitudinally, the three leaflets guard the septal, inferior, and antero-superior components of the right atrioventricular junction (Figures 7.5 panel B, 7.14). The most prominent ***papillary muscle*** of the tricuspid valve, the *anterior* muscle, is most frequently attached to, and supports, the middle of the antero-superior leaflet (Figure 7.5). In other instances, it provides tendinous cords for both the antero-superior and -inferior leaflets of the valve (Figure 7.14). The zone of apposition between the antero-superior leaflet, which is the largest leaflet of the valve, and the septal leaflet is supported by the characteristic *medial papillary muscle*. This structure is also known as the *conal papillary muscle*, the *papillary muscle of the septum*, or the *muscle of Lancisi* (Figures 7.6, 7.14). The septal leaflet itself has multiple tendinous cords attaching it directly to the inferior part of the ventricular septum. These septal attachments are the most consistent feature of the tricuspid valve. There is usually a smaller inferior papillary muscle supporting the zone of apposition between the inferior and septal leaflets, although this muscle is frequently duplicated.[12]

The ***apical*** component of the ventricle is dominated by its coarse trabeculations, which occupy the entirety of the ventricular

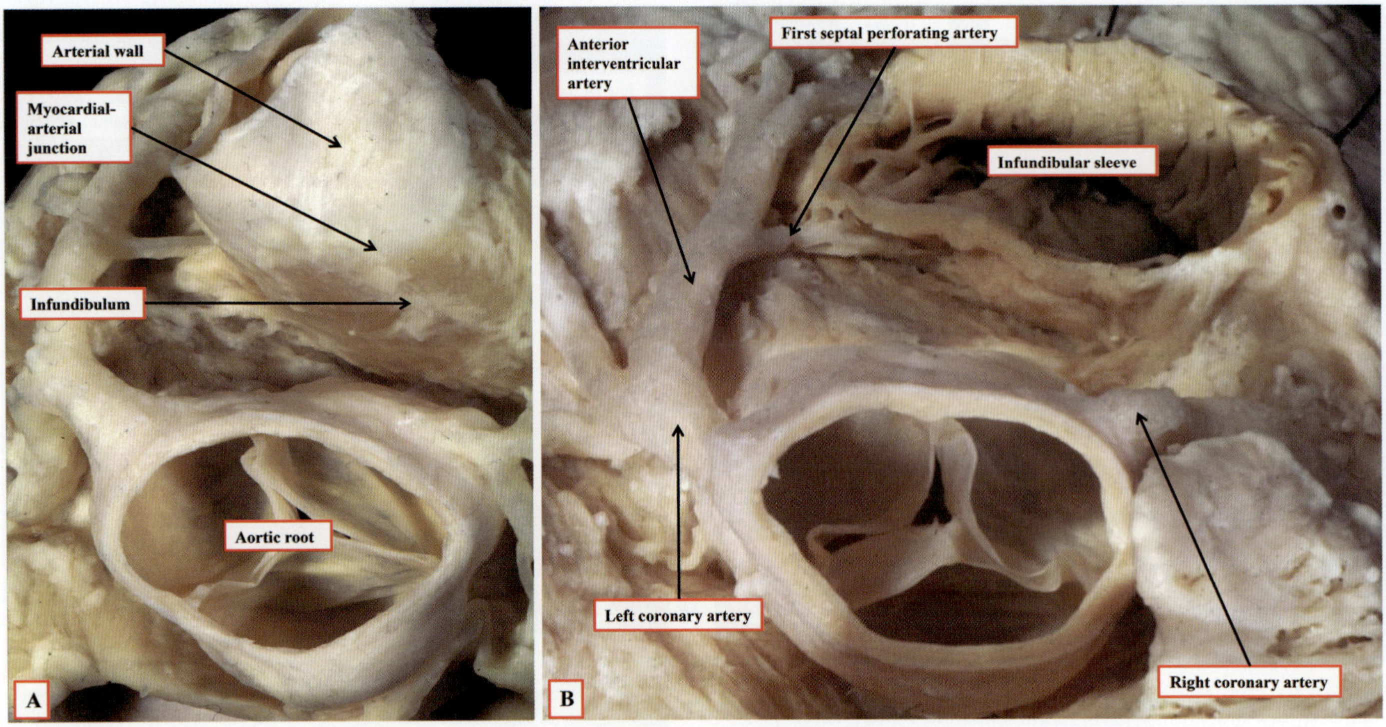

Figure 7.12. The dissections show the infundibular sleeve which lifts the pulmonary root away from the base of the ventricular mass. In panel A, the arterial wall of the pulmonary root has been reflected anteriorly to show the myocardial–arterial junction. In panel B, the sleeve has been transected to reveal the deep groove that interposes between the base of the infundibulum and the sinuses of the aortic root. Note the location of the first septal perforating artery. It is the presence of the infundibular sleeve that makes possible the Ross procedure.

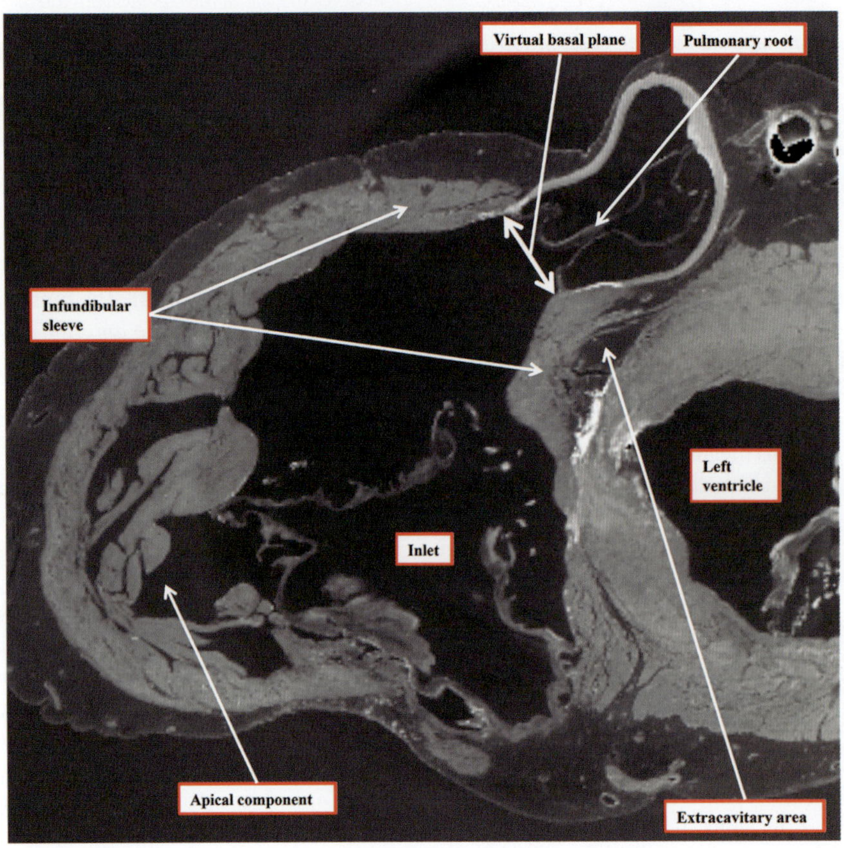

Figure 7.13. The image is a two-dimensional section taken from a three-dimensional dataset of an adult human heart prepared by Synchrotron scanning. The section was specifically chosen to reveal the extent of the free-standing infundibular sleeve that lifts the leaflets of the pulmonary valve away from the base of the ventricular cone. Note the extensive extracavitary area interposing between the infundibular sleeve and the wall of the left ventricle.

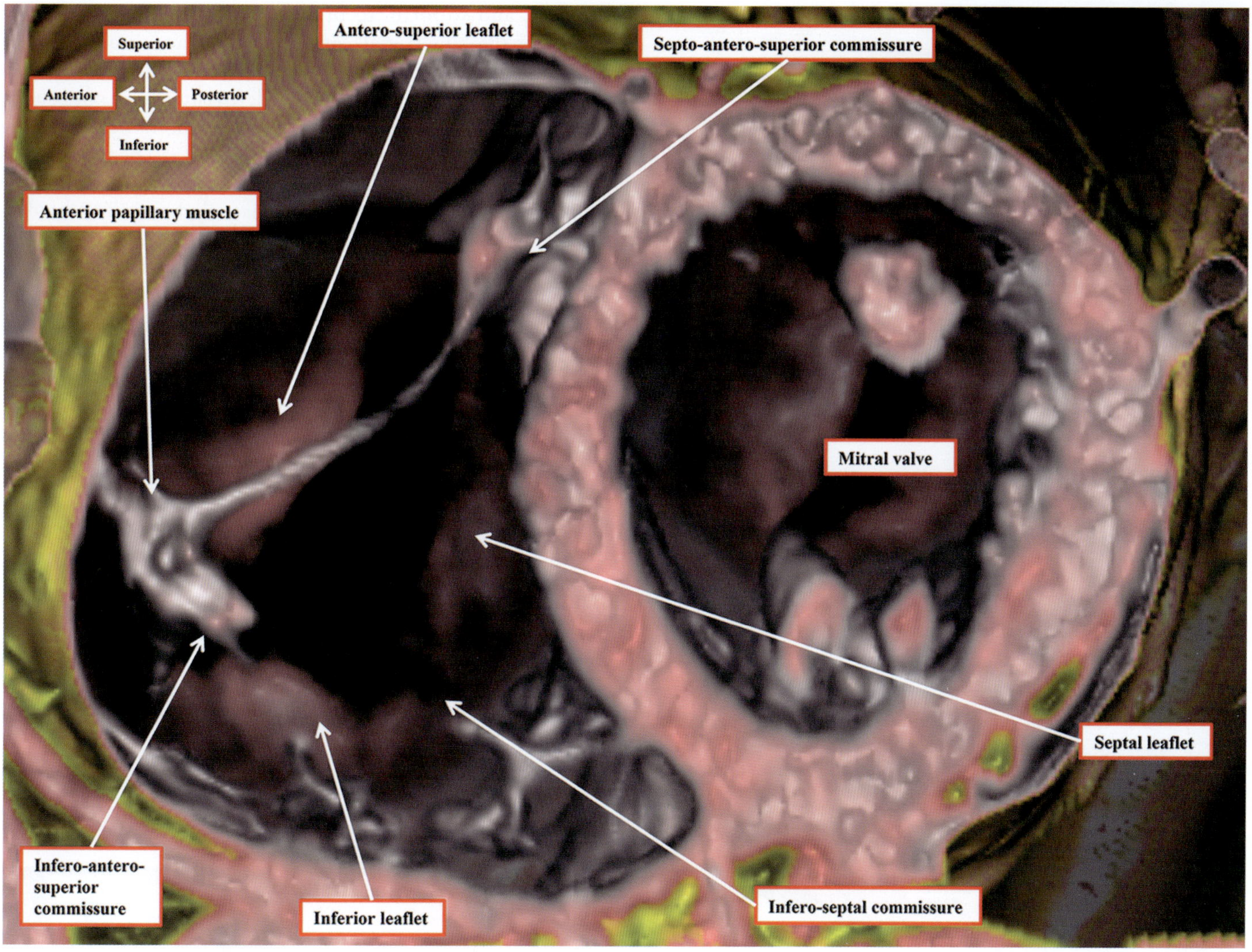

Figure 7.14. The virtual dissection of a computed tomographic dataset, viewed in left anterior oblique projection, confirms that the leaflets of the tricuspid valve are located septally, antero-superiorly, and inferiorly. In this heart, the anterior papillary muscle supported the infero-antero-superior commissure of the valve. The septo-antero-superior commissure is supported by the medial papillary muscle.

outer curvature (Figure 7.2). During development, some of the trabeculations coalesce to form the papillary muscles of the tricuspid valve and additional characteristic trabecular structures. Of these latter trabeculations, one is particularly well formed. It reinforces the surface of the septum and is known as the septomarginal trabeculation or the septal band (Figure 7.15).[15] It has an obvious body, which extends along the septal surface to the apex, where it gives rise to the most prominent of the septoparietal trabeculations, known as the ***moderator band*** (Figure 7.15). This structure, which carries a fascicle of the right bundle branch, may be an arrhythmic substrate, and should be considered for specific mapping and targeted ablation.[16] The most cranial of the series of septoparietal trabeculations is usually found at the mouth of the infundibulum, but trabeculations can extend within the infundibular sleeve. At the ventricular base, the septomarginal trabeculation itself divides into cranial and caudal limbs. These clasp the inner curvature of the right ventricle. This fold, well described as being a part of the ***supraventricular crest***, or ***crista supraventricularis***, separates the leaflets of the tricuspid and pulmonary valves (Figures 7.6, 7.15).[15] Its distal component forms part of the free-standing infundibulum, specifically the part directly adjacent to the aortic root (Figure 7.12 panel B).

Within the ventricular walls, the cardiomyocytes are aggregated together as a three-dimensional mesh within a supporting matrix of fibrous tissue.[17] When the walls are dissected carefully, it is possible to discern a particular “grain”, produced by the longitudinal alignment of chains of aggregated cardiomyocytes (Figure 7.16). The orientation of the grain of the aggregated cardiomyocytes changes when traced transmurally, albeit that the chains are not themselves separated by cleavage planes or sheets of fibrous tissue. Cardiomyocytes of one component within the wall interconnect with those of

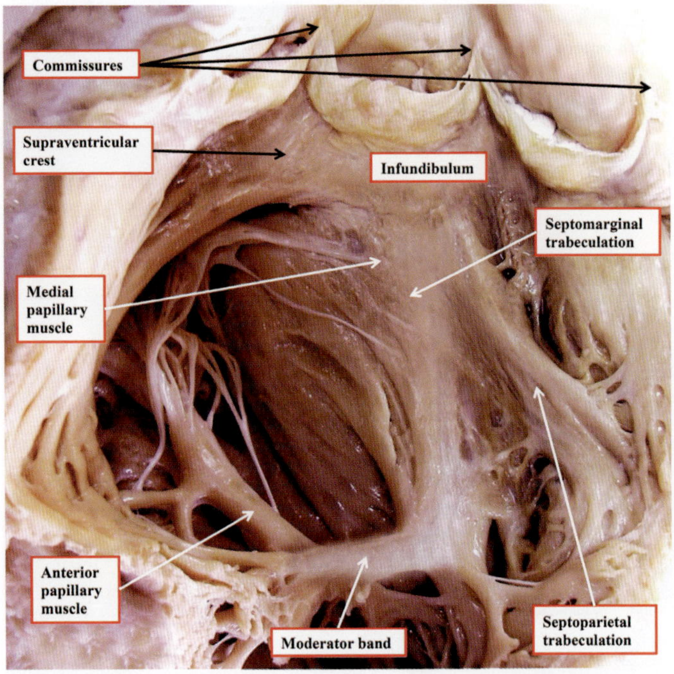

Figure 7.15. The parietal wall of the right ventricle has been reflected to show the arrangement of the papillary muscles supporting the anterior-superior leaflet of the tricuspid valve and the location of the prominent septomarginal trabeculation. A series of septoparietal trabeculations extend from the anterior surface of the septomarginal trabeculation. One of these is the moderator band, which crosses the cavity of the ventricle and supports the origin of the anterior papillary muscle.

the next, and so forth, to produce a continuum. In the right ventricle, the superficial cardiomyocytes are arranged more circumferentially than in the left ventricle. A relatively distinct middle component, as found in the left ventricle, is not usually present in the right ventricle, but can be found in the setting of malformations such as tetralogy of Fallot.[18] The fashion and significance of aggregation of the cardiomyocytes within the walls of the cardiac chambers are discussed and illustrated in greater detail in Chapter 9.

The ***pulmonary valve***, which guards the ventricular outlet and is housed in the ***pulmonary root***, has three leaflets (Figure 7.15). Each leaflet is supported proximally by the free-standing infundibular sleeve (Figure 7.12).[4,5] Their characteristic feature is the crossing of their semilunar hinges over the myocardial–arterial junction (Figure 7.16). This results in crescents of ventricular myocardium being incorporated at the base of each of the pulmonary valvar sinuses. Fibrous arterial tissues then fill the interleaflet triangles between the sinuses, albeit enclosing the distal parts of the ventricular cavity. They extend between the pulmonary valvar sinuses to the level of the sinutubular junction (Figure 7.17).[5]

It is the attachments of the adjacent leaflets at the ***sinutubular junction***, therefore, that mark the distal extent of the ventricular cavity when the leaflets of the pulmonary valve are in their closed positions. The sinutubular junction itself, when defined as the distal extent of the right ventricular cavity, does not form the narrowest

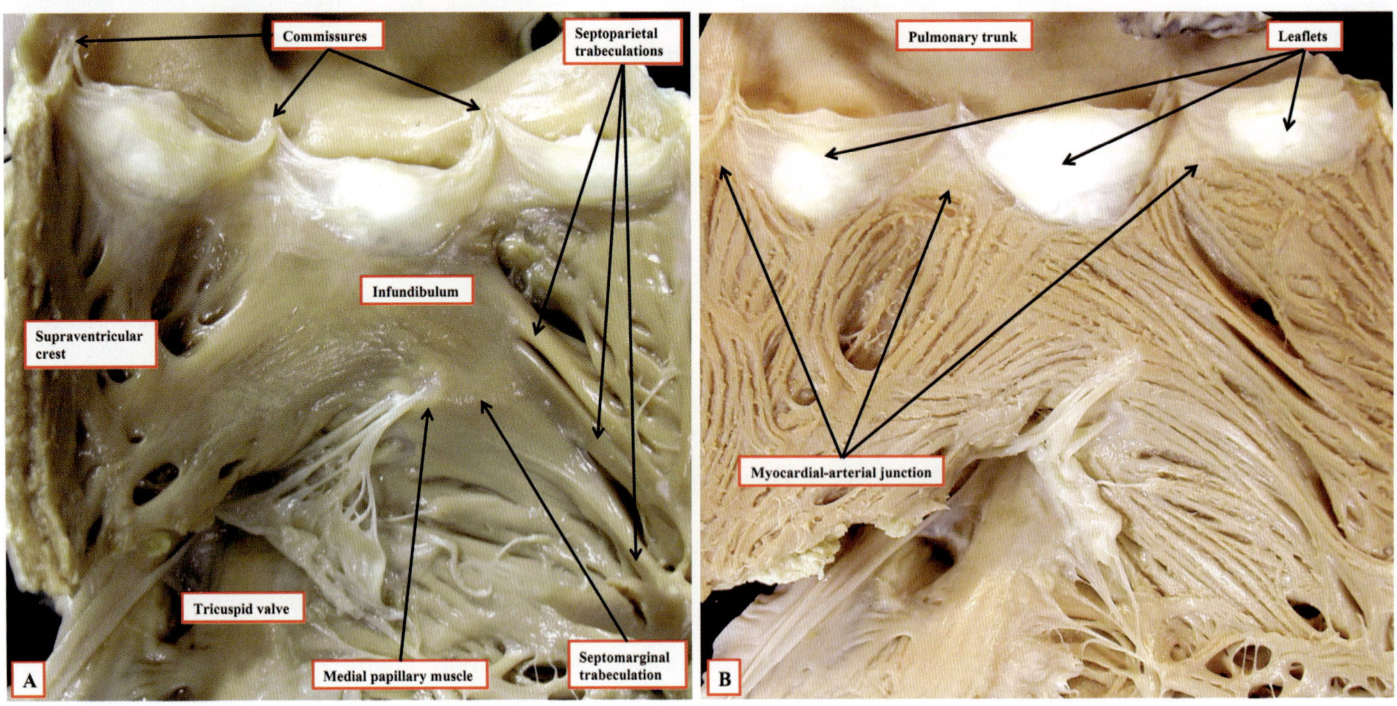

Figure 7.16. The images show how the leaflets of the pulmonary valve are supported by the muscular infundibular sleeve, which lifts them away from the base of the ventricular mass. In panel A, the outflow tract has been opened to show the arrangement of the three leaflets of the valve. In panel B, the endocardial surface has been removed and the subendocardial myocardium dissected to show how the cardiomyocytes are aggregated in parallel arrangement within the walls and trabeculations of the outflow tract. Panel B also shows how each leaflet of the valve is hinged such that its nadir is located proximal to the myocardial–arterial junction, with the semilunar hinges coming together at the commissure, incorporating triangles of arterial wall as the distal extent of the ventricular cavity.

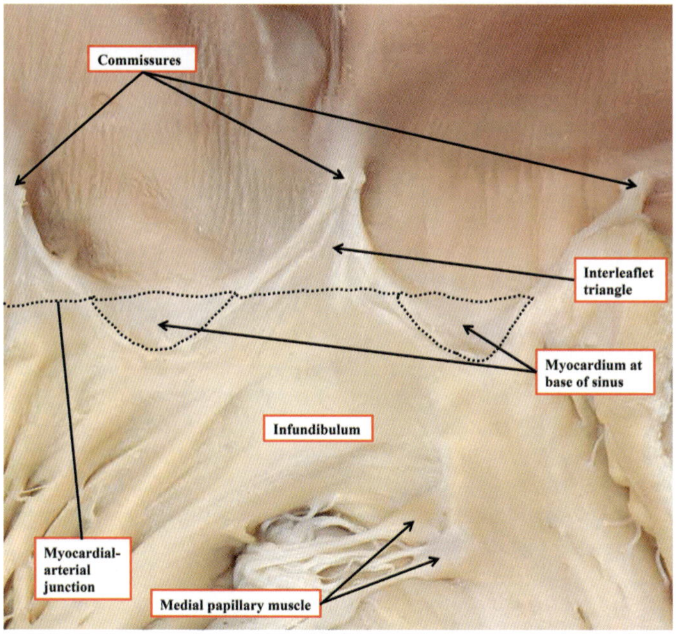

Figure 7.17. The image shows a close-up of two of the leaflets of the trifoliate pulmonary valve. The leaflets themselves have been removed to show how the hinges cross the myocardial–arterial junction. This results in myocardium being incorporated at the base of each of the valvar sinuses, with arterial wall forming the wall of the ventricle directly beneath the valvar commissures.

part of the right ventricular outflow tract. The narrowest area is distal to the plane created by joining together the three commissures at the sinutubular junction.[3] It is the more distal ***tubular plane*** that is usually taken by echocardiographers to mark the distal extent of the pulmonary root (Figure 7.18).

In terms of its electrophysiology, the myocardial components of the ***right ventricular outflow tract*** are characterized by the shorter durations of their action potentials relative to the right ventricular apical region. It is the outflow tract myocardium that drives the transmural dispersion of repolarization and action potentials under normal physiological conditions.[19] Defects of connexins, the proteins involved in cell-to-cell connections, may also be responsible.[20] Thus, the right ventricular outflow myocardium is a dominant site of origin of premature ventricular contractions and ventricular tachyarrhythmias, including the ***Brugada syndrome***.[22] The majority of ***idiopathic outflow tract arrhythmias*** arise from the ventriculo-arterial junctions of the pulmonary trunk and the aorta.[23] The right ventricular outflow tract is also most frequently diseased in the setting of ***arrhythmogenic right ventricular cardiomyopathy***.[19–21,]

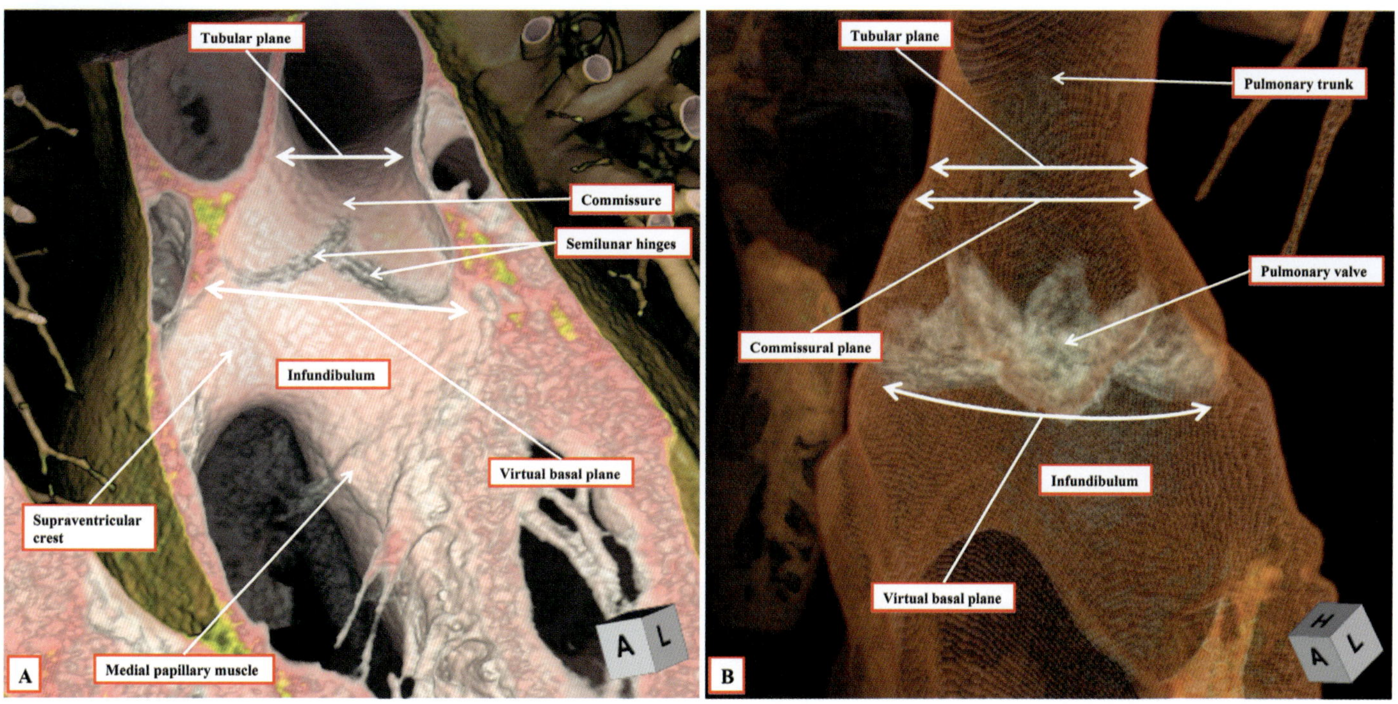

Figure 7.18. The images are taken from a computed tomographic dataset from a child with a volume-overloaded right ventricle. They show the planes that can be measured to reveal the dimensions of the pulmonary root. In panel B, the leaflets of the pulmonary valve have been segmented such that they can be "ghosted" within the root. The images show that the narrowest diameter at the junction between the pulmonary root and the intrapericardial arterial trunk is distal to the plane that can be created by joining together the commissures formed by the attachments of the semilunar hinge lines of the leaflets of the pulmonary valve at the sinutubular junction. This narrowest diameter has been described as the tubular plane.

REFERENCES

1. Crucean A, Spicer DE, Tretter JT, Mohun TJ, Anderson RH. Revisiting the anatomy of the right ventricle in the light of knowledge of its development. *J Anat*. 2024;**244**:297–311. doi: 10.1111/joa.13960
2. Toh H, Mori S, Izawa Y, Fujita H, Miwa K, Suzuki M, Takahashi Y, Toba T, Watanabe Y, Kono AK, et al. Prevalence and extent of mitral annular disjunction in structurally normal hearts: comprehensive 3D analysis using cardiac computed tomography. *Eur Heart J Cardiovasc Imaging*. 2021;**22**:614–622. doi: 10.1093/ehjci/jeab022
3. Lis M, Krawczyk-Ozog A, Holda J, Tyrak K, Dudkiewicz D, Yakovliev A, Strona M, Bolechala F, Jakiel R, Jakiel M, et al. Pulmonary valve morphometry revisited: clinical implications for valvular and supravalvular interventions. *Clin Anat*. 2023;**36**:234–241. doi: 10.1002/ca.23959
4. Merrick AF, Yacoub MH, Ho SY, Anderson RH. Anatomy of the muscular subpulmonary infundibulum with regard to the Ross procedure. *Ann Thorac Surg*. 2000;**69**:556–561. doi: 10.1016/s0003-4975(99)01300-4
5. Stamm C, Anderson RH, Ho SY. Clinical anatomy of the normal pulmonary root compared with that in isolated pulmonary valvular stenosis. *J Am Coll Cardiol*. 1998;**31**:1420–1425. doi: 10.1016/s0735-1097(98)00089-8
6. Amofa D, Mori S, Toh H, Ta HT, Du Plessis M, Davis N, Izawa Y, Spicer DE, Anderson RH, Tretter JT. The rotational position of the aortic root related to its underlying ventricular support. *Clin Anat*. 2019;**32**:1107–1117. doi: 10.1002/ca.23462
7. Tretter JT, Koneru JN, Spicer DE, Ellenbogen KA, Anderson RH, Ben-Haim S. A new dimension in cardiac imaging: three-dimensional exploration of the atrioventricular conduction axis with hierarchical phase-contrast tomography. *Heart Rhythm*. 2024;**21**:2388–2396. doi: 10.1016/j.hrthm.2024.10.002
8. Li A, Zuberi Z, Bradfield JS, Zarif JK, Ward DE, Anderson RH, Shivkumar K, Saba MM. Endocardial ablation of ventricular ectopic beats arising from the basal inferoseptal process of the left ventricle. *Heart Rhythm*. 2018;**15**:1356–1362. doi: 10.1016/j.hrthm.2018.04.029
9. Tretter JT, Izawa Y, Spicer DE, Okada K, Anderson RH, Quintessenza JA, Mori S. Understanding the aortic root using computed tomographic assessment: a potential pathway to improved customized surgical repair. *Circ Cardiovasc Imaging*. 2021;**14**:e013134. doi: 10.1161/CIRCIMAGING.121.013134
10. Tretter JT, Spicer DE, Sanchez-Quintana D, Back Sternick E, Farre J, Anderson RH. Miniseries 1—Part III: 'Behind the scenes' in the triangle of Koch. *Europace*. 2022;**24**:455–463. doi: 10.1093/europace/euab285
11. Anderson RH, Tretter JT, Spicer DE, Mori S. The fate of the outflow tract septal complex in relation to the classification of ventricular septal defects. *J Cardiovasc Dev Dis*. 2019;**6**:9. doi: 10.3390/jcdd6010009
12. Tretter JT, Sarwark AE, Anderson RH, Spicer DE. Assessment of the anatomical variation to be found in the normal tricuspid valve. *Clin Anat*. 2016;**29**:399–407. doi: 10.1002/ca.22591
13. Hahn RT, Weckbach LT, Noack T, Hamid N, Kitamura M, Bae R, Lurz P, Kodali SK, Sorajja P, Hausleiter J, et al. Proposal for a standard echocardiographic tricuspid valve nomenclature. *JACC Cardiovasc Imaging*. 2021;**14**:1299–1305. doi: 10.1016/j.jcmg.2021.01.012
14. Victor S, Nayak VM. Tricuspid valve is bicuspid. *Ann Thorac Surg*. 2000;**69**:1989–1990. doi: 10.1016/s0003-4975(00)01396-5
15. Anderson RH, Becker AE, Van Mierop LH. What should we call the 'crista'? *Br Heart J*. 1977;**39**:856–859. doi: 10.1136/hrt.39.8.856
16. Abouezzeddine O, Suleiman M, Buescher T, Kapa S, Friedman PA, Jahangir A, Mears JA, Ladewig DJ, Munger TM, Hammill SC, et al. Relevance of endocavitary structures in ablation procedures for ventricular tachycardia. *J Cardiovasc Electrophysiol*. 2010;**21**:245–254. doi: 10.1111/j.1540-8167.2009.01621.x
17. Anderson RH, Smerup M, Sanchez-Quintana D, Loukas M, Lunkenheimer PP. The three-dimensional arrangement of the myocytes in the ventricular walls. *Clin Anat*. 2009;**22**:64–76. doi: 10.1002/ca.20645
18. Sanchez-Quintana D, Anderson RH, Ho SY. Ventricular myoarchitecture in tetralogy of Fallot. *Heart*. 1996;**76**:280–286. doi: 10.1136/hrt.76.3.280
19. Aras K, Gams A, Faye NR, Brennan J, Goldrick K, Li J, Zhong Y, Chiang CH, Smith EH, Poston MD, et al. Electrophysiology and arrhythmogenesis in the human right ventricular outflow tract. *Circ Arrhythm Electrophysiol*. 2022;**15**:e010630. doi: 10.1161/CIRCEP.121.010630
20. Boukens BJ, Christoffels VM, Coronel R, Moorman AF. Developmental basis for electrophysiological heterogeneity in the ventricular and outflow tract myocardium as a substrate for life-threatening ventricular arrhythmias. *Circ Res*. 2009;**104**:19–31. doi: 10.1161/CIRCRESAHA.108.188698104/1/19 [pii]
21. Zhang J, Sacher F, Hoffmayer K, O'Hara T, Strom M, Cuculich P, Silva J, Cooper D, Faddis M, Hocini M, et al. Cardiac electrophysiological substrate underlying the ECG phenotype and electrogram abnormalities in Brugada syndrome patients. *Circulation*. 2015;**131**:1950–1959. doi: 10.1161/CIRCULATIONAHA.114.013698
22. Enriquez A, Muser D, Markman TM, Garcia F, Mapping and Ablation of Premature Ventricular Complexes: State of the Art. *JACC Clin Electrophysiol*. 2024;**10**:1206–1222. doi: 10.1016/j.jacep.2024.02.008

8 The Left Ventricle

As is the case with the morphologically right ventricle, the left ventricle can be described in terms of possessing inlet, apical, and outlet components, with the outlet component supporting the aortic root (Figure 8.1). And, as was shown in Chapter 1, although termed the "left", the ventricle is positioned, for the most part, posteriorly relative to its morphologically right partner.[1] In terms of its development, the larger part of the initial linear primary heart tube persists as the definitive left ventricle.[2] As in the right ventricle, ballooning of the apical component from the inlet of the ventricular loop provides the ventricle with its morphological identity.[3] From the outset, the left ventricle possesses its inlet component. It is with the acquisition of the aortic root during the latter part of embryonic life and the beginning of the fetal period that the ventricle obtains its outlet. Since the outlet is the new part of the chamber, it is not surprising that there should, potentially, be significant variability postnatally in the precise relationships of the outlet component relative to the remainder of the ventricle.[4]

The overall walls enclosing the cavity of the left ventricle extend from the ***atrioventricular*** to the ***sinutubular junctions*** (Figure 8.2). Not all of these walls are myocardial. This is because, as in the right ventricle, the myocardial walls of the left ventricle do not reach the sinutubular junction. Significant parts of the walls of its ***outlet*** component, which incorporates the ***aortic root***, are made up of fibrous tissue. These are the ***triangles*** that interpose between the aortic valvar sinuses, with the arterial walls of the sinuses supporting the semilunar leaflets of the aortic valve (Figure 8.3).[5,6] Unlike the right ventricle, where myocardium is found at the bases of all three pulmonary valvar sinuses (Figure 7.17), the myocardium of the ventricular septum is found only at the bases of the aortic valvar sinuses which give rise to the coronary arteries, and also at the base of the intervening interleaflet triangle (Figure 8.3). This means that the left ventricle, unlike its morphologically right counterpart, does not possess a complete infundibulum (Figure 8.1).

Very rarely, however, it is possible to find the arrangement with myocardium interposing between the leaflets of the aortic and mitral valves.[5] Except in these very rare instances, the leaflet supported by the non-coronary sinus of the aortic root, along with part of the left coronary aortic leaflet, is in fibrous continuity in

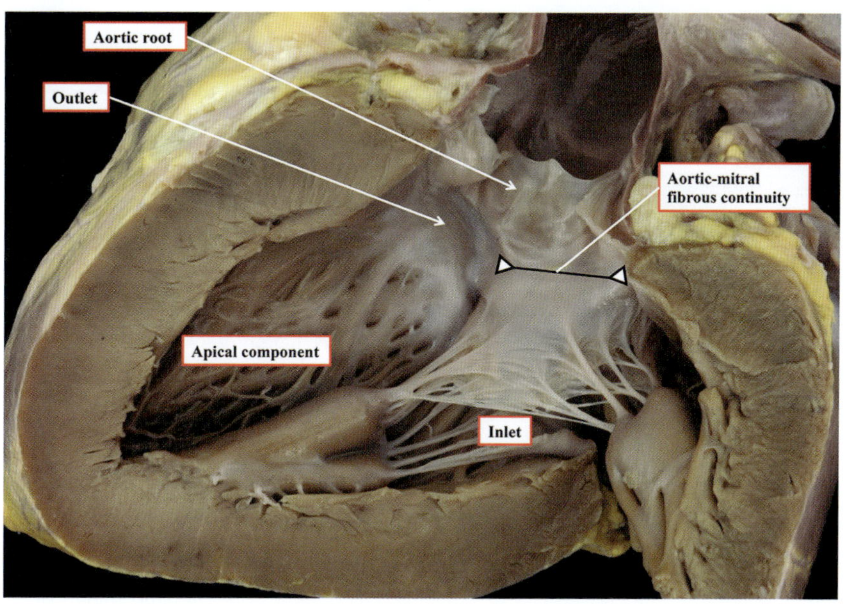

Figure 8.1. The left ventricle has been opened by making a cut parallel to the septum and opening the cavity in clam-like fashion. The cavity is made up of the inlet, supporting the tension apparatus of the mitral valve, the finely trabecular apical component, and the outlet supporting the aortic root. The roof of the cavity is formed by the area of fibrous continuity between the leaflets of the aortic and mitral valves.

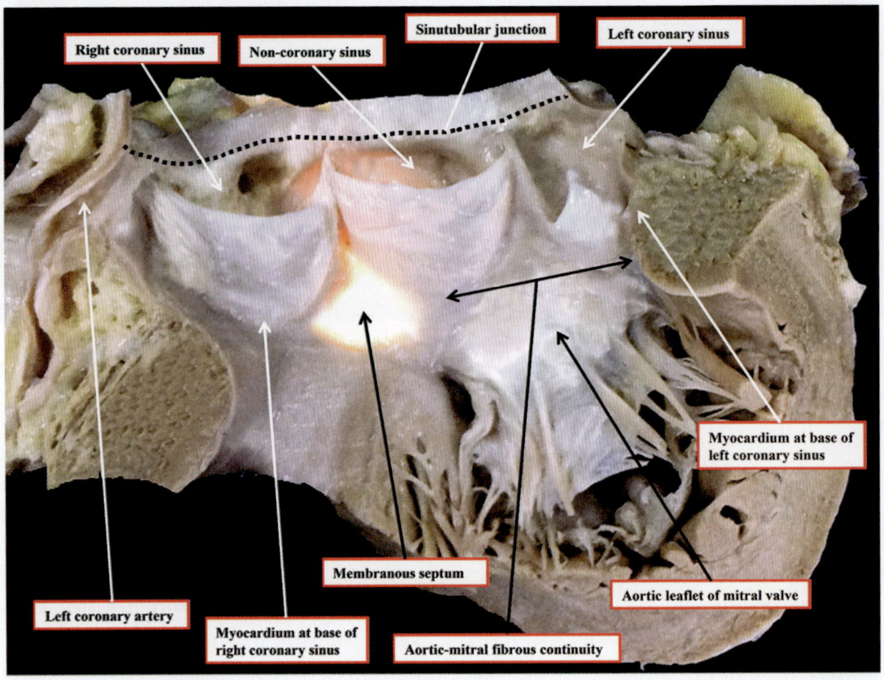

Figure 8.2. The aortic root has been opened and spread to show how the ventricular cavity extends to the level of the sinutubular junction, with the interleaflet triangles forming the fibrous walls of the distal part of the cavity. The myocardial walls support only the leaflets of the valvar sinuses that give rise to the coronary arteries.

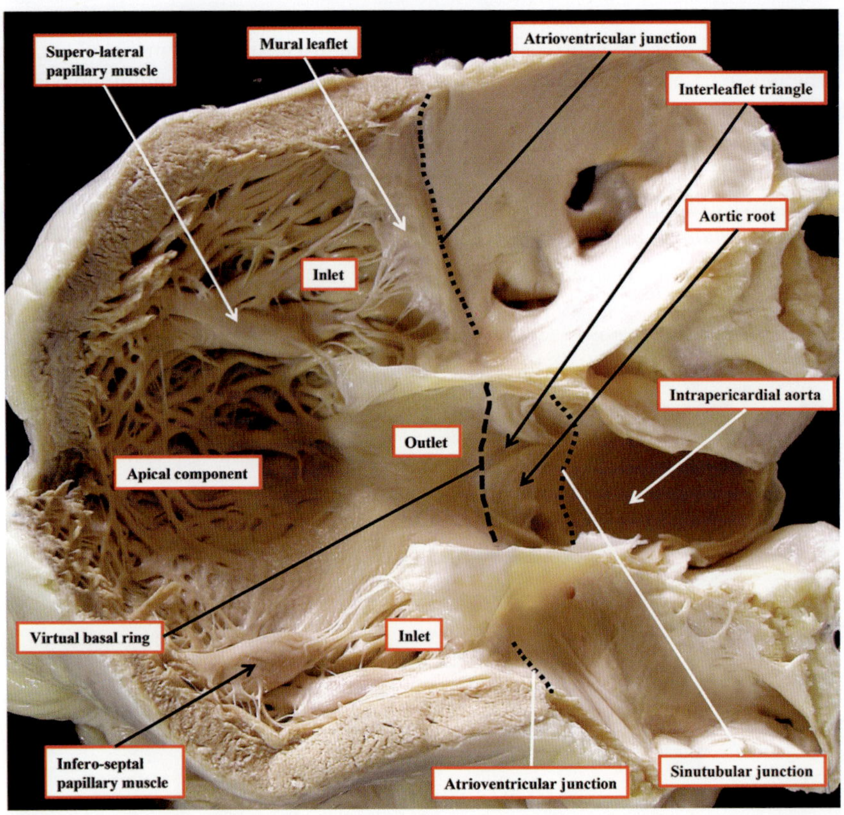

Figure 8.3. The left ventricle has been opened by making a cut through its inlet adjacent to the inferior part of the ventricular septum. An additional cut has then been made through the aortic leaflet of the mitral valve, with the two components of the leaflet opened to show the outlet part of the cavity. The dissection shows how the cavity extends from the atrioventricular to the sinutubular junctions. As shown in Figure 8.2, the myocardial walls of the ventricle do not reach the sinutubular junction. Because of the fibrous continuity between the leaflets of the aortic and mitral valves, myocardial support is provided only to the two leaflets of the aortic valve which guard the sinuses giving rise to the right and left coronary arteries. The sinutubular junction also forms the distal boundary of the aortic root. Its proximal boundary is formed by the virtual ring constructed by joining together the nadirs of attachment of the semilunar leaflets of the aortic valve.

the inner heart curvature with one of the leaflets of the mitral valve (Figure 8.3). Because of the fibrous continuity between the inlet and outlet components in the inner heart curvature, only part of the left atrioventricular junction has myocardial support. When the left ventricular cavity is viewed from the apex looking towards the base, the fibrous continuity between the leaflets of its inlet and outlet valves can be seen to form its roof (Figure 8.4). The orifices of the two valves overlap within the short axis of the ventricular cone.[7]

The valvar orifices, however, do not fully occupy the base of the left ventricular cone. This is because the extensive ***infero-septal recess*** of the subaortic outflow tract interposes between the ***aortic***, or anterior, leaflet of the mitral valve and the inferior extension of the muscular ventricular septum (Figure 8.5).[8] The fibrous roof of the recess, which is formed by an area of fibrous continuity between the leaflets of the tricuspid and mitral valves, supports the base of the antero-inferior buttress of the atrial septum. The right border of the recess is formed by the atrioventricular component of the membranous septum. The fibrous roof is then itself continuous with the rightward end of the area of fibrous continuity between the leaflets of the mitral and aortic valves (Figure 8.6).

Although the entirety of the area of fibrous continuity has previously been defined as the ***right fibrous trigone***, it is preferable to restrict the term ***right trigone*** to the rightward end of the area of aortic-to-mitral fibrous continuity. This definition then matches the one used for the leftward end of this area of fibrous continuity, which is recognized as the ***left fibrous trigone***. Taken together, these fibrous tissues serve to anchor the aortic–mitral unit within the base of the ventricular cone (Figure 8.4). When considered as an overall entity, the tissues at the rightward end of the area of aortic-to-mitral continuity can be defined as the ***central fibrous body***.[9] This fibrous area makes up the largest part of the so-called "fibrous skeleton" of the heart. The fibrous component, nonetheless, remains relatively small when considered in the overall context of the ventricular mass. When traced inferiorly, the apex of the infero-septal recess overlaps the superiorly directed apex of the inferior pyramidal space.[9] This latter space is the area on the atrial side of the atrioventricular junctions, enclosed by the diverging vestibules of the right and left atrial chambers. By virtue of the overlap, the atrioventricular conduction axis is able to penetrate the fibrous insulating tissues of the atrioventricular junctions, thus reaching its position on the crest of the superior part of the muscular ventricular septum (Figure 8.7). When traced forward, the conduction axis branches to give rise to its right and left fascicles.

The ventricular ***inlet*** is guarded by the ***mitral valve***. Its components extend from the atrioventricular junction to the distal attachments of its papillary muscles within the left ventricular myocardial cone. When functioning in appropriate fashion, its parts work together as a valvar complex (Figure 8.8).[10] The leaflets are frequently described as being supported within the atrioventricular junction by an "*annulus*". If interpreted on the basis of presence of a continuous zone of collagen hinging the mural leaflet within the junction, which also separates the atrial myocardium from the crest of the ventricular cone, then this is a gross exaggeration. Such an arrangement

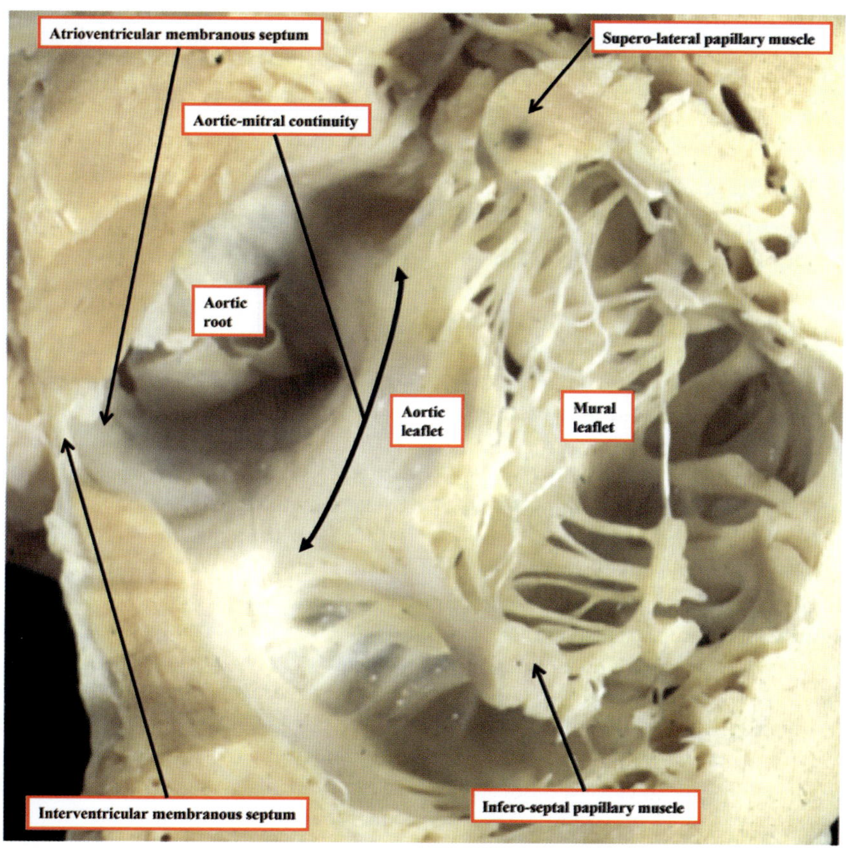

Figure 8.4. The roof of the left ventricle is shown as seen from the apex. The orifices of the aortic root and mitral valve overlap within the short axis of the ventricular cavity, with the continuity between the leaflets of the valves forming its fibrous roof.

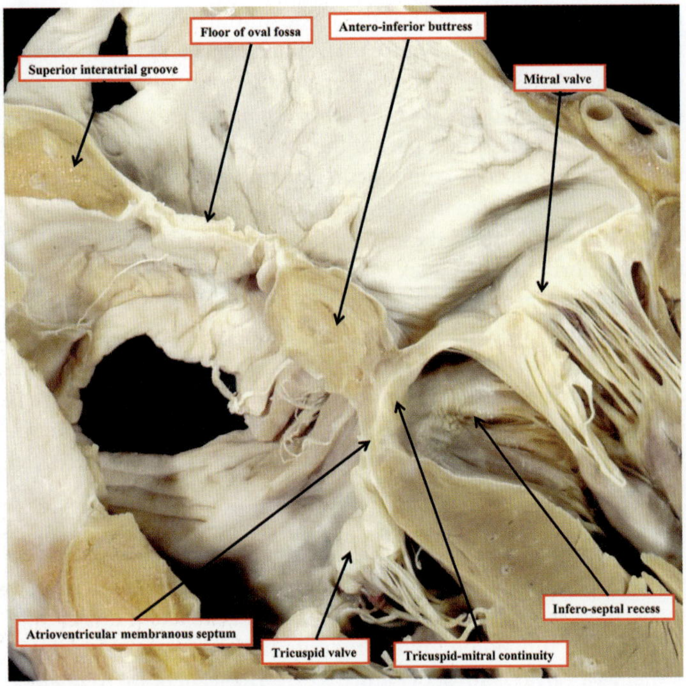

Figure 8.5. The "four-chamber" cut though the ventricular inlets reveals the deep infero-septal recess of the left ventricular outflow tract that interposes between the leaflets of the mitral valve and the inferior component of the ventricular septum. The roof of the recess, formed by an area of fibrous continuity between the leaflets of the mitral and tricuspid valves, and incorporating the atrioventricular part of the membranous septum as part of its rightward wall, supports the antero-inferior buttress of the atrial septum.

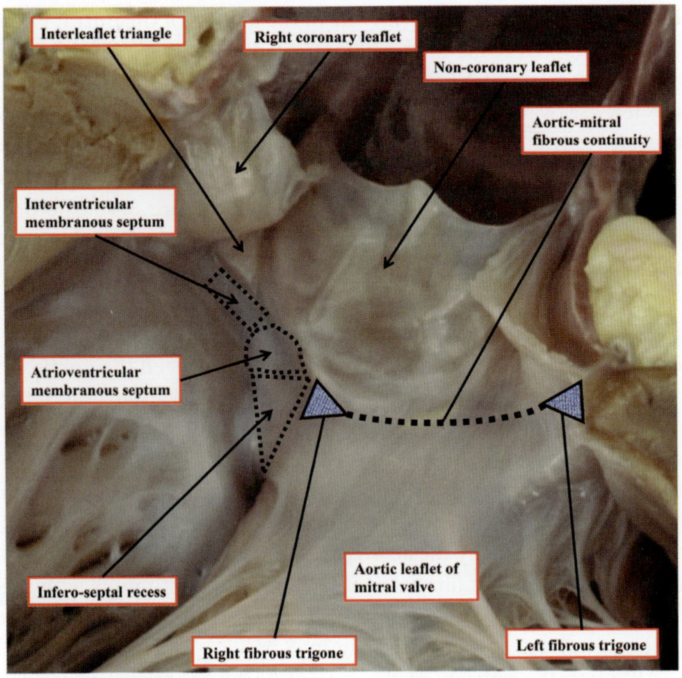

Figure 8.6. The image shown in Figure 8.1 has been enlarged so as to show the components of the fibrous tissues that form the roof of the left ventricular cavity. The rightward and leftward ends of the area of fibrous continuity between the leaflets of the aortic and mitral valves are thickened to form the right and left fibrous trigones. The right trigone is then continuous with the fibrous roof of the infero-septal recess, which as shown in Figure 8.5 supports the buttress of the atrial septum. This area is then continuous with the membranous part of the septum, crossed on its right side to separate the atrioventricular and interventricular parts. The interventricular part is itself continuous with the fibrous triangle separating the right and non-coronary sinuses of the aortic root. Taken together, the right fibrous trigone, the roof of the infero-septal recess, and the fibrous membranous septum produce the so-called central fibrous body.

has been illustrated by those promoting the notion of an extensive "*fibrous skeleton*".[11]

As explained in Chapter 6, such continuity of the fibrous components is not to be found throughout the junctional areas. When attention is paid to the overall hinge of the mural leaflet within the junction, it is possible at some sites to find support provided by a fibrous cord, which also provides the atrioventricular insulation. In other parts of the junction in the same heart, the leaflet can be tethered by a fibrous sheet, which separates the leading edge of the left atrial vestibule from the crest of the parietal wall of the ventricle (Figure 6.13 panel A). In still other parts of the same junction, the leaflet can be hinged directly to the ventricular wall. The fibro-adipose tissue of the junction then provides the atrioventricular insulation (Figure 6.13 panel B).[12] The arrangement in which the hinge is provided by a fibrous sheet is described as a ***mitral annular disjunction***.[13] The mere finding of the separation between the atrial vestibular myocardium and the crest of the ventricular wall is a normal finding (**Figure 8.9**).[14] As was discussed in Chapter 6, the presence of such disjunction has achieved clinical importance because of a potential association with mitral valvar prolapse, arrhythmias, and sudden cardiac death.[15,16] As yet, however, the distinction between the normal findings and their potential pathological significance remains to be proven.[17]

The hinging of the aortic leaflet of the mitral valve is more complex. It takes its support from the extensive area of fibrous tissue making up the region of aortic-to-mitral continuity. When viewed from the ventricular aspect, it is not possible to recognize a discrete linear junctional zone within this area. It is inspection from the atrial aspect that reveals the linear insertion of the atrial myocardium. Its distal margin can then be taken to represent the atrioventricular junction (**Figure 8.8**). When considered in three dimensions, this distal extent of the atrial myocardium is saddle-shaped, with the peak of the saddle found in the area adjacent to the aortic root.

Due to the variation noted in the hinging of the leaflets, it is much better to describe the area of union between the atrial and ventricular myocardial components as the ***atrioventricular junction***, rather than the "annulus" (**Figure 8.8**). The overall skirt of leaflet tissue is attached within the junction, with its pattern of closure showing but a single ***zone of apposition*** between two major leaflets.[17] When viewed in closed position from the atrial aspect, one of the leaflets can be seen to guard two-thirds of the valvar perimeter, with the other guarding but one-third (**Figure 8.10**).

Opening the valve and spreading the junction shows that the leaflet guarding the short part of the perimeter is much deeper than its partner. This means that the surface area of the leaflets is relatively equal (**Figure 8.10**). The leaflet with a larger length but a shorter depth is tethered within the mural part of the atrioventricular

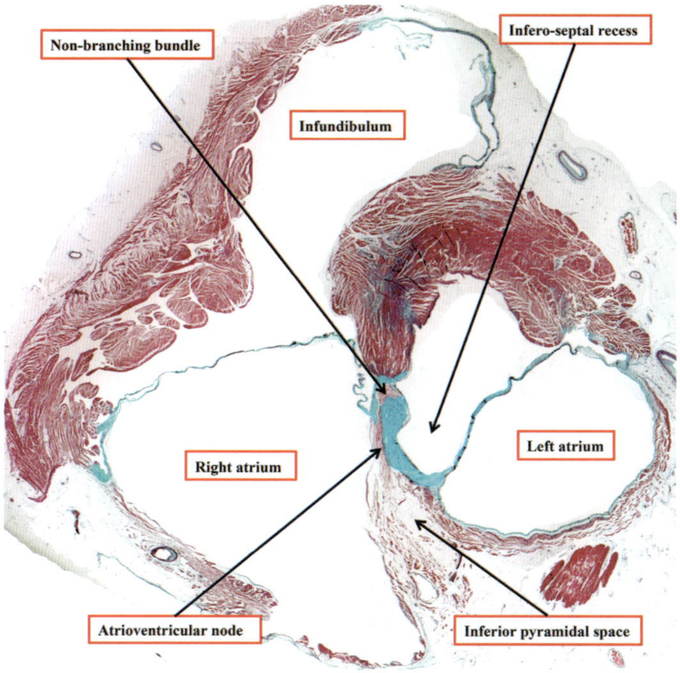

Figure 8.7. The short axis section, stained using the trichrome technique, shows how, by virtue of the overlap of the apexes of the inferior pyramidal space and the infero-septal recess of the left ventricle, the atrioventricular conduction axis is able to penetrate the insulating plane to reach the crest of the superior part of the muscular ventricular septum.

junction (Figure 8.11). The other leaflet is in fibrous continuity with the non-coronary and left coronary leaflets of the aortic valve (Figure 8.10).

It is the manner of hinging of the leaflets within the junction that provides the optimal means of distinguishing between them. Thus, in the normal human heart, by virtue of the relation of one of the leaflets to the aortic root, it can be described as the ***aortic leaflet*** of the mitral valve. It is more usually described as being "*anterior*". The second ***mural leaflet*** is then described as being "posterior". But when viewed attitudinally, the mural leaflet extends around the aortic leaflet at the ends of the zone of apposition between them (Figures 8.4, 8.10). This means that not all parts of the leaflet are strictly "*posterior*".[17] It has now also become conventional to describe the mural leaflet as having three "***scallops***" (Figure 8.12).[18] Some suggest that the scallops should be elevated to the state of individual leaflets. Others, pointing to the presence of additional components of leaflet tissues at the ends of the zone of apposition, argue in favour of the mural leaflet having five parts.[19] In reality, there is marked individual variation in the arrangement of these component parts, although most usually it is possible to find the anticipated three scallops (Figure 8.12).

It is the presence of three such scallops that has resulted in the description, for the mural leaflet, of scallops P1 through P3, with the scallop positioned supero-laterally numbered as ***P1*** and the infero-medial scallop identified as ***P3***.[18] The opposing components of the aortic leaflet are then conventionally numbered as A1 through A3 (Figure 8.13). This system is valid in the majority but not all

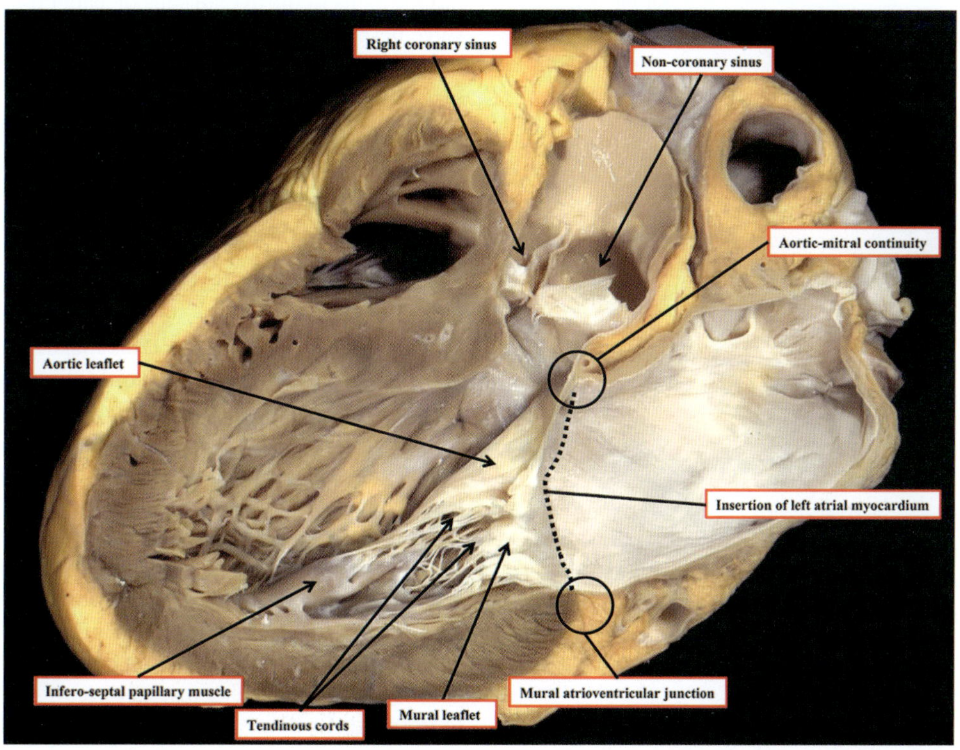

Figure 8.8. The mitral valve guards the inlet component of the left ventricle, extending from the atrioventricular junction to the insertion of its papillary muscles. As shown by the echocardiographic parasternal long axis equivalent section, the valve has various components that work together in harmony to form the valvar complex. The components are the junction, the leaflets, the tendinous cords, and the papillary muscles. Only one of the muscles can be seen in this section.

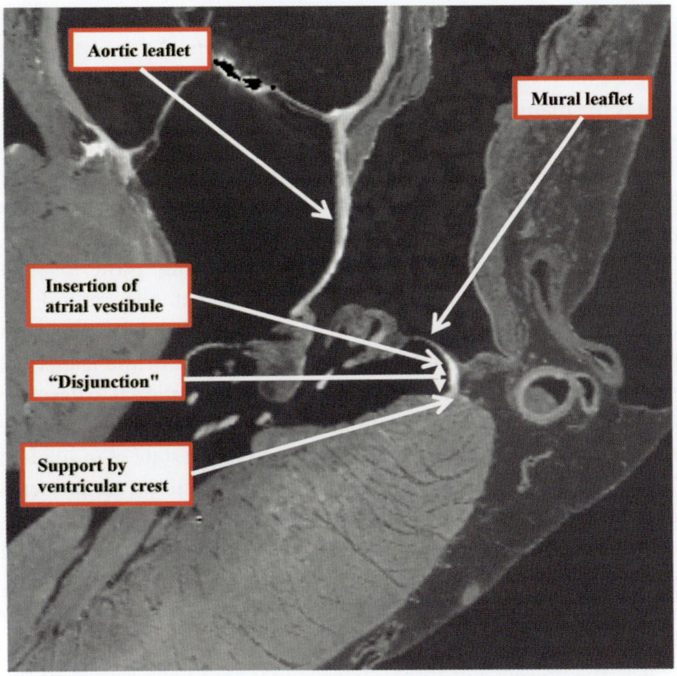

Figure 8.9. The image is taken from a postmortem heart imaged using Synchrotron scanning. It shows a section across the hinge of the mural leaflet of the mitral valve. The shelf-like support of the leaflet produces separation between the insertion of the left atrial vestibule and the crest of the parietal wall of the left ventricle. This is the arrangement that has achieved prominence as "disjunction". It is a normal feature, albeit with other parts of the same mural atrioventricular junction lacking such separation.

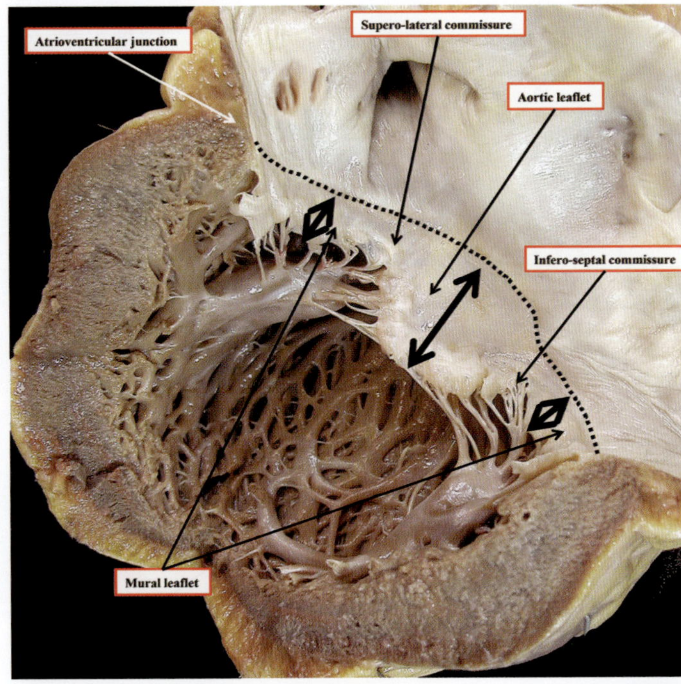

Figure 8.11. When the mitral valve is opened by making a cut through the middle of the mural leaflet, as shown in this image, it can be seen that the aortic leaflet (long double-headed arrow), although guarding only one-third of the perimeter, is much deeper than the mural leaflet (short double-headed arrows). The surface area of the two leaflets is more-or-less the same.

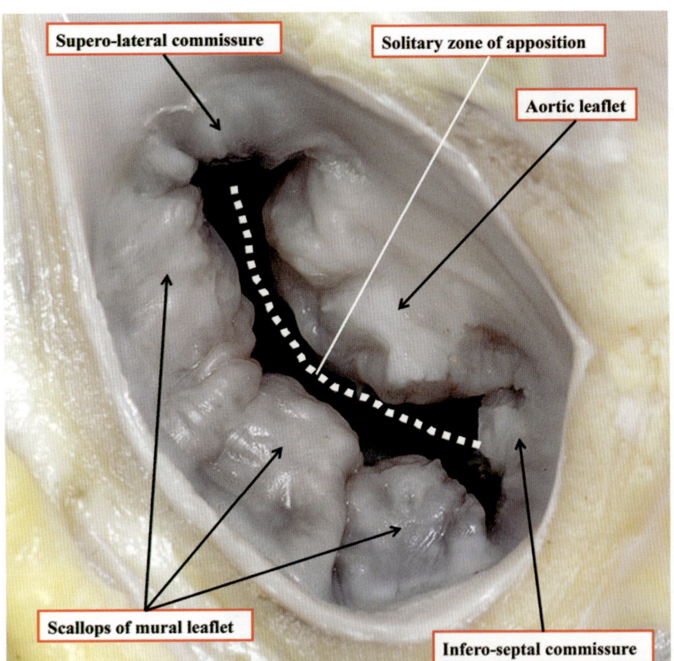

Figure 8.10. The mitral valve has been photographed from the atrial aspect in its closed position. There is but a solitary zone of apposition within the skirt of leaflet tissue hinged from the atrioventricular junction. Note that the line of apposition does not reach to the margins of the junction. The two leaflets joining along this zone guard markedly dissimilar components of the valvar periphery. The leaflet guarding one-third is in fibrous continuity with the aortic root and is best termed the aortic leaflet. The leaflet guarding two-thirds of the periphery is hinged within the mural part of the junction.

individuals. Irrespective of the individual variability, the presence of multiple slits in the overall skirt of leaflet tissue forming the normal valve permits the two leaflets to fit snugly when closed along their solitary zone of apposition.[20] It is the ends of this solitary zone of apposition that are nominated as the ***commissures***. They are positioned supero-laterally and infero-medially when the valve is viewed in attitudinally appropriate fashion.[17]

The leaflets are supported by ***tendinous cords*** along the entirety of their free edges (Figure 8.11). Of the free-edge cords, the ones at the ends of the zone of apposition diverge to support both leaflets. Some have defined these diverging entities as commissural cords.[21] Other free-edge cords diverge in comparable fashion to support the adjacent ends of the scallops. This makes it difficult to distinguish between commissural and cleft cords. It is sufficient simply to recognize the cords as supporting the free edges of the leaflets. The cords from both leaflets then converge to insert into the paired ***papillary muscles***. Like the ends of the zone of apposition between the leaflets, they are located ***infero-medially*** and ***supero-laterally*** within the short axis of the ventricular cone (Figure 8.14). It is a mistake to describe the muscles as being "*postero-medial*" and "*antero-lateral*". The muscles can be viewed in this fashion only when the heart is removed from the chest and assessed in "Valentine" fashion.

With regard to the tendinous cords, additional strut cords extend from the papillary muscles to reinforce the support provided to the aortic leaflet on its ventricular surface (Figure 8.15 panel A). Multiple basal cords then extend from the parietal wall of the ventricle to the ventricular surfaces of the components of the mural leaflet, usually with each individual cord supported by its own miniature papillary muscle (Figure 8.15 panel B). The papillary muscles

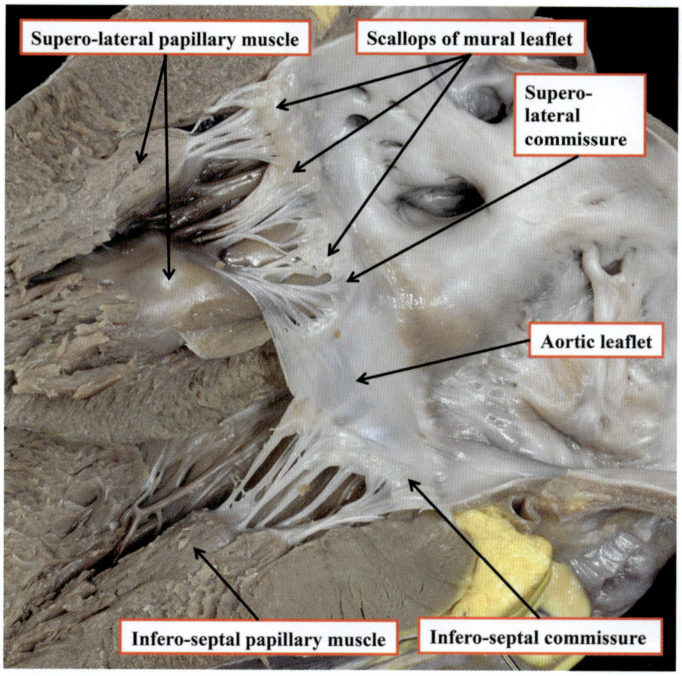

Figure 8.12. The atrioventricular junction has been opened through the infero-septal commissure. Having spread the junction, it is possible to recognize the components of the mural leaflet. As in this heart, there are usually three such "scallops", located infero-medially, posteriorly and laterally, and supero-laterally. In addition, small components of the leaflet tissue are found at the ends of the zone of apposition between the leaflets.

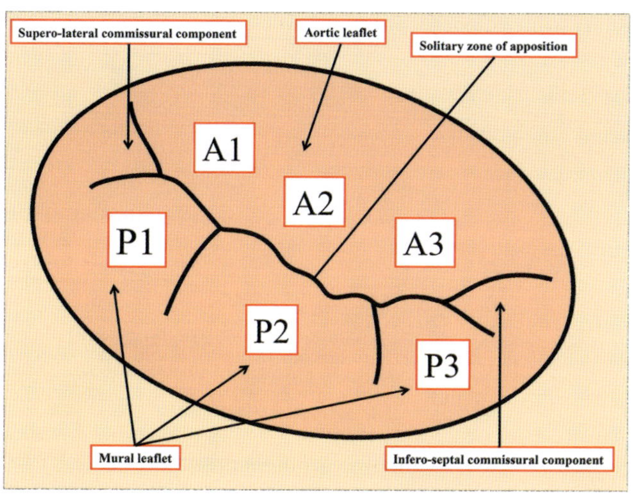

Figure 8.13. The drawing shows the idealized configuration of the components of the skirt of valvar tissue guarding the orifice of the mitral valve as it would be seen from the atrial aspect with the leaflets closed (compare with Figure 8.11). The three scallops typically found within the mural leaflet have become known as P1, P2, and P3, with the apposing components of the aortic leaflet labelled as A1, A2, and A3. As can be seen, the components positioned supero-laterally are numbered 1, with the infero-septal components numbered as 3. Note also the presence of the commissural components at the margins of the solitary zone of apposition. Some have suggested that the scallops, and the commissural components, should be elevated to the state of leaflets, but it remains conventional still to consider the valve as having but two leaflets.

themselves are anchored to the parietal ventricular walls, usually with trabeculations interposed at the junction of the muscles with the compact ventricular wall.[22] Idiopathic tachycardias may originate from the papillary muscles.[23–27] Increased echogenicity, late gadolinium enhancement, and calcifications are often seen on papillary muscles in patients with focal arrhythmias, and can indicate the site of origin.[28] Catheter ablation of tachycardias from the papillary muscles may be difficult due to the contraction of the muscle, and cryoablation may be preferable in this setting. Intracardiac echocardiography allows assessment of catheter–tissue contact and optimal alignment of the catheter with the papillary muscle axis[29] and is helpful in avoiding ablation-induced damage to the mitral valve.[30]

The ***apical*** part of the ventricle, as the name suggests, extends beyond the ventricular inlet to the apex of the ventricular myocardial cone. Its wall is very thin at the apical point. It has characteristic fine criss-crossing trabeculations, but a smooth septal surface. The branches of the conduction axis cascade down the septal surface, with the superior and inferior fascicles running from the branching part of the central conduction axis. As was initially illustrated by Tawara,[31] they extend towards the papillary muscles (Figure 8.16). Branches of the fascicles cross the ventricular cavity from the septum to the papillary muscles as the ***false tendons***.[32] These structures are of clinical relevance since they may give rise to arrhythmia. They should be considered for specific mapping and targeted ablation.[26,27]

The apical part continues without any obvious anatomical boundary to become the ventricular outlet, which is limited inferiorly by the aortic leaflet of the mitral valve. An extensive recess of the outflow tract extends inferiorly towards the crux of the heart, intervening between the aortic leaflet of the mitral valve and the septum (Figure 8.17).

The outflow component continues as the ***aortic root***, which extends distally to the level of the sinutubular junction.[33] The larger parts of its walls are fibrous rather than myocardial. Its proximal border is a virtual basal ring, constructed by joining together the nadirs of the leaflets of the aortic valve. The valve itself is another complex, made up of the semilunar leaflets and their supporting valvar sinuses (Figure 8.18).

In the normal valve, there are three ***sinuses***, supporting three leaflets. Of the sinuses, it is usually only two that give rise to coronary arteries. This permits the sinuses, and the leaflets they support, to be named as being right coronary, left coronary, and non-coronary (Figure 8.19). On occasion, however, a coronary artery can arise from the sinus that usually is non-coronary.[34] In such settings, the third sinus can be described as being non-adjacent, being separated by the other sinuses from the pulmonary root.

The semilunar nature of the hinges of the valvar leaflets (Figure 8.20) has created great confusion with regard to the description of a valvar "***annulus***".[35] Echocardiographers define the "annulus" in terms of the level that can be constructed by joining together the nadirs of attachment of the semilunar leaflets. This is no more than the virtual plane forming the proximal boundary of the root. In contrast, many cardiac surgeons define the semilunar remnants used for the anchorage of sutures subsequent to the removal of the leaflets during valvar replacement as the "annulus". At the least, these remaining structures are real anatomical entities (Figure 8.20).

Further confusion exists with the use of '***cusp***'. Although initially used to describe the valvar leaflets, the word is increasingly used by electrophysiologists to account for the valvar sinuses. As was pointed

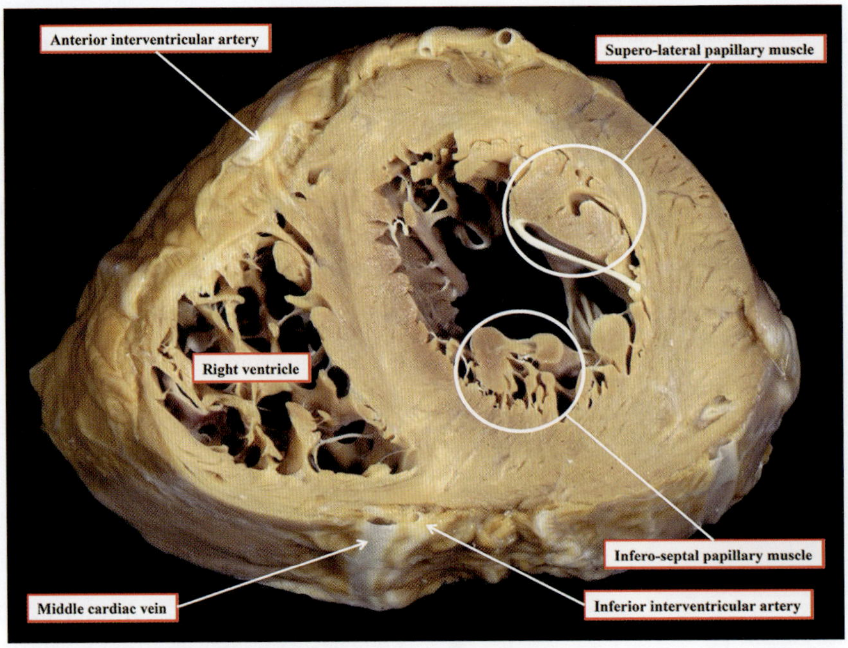

Figure 8.14. The ventricular cone has been sectioned in its short axis and photographed from the apex looking towards the base in attitudinally appropriate fashion. As can be seen, when viewed in this fashion the papillary muscles supporting the ends of the zone of apposition of the leaflets of the mitral valve are positioned infero-medially, or infero-septally, and supero-laterally within the ventricular cavity. It is a mistake to consider them as being "postero-medial" and "antero-lateral".

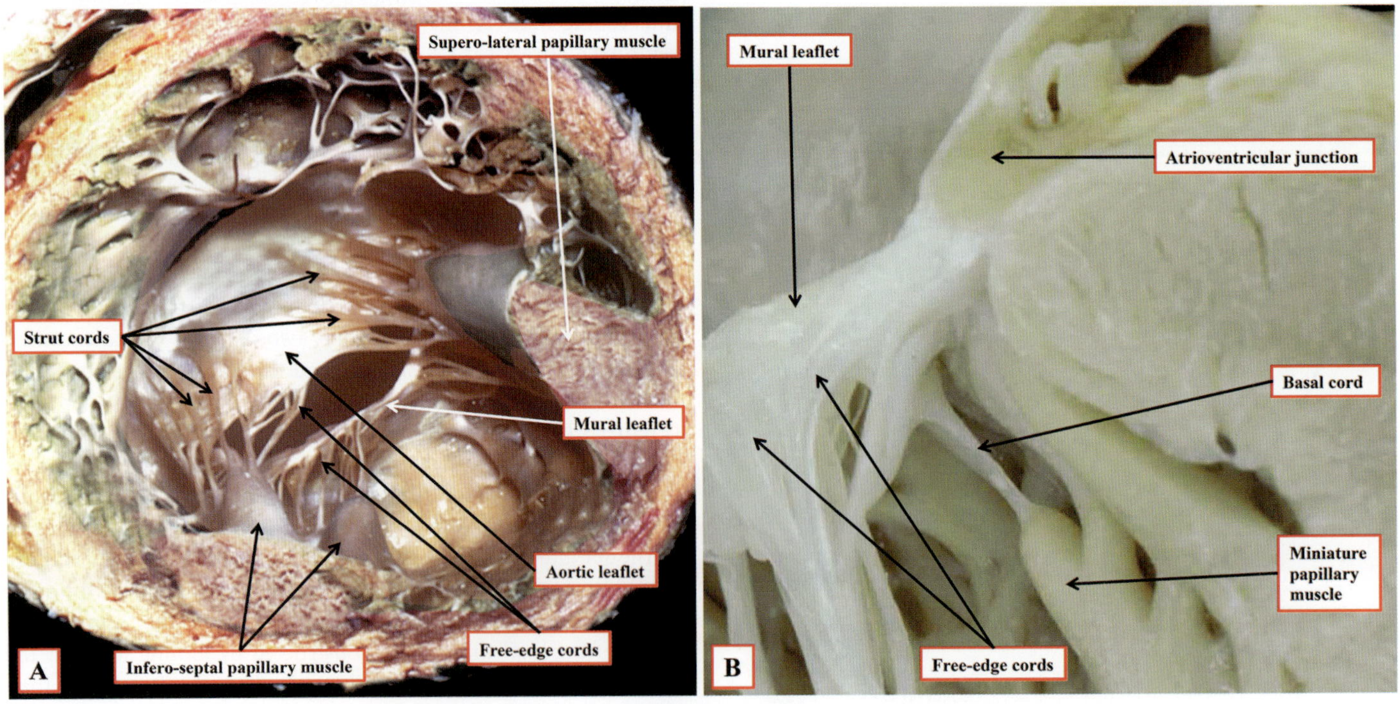

Figure 8.15. Panel A shows a view of the mitral valve as seen from the front, having removed the anterior wall of the left ventricle. It shows how strut cords reinforce the ventricular aspect of the aortic leaflet of the valve. Panel B shows the upturned mural leaflet of a different heart, revealing the presence of a basal cord, supported by its own miniaturized papillary muscle.

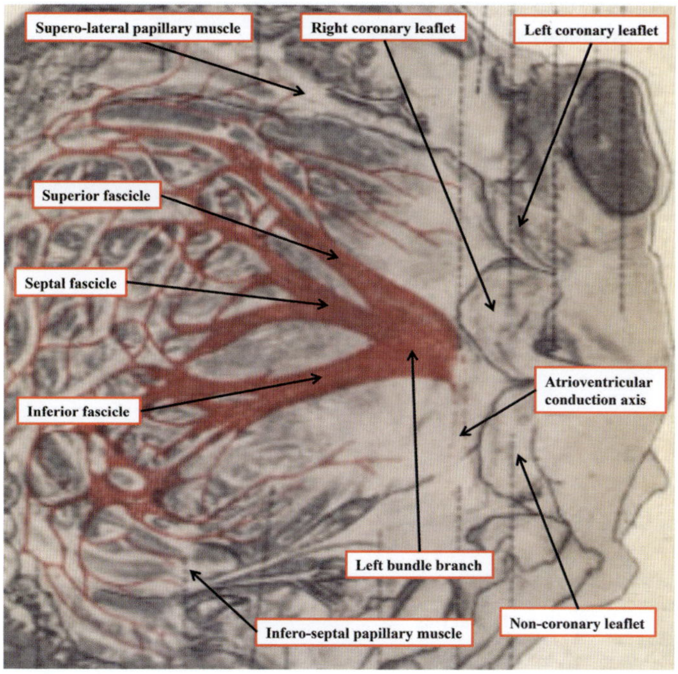

Figure 8.16. The drawing is taken from the initial monograph published by Tawara.[31] It has been reorientated so as to be seen in relatively correct attitudinal fashion, comparable to the heart shown in Figure 8.3. The reconstructions made by Tawara show how the superior and inferior fascicles of the left bundle branch extend towards the supero-lateral and infero-septal, or infero-medial, papillary muscles. Note also the proximity of the main stem of the left bundle to the nadir of the right coronary leaflet.

out in Chapter 6, the solution to this problem is to avoid using 'cusp', and to describe separately the leaflets and the ***sinuses***.[36] It is less easy to adjudicate on which entity should be defined as the "annulus", the more so since the most obvious ring within the aortic root is the sinutubular junction. It is likely that different constituencies will continue to use different definitions. It is probably the dimensions of the virtual basal ring, however, that are of most overall clinical significance. During diastole, when the leaflets come together to produce valvar competency, this plane is oval rather than circular.[37] The semilunar nature of the hinges permits the leaflets to close in perfect fashion to achieve valvar competence (Figure 8.21).

Since the leaflets come together during diastole under the influence of the arterial pressure exceeding the ventricular pressure, they do not require the extensive tension apparatus that retains the leaflets of the atrioventricular valves in their closed position during ventricular systole. The interaction between the leaflets, the walls of the sinuses, and their ventricular support is just as complex, nonetheless, as the arrangement to be found in the ventricular inlet. When the leaflets are in their closed position, the centroid of the valvar complex lies well below the level of the sinutubular junction (Figure 8.22). This does not disguise the fact that the ventricular cavity itself extends to the level of the sinutubular junction. It is the peripheral attachments of the leaflets at the sinutubular junction that are defined as the valvar ***commissures*** (Figure 8.21).

The line of closure of the leaflets along their zones of apposition is itself away from their free edge (Figure 8.23). This means that the fenestrations often found within the lunules of the leaflets towards their edges do not produce any valvar regurgitation. The assessment

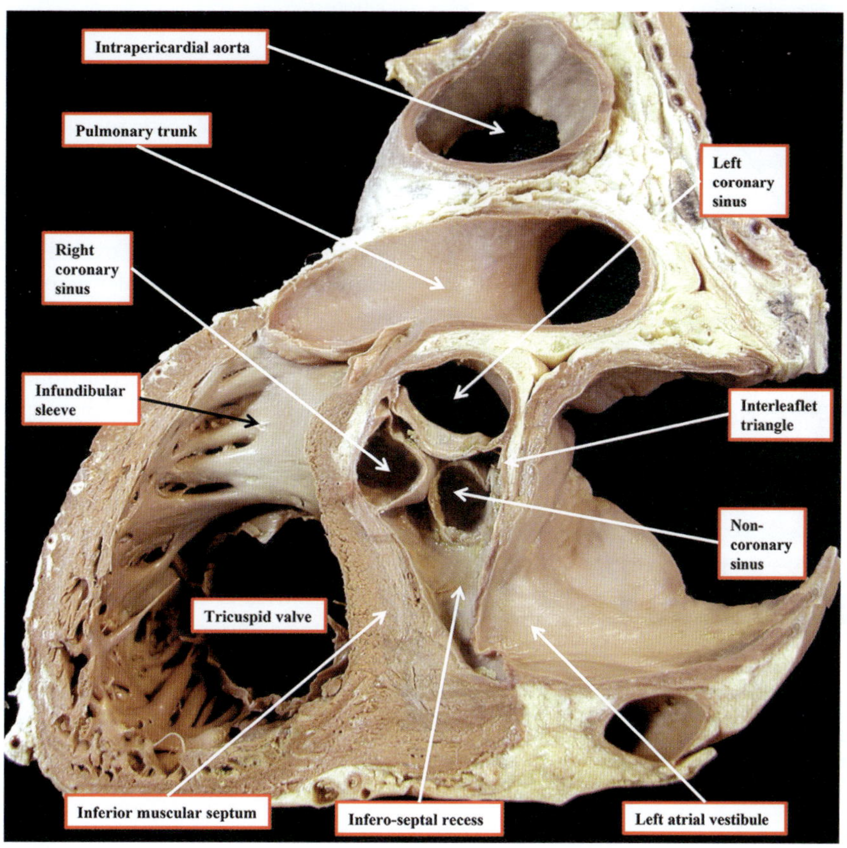

Figure 8.17. The image shows the short axis of the base of the ventricular cone, viewed from the apex, with the section passing obliquely through the left atrial vestibule. The roof of the infero-septal recess of the left ventricular outflow tract is shown extending towards the crux of the heart. Note also the predominantly fibrous walls of the aortic root, albeit with myocardium at the base of the right coronary sinus.

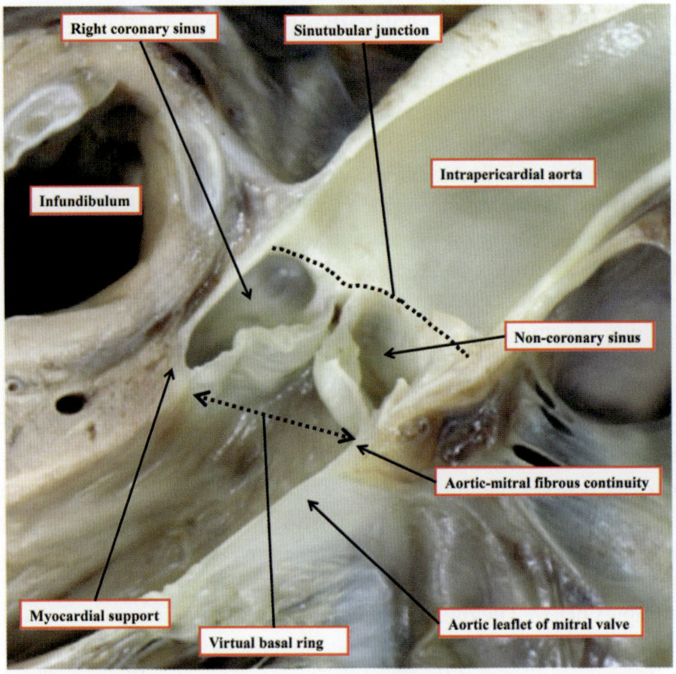

Figure 8.18. The image shows a close-up view of the aortic root as revealed by making a section across the ventricular mass to parallel the echocardiographic four-chamber projection. The aortic root extends distally to the sinutubular junction. Its proximal border is a virtual plane made by joining together the nadirs of the semilunar hinges of the leaflets of the aortic valve. Note that the base of the right coronary leaflet is supported by myocardium, whereas the non-coronary leaflet is in fibrous continuity with the aortic leaflet of the mitral valve.

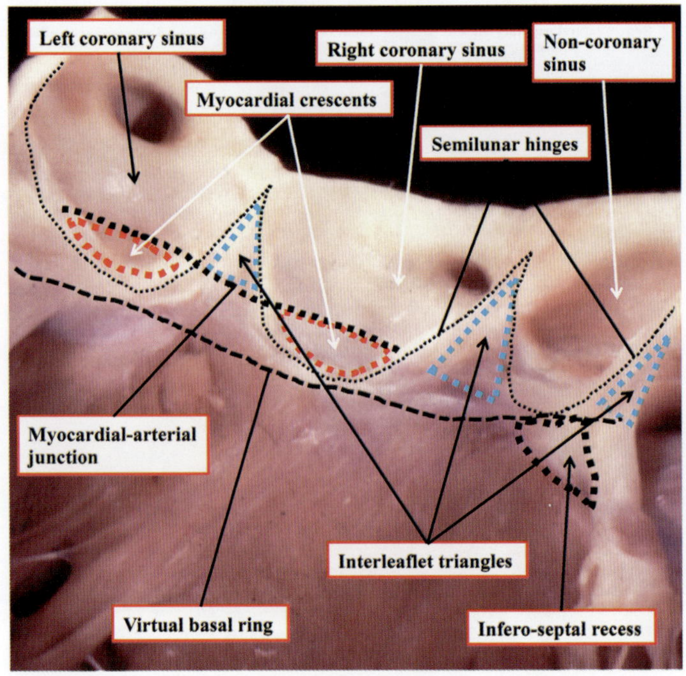

Figure 8.20. The aortic root has been opened by making a cut between the left coronary and non-coronary sinus. Having spread the root, the valvar leaflets have then been removed, revealing their semilunar support within the root. It is the semilunar remnants that are considered by some surgeons to represent the valvar "annulus". Other surgeons, however, join with echocardiographers in defining the virtual basal ring as the "annulus". Note also the myocardium incorporated at the bases of the sinuses giving rise to the coronary arteries, and the fibrous interleaflet triangles extending to the level of the sinutubular junction.

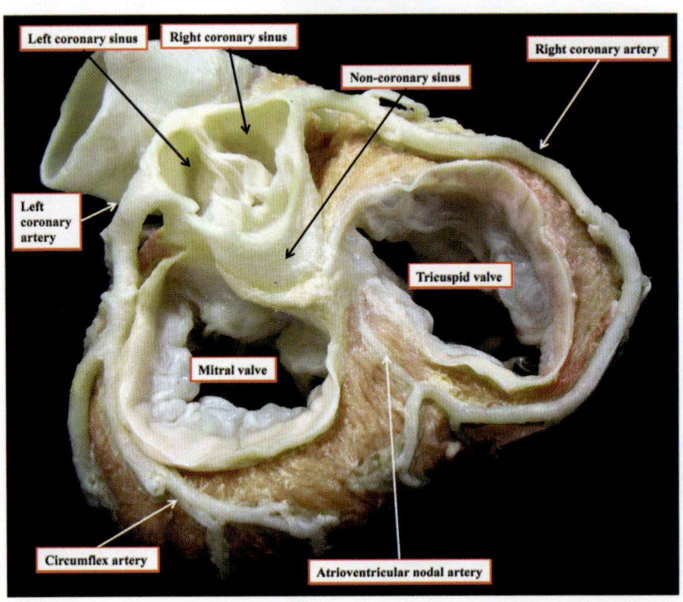

Figure 8.19. The base of the ventricular mass is viewed from the atrial aspect, having removed the intrapericardial arterial trunks and the walls of the atrial chambers. The dissection shows how the sinuses of the aortic root can be distinguished as supporting the right and left coronary arteries, with the third sinus being non-coronary.

of the long axis of the aortic root with the leaflets in their closed position also permits measurements to be made to assist the surgeon contemplating repair rather than replacement of the diseased valve (Figure 8.23).[37,38]

An understanding of the overall anatomy of the left ventricular outflow tract is of particular importance because of its association with ***idiopathic ventricular arrhythmias***. These may arise from the myocardium found at the bases of the sinuses that give rise to the coronary arteries, or from the margin of the summit of the left ventricular cone which supports the left coronary sinus. As was explained in Chapter 6, the latter region is identified by electrophysiologists as the left ventricular summit (Figure 6.17).[39] Arrhythmias arising from the left ventricular summit may be epicardial, but may sometimes be successfully ablated from adjacent endocardial structures, such as the left coronary sinus of Valsalva, the left ventricular endocardium below the aortic valve, and occasionally the anterior aspect of the right ventricular outflow tract.[40] The basal inferior component of the muscular ventricular septum may also be the origin of idiopathic ventricular arrhythmia. Such substrates can successfully be ablated using an endocardial approach through the infero-septal recess.[8]

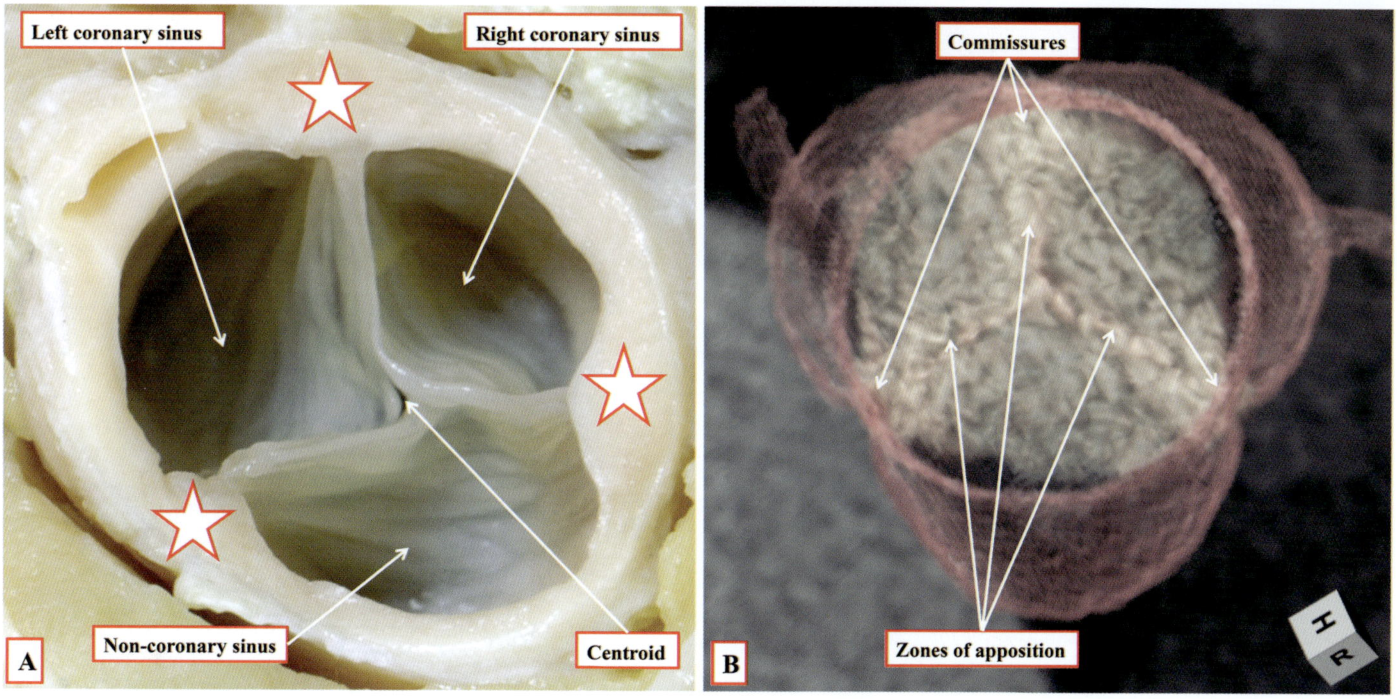

Figure 8.21. In panel A, the closed aortic valve has been photographed from its arterial aspect with the leaflets in their closed position. The white stars with red borders shows the peripheral attachments of the zones of apposition between the leaflets. They meet at the valvar centroid. Panel B, which is a computed tomographic image, shows how their peripheral attachments are defined as the valvar commissures.

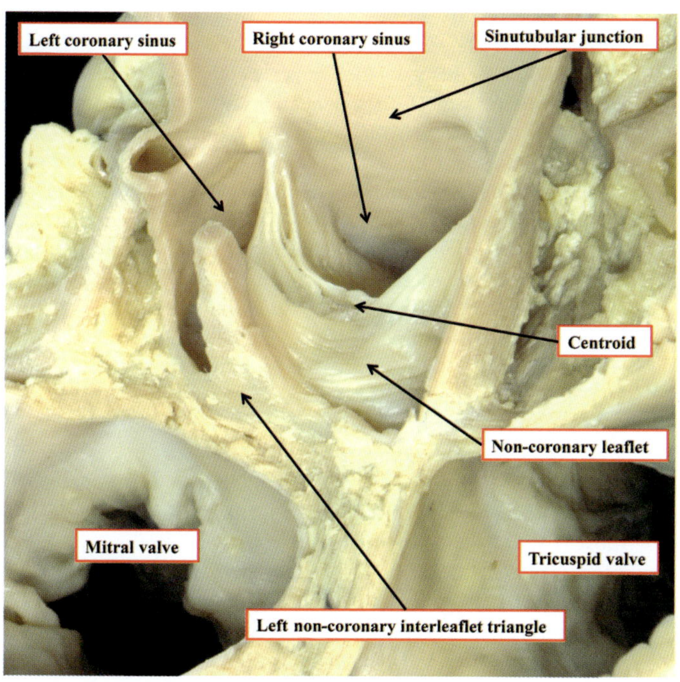

Figure 8.22. Having removed the atrial walls, the aortic root has been dissected by removing the walls of the left coronary and non-coronary sinuses. The dissection is photographed from above and behind. The leaflets come together at the centroid when closed, with the centroid being well below the level of the sinutubular junction.

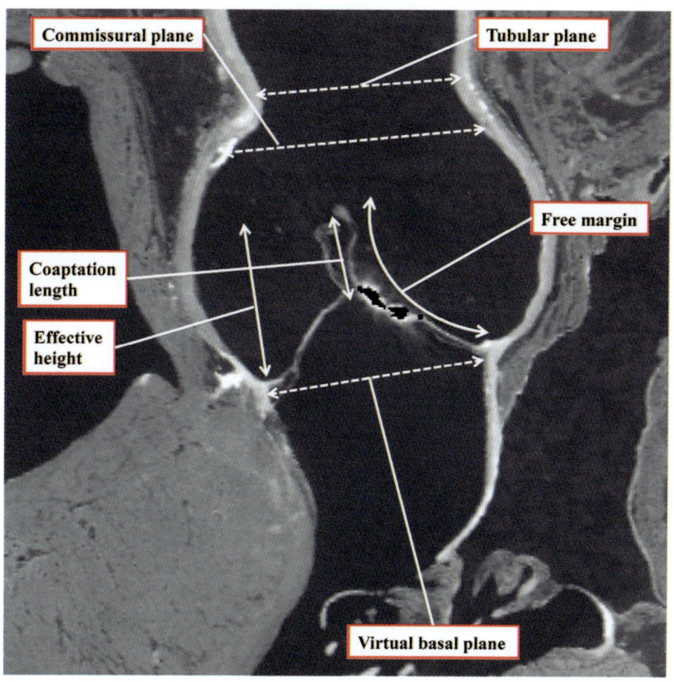

Figure 8.23. The image is taken from the same dataset prepared using Synchrotron scanning as was used to prepare Figure 8.9. This image shows that when the leaflets of the aortic valve are in their closed position, the line of their apposition is proximal to the distal extent of their free margins. This is known as the coaptation length of the valve. Fenestrations in this part of the leaflets would not produce valvar regurgitation. The image also shows the metrics that are now provided for surgeons contemplating repair rather than replacement for diseased aortic valves.

REFERENCES

1. Mori S, Tretter JT, Spicer DE, Bolender DL, Anderson RH. What is the real cardiac anatomy? *Clin Anat*. 2019;**32**:288–309. doi: 10.1002/ca.23340
2. Aanhaanen WT, Brons JF, Dominguez JN, Rana MS, Norden J, Airik R, Wakker V, de Gier-de Vries C, Brown NA, Kispert A, et al. The Tbx2+ primary myocardium of the atrioventricular canal forms the atrioventricular node and the base of the left ventricle. *Circ Res*. 2009;**104**:1267–1274. doi: 10.1161/CIRCRESAHA.108.192450
3. Moorman AF, Christoffels VM. Cardiac chamber formation: development, genes, and evolution. *Physiol Rev*. 2003;**83**:1223–1267. doi: 10.1152/physrev.00006.2003
4. Amofa D, Mori S, Toh H, Ta HT, Du Plessis M, Davis N, Izawa Y, Spicer DE, Anderson RH, Tretter JT. The rotational position of the aortic root related to its underlying ventricular support. *Clin Anat*. 2019;**32**:1107–1117. doi: 10.1002/ca.23462
5. Rosenquist GC, Clark EB, Sweeney LJ, McAllister HA. The normal spectrum of mitral and aortic valve discontinuity. *Circulation*. 1976;**54**:298–301. doi: 10.1161/01.cir.54.2.298
6. Sutton JP, 3rd, Ho SY, Anderson RH. The forgotten interleaflet triangles: a review of the surgical anatomy of the aortic valve. *Ann Thorac Surg*. 1995;**59**:419–427. doi: 10.1016/0003-4975(94)00893-c
7. Crucean A, Spicer DE, Tretter JT, Mohun TJ, Cook AC, Sanchez-Quintana D, Hikspoors J, Lamers WH, Anderson RH. Revisiting the anatomy of the left ventricle in the light of knowledge of its development. *J Anat*. 2024;**245**:201–216. doi: 10.1111/joa.14048
8. Li A, Zuberi Z, Bradfield JS, Zarif JK, Ward DE, Anderson RH, Shivkumar K, Saba MM. Endocardial ablation of ventricular ectopic beats arising from the basal inferoseptal process of the left ventricle. *Heart Rhythm*. 2018;**15**:1356–1362. doi: 10.1016/j.hrthm.2018.04.029
9. Tretter JT, Spicer DE, Sanchez-Quintana D, Back Sternick E, Farre J, Anderson RH. Miniseries 1–Part III: 'Behind the scenes' in the triangle of Koch. *Europace*. 2022;**24**:455–463. doi: 10.1093/europace/euab285
10. Perloff JK, Roberts WC. The mitral apparatus. Functional anatomy of mitral regurgitation. *Circulation*. 1972;**46**:227–239. doi: 10.1161/01.cir.46.2.227
11. Saremi F, Sanchez-Quintana D, Mori S, Muresian H, Spicer DE, Hassani C, Anderson RH. Fibrous skeleton of the heart: anatomic overview and evaluation of pathologic conditions with CT and MR imaging. *Radiographics*. 2017;**37**:1330–1351. doi: 10.1148/rg.2017170004
12. Angelini A, Ho SY, Anderson RH, Davies MJ, Becker AE. A histological study of the atrioventricular junction in hearts with normal and prolapsed leaflets of the mitral valve. *Br Heart J*. 1988;**59**:712–716. doi: 10.1136/hrt.59.6.712
13. Hutchins GM, Moore GW, Skoog DK. The association of floppy mitral valve with disjunction of the mitral annulus fibrosus. *N Engl J Med*. 1986;**314**:535–540. doi: 10.1056/NEJM198602273140902
14. Toh H, Mori S, Izawa Y, Toba T, Nishii T, Hirata KI. Revival of mitral and tricuspid annular disjunctions: are these really abnormal findings? *JACC Cardiovasc Imaging*. 2021;**14**:1682–1684. doi: 10.1016/j.jcmg.2021.05.026
15. Dejgaard LA, Skjolsvik ET, Lie OH, Ribe M, Stokke MK, Hegbom F, Scheirlynck ES, Gjertsen E, Andresen K, Helle-Valle TM, et al. The mitral annulus disjunction arrhythmic syndrome. *J Am Coll Cardiol*. 2018;**72**:1600–1609. doi: 10.1016/j.jacc.2018.07.070
16. Essayagh B, Sabbag A, Antoine C, Benfari G, Yang LT, Maalouf J, Asirvatham S, Michelena H, Enriquez-Sarano M. Presentation and outcome of arrhythmic mitral valve prolapse. *J Am Coll Cardiol*. 2020;**76**:637–649. doi: 10.1016/j.jacc.2020.06.029
17. Anderson RH, Garbi M, Zugwitz D, Petersen SE, Nijveldt R. Anatomy of the mitral valve relative to controversies concerning the so-called annular disjunction. *Heart*. 2023;**109**:734–739. doi: 10.1136/heartjnl-2022-322043
18. Carpentier A. Cardiac valve surgery—the "French correction". *J Thorac Cardiovasc Surg*. 1983;**86**:323–337. PMID: 6887954
19. Kumar N, Kumar M, Duran CM. A revised terminology for recording surgical findings of the mitral valve. *J Heart Valve Dis*. 1995;**4**:70–75; discussion 76–77. PMID: 7742993
20. Victor S, Nayak VM. Definition and function of commissures, slits and scallops of the mitral valve: analysis in 100 hearts. *Asia Pacific J Thoracic Cardiovasc Surg*1994;**3**:10–16. doi: 10.1016/1324-2881(94)90050-7
21. Lam JH, Ranganathan N, Wigle ED, Silver MD. Morphology of the human mitral valve. I. Chordae tendineae: a new classification. *Circulation*. 1970;**41**:449–458. doi: 10.1161/01.cir.41.3.449
22. Axel L. Papillary muscles do not attach directly to the solid heart wall. *Circulation*. 2004;**109**:3145–3148. doi: 10.1161/01.CIR.0000134276.06719.F3
23. Ip JE, Liu CF, Thomas G, Cheung JW, Markowitz SM, Lerman BB. Unifying mechanism of sustained idiopathic atrial and ventricular annular tachycardia. *Circ Arrhythm Electrophysiol*. 2014;**7**:436–444. doi: 10.1161/CIRCEP.113.001368CIRCEP.113.001368 [pii]
24. Al'Aref SJ, Ip JE, Markowitz SM, Liu CF, Thomas G, Frenkel D, Panda NC, Weinsaft JW, Lerman BB, Cheung JW. Differentiation of papillary muscle from fascicular and mitral annular ventricular arrhythmias in patients with and without structural heart disease. *Circ Arrhythm Electrophysiol*. 2015;**8**:616–624. doi: 10.1161/CIRCEP.114.002619
25. Dukkipati SR, Choudry S, Koruth JS, Miller MA, Whang W, Reddy VY. Catheter ablation of ventricular tachycardia in structurally normal hearts: indications, strategies, and outcomes—Part I. *J Am Coll Cardiol*. 2017;**70**:2909–2923. doi: 10.1016/j.jacc.2017.10.031
26. Abouezzeddine O, Suleiman M, Buescher T, Kapa S, Friedman PA, Jahangir A, Mears JA, Ladewig DJ, Munger TM, Hammill SC, et al. Relevance of endocavitary structures in ablation procedures for ventricular tachycardia. *J Cardiovasc Electrophysiol*. 2010;**21**:245–254. doi: 10.1111/j.1540-8167.2009.01621.x
27. Zhang J, Liang M, Wang Z, Zhang X, Fan J, Jia Y, Xiao F, Fu B, Zhang H, Huang J. Catheter ablation of premature ventricular complexes associated with left ventricular false tendons. *Heart Rhythm*. 2021;**18**:1968–1975. doi: 10.1016/j.hrthm.2021.06.1197
28. Tokavanich N, Huntrakul A, Yokokawa M, Kovacs B, Ghannam M, Liang JL, Attili A, Cochet H, Latchamsetty R, Jongnarangsin K, et al. Relationship of structural abnormalities of papillary muscles to the site of origin of ventricular arrhythmias. *JACC Clin Electrophysiol*. 2025;**11**:259–269. doi: 10.1016/j.jacep.2024.10.004
29. Kautzner J, Peichl P. Papillary muscle ventricular tachycardia or ectopy: diagnostics, catheter ablation and the role of intracardiac echocardiography. *Arrhythm Electrophysiol Rev*. 2019;**8**:65–69. doi: 10.15420/aer.2018.80.2
30. Chee J, Lin AN, Julien H, Lin D, Schaller RD, Frankel DS, Supple GE, Santangeli P, Riley MP, Nazarian S, et al. Impact of left ventricular papillary muscle ventricular arrhythmia ablation on

mitral valve function. *JACC Clin Electrophysiol.* 2022;**8**:1475–1483. doi: 10.1016/j.jacep.2022.07.025

31. Tawara S. Das Reizleitungssystem des Säugetierherzens. Jena: G. Fischer; 1906.
32. Luetmer PH, Edwards WD, Seward JB, Tajik AJ. Incidence and distribution of left ventricular false tendons: an autopsy study of 483 normal human hearts. *J Am Coll Cardiol.* 1986;**8**:179–183. doi: 10.1016/s0735-1097(86)80110-3
33. Anderson RH. Clinical anatomy of the aortic root. *Heart.* 2000;**84**:670–673. doi: 10.1136/heart.84.6.670
34. Liberman L, Pass RH, Kaufman S, Hordof AJ, Printz BF, Prakash A. Left coronary artery arising from the non-coronary sinus: a rare congenital coronary anomaly. *Pediatr Cardiol.* 2005;**26**:672–674. doi: 10.1007/s00246-004-0847-6
35. Anderson RH, Spicer DE, Quintessenza JA, Najm HK, Tretter JT. Words and how we use them—which is to be the master? *J Card Surg.* 2022;**37**:2481–2485. doi: 10.1111/jocs.16620
36. Tretter JT, Spicer DE, Franklin RCG, Beland MJ, Aiello VD, Cook AC, Crucean A, Loomba RS, Yoo SJ, Quintessenza JA, et al. Expert consensus statement: anatomy, imaging, and nomenclature of congenital aortic root malformations. *Ann Thorac Surg.* 2023;**116**:6–16. doi: 10.1016/j.athoracsur.2023.03.023
37. Tretter JT, Izawa Y, Spicer DE, Okada K, Anderson RH, Quintessenza JA, Mori S. Understanding the aortic root using computed tomographic assessment: a potential pathway to improved customized surgical repair. *Circ Cardiovasc Imaging.* 2021;**14**:e013134. doi: 10.1161/CIRCIMAGING.121.013134
38. Tretter JT, Burbano-Vera NH, Najm HK. Multi-modality imaging evaluation and pre-surgical planning for aortic valve-sparing operations in patients with aortic root aneurysm. *Ann Cardiothorac Surg.* 2023;**12**:295–317. doi: 10.21037/acs-2023-avs2-0040
39. Mori S, Bradfield JS, Fukuzawa K, Shivkumar K. Comprehensive anatomy of the summit of the left ventricle. *JACC Clin Electrophysiol.* 2024;**10**:168–184. doi: 10.1016/j.jacep.2023.09.022
40. Guandalini GS, Santangeli P, Schaller R, Pothineni NVK, Briceno DF, Enriquez A, Razminia P, Tung R, Marchlinski FE, Garcia FC. Intramyocardial mapping of ventricular premature depolarizations via septal venous perforators: differentiating the superior intraseptal region from left ventricular summit origins. *Heart Rhythm.* 2022;**19**:1475–1483. doi: 10.1016/j.hrthm.2022.03.004

9

Mural Architecture of the Heart

Despite the huge advances that have been made in elucidating the anatomy of the various chambers of the heart, there still remains no consensus with regard to the precise architecture of their walls. Much of this reflects the continuing approach of investigators who make direct comparisons between cardiac and skeletal muscle.[1] Almost all voluntary muscles have discrete origins and insertions and are enclosed within fibrous sheaths. The working unit of skeletal muscle is the myocyte, with each individual myocyte also described as a "***fibre***". This is justifiable for skeletal muscles, since each fibre, or myocyte, can extend over several centimetres when measured from its origin to its insertion. The skeletal myocytes are not electrically connected, but rather each cell is supplied with a discrete motor end plate. It is this feature that permits fine control of movement. When each individual myocyte is stimulated to contract, the contraction does not spread to the adjacent myocytes. Control of force, therefore, is achieved by recruitment of more or less motor units within an individual muscle.

The arrangement is quite different in the myocardium, where the overall myocardial mass is activated via the impulse created in the sinus node. The walls of the cardiac chambers, therefore, must not only contract, but also conduct the cardiac impulse. Despite having to assume the dual roles of conduction and contraction within the walls of the cardiac chambers, the individual cardiomyocyte remains the working unit of the myocardium. Unlike the individual skeletal myocytes, however, which have considerable length, the cardiomyocytes are no longer than 0.1 mm. They are joined together at their ends to form continuous branching chains (**Figure 9.1**).

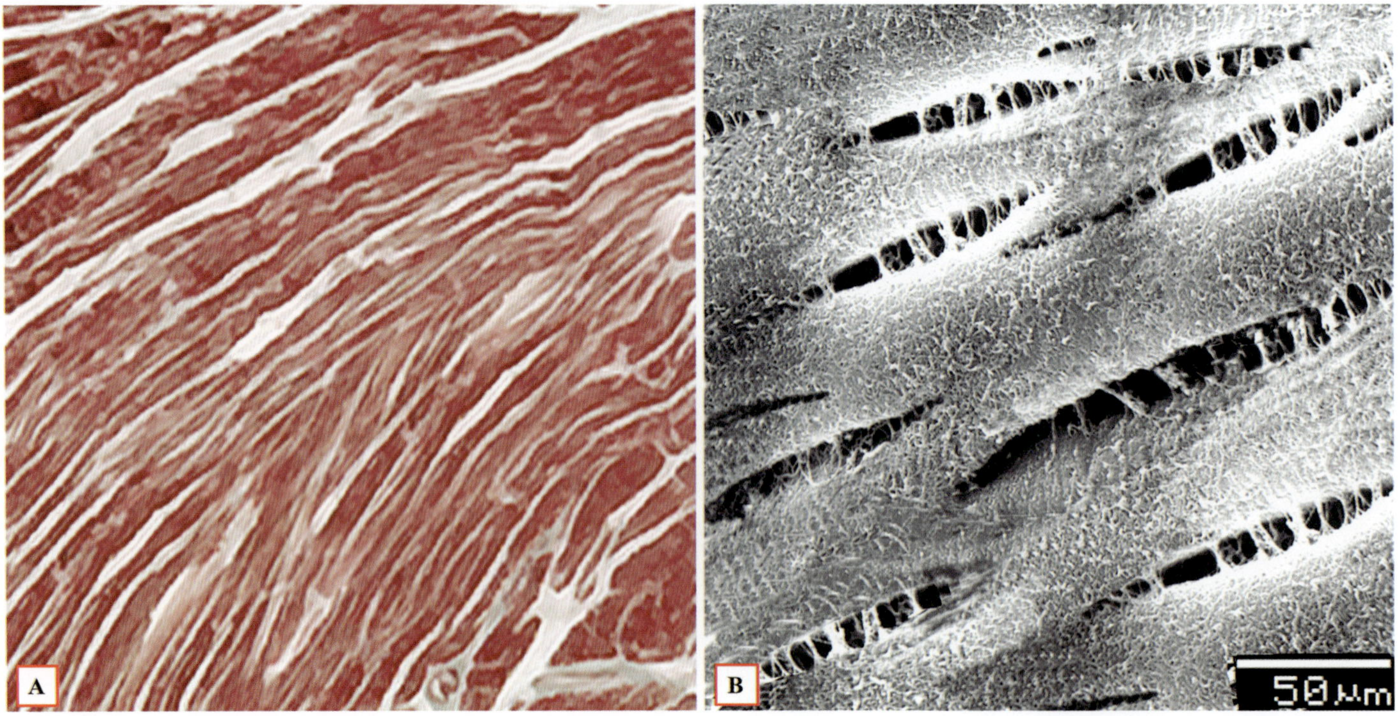

Figure 9.1. The panels show the fashion in which individual cardiomyocytes are joined together so as to produce chains. It is the individual cardiomyocyte that is the working unit of the myocardium. Panel A is a histological section of ventricular myocardium stained using the trichrome technique, whilst panel B shows a scanning electron micrograph, again showing ventricular myocardium. Note the endomysial strands on panel B that support the adjacent cells.

Unlike the skeletal myocytes, furthermore, the cardiomyocytes are not activated individually. They contract collectively, as influenced by the activities of the conduction system. In the atrial chambers, it is the manner of their aggregation into chains that underscores the preferential conduction between the sinus and atrioventricular nodes (Figure 9.2). In the ventricles, in contrast, the individual cardiomyocytes are aggregated together so as to optimize systolic emptying of the chambers. This requires a particular manner of aggregation, since when an individual cardiomyocyte contracts, its width increases by no more than one-tenth. In contrast, the ventricular walls during systolic emptying thicken by significantly more than one-tenth. This means that the aggregation of the individual cells must be such as to permit their re-packing during mural thickening.[2]

Those seeking to explain the basis of the re-packing have suggested that the aggregation is such as to produce lamellar entities that are able to slide against one another.[3] A drawing used to illustrate the concept showed fibrous partitions creating discrete laminar units, with the alleged units then occupying the full thickness of the ventricular walls (Figure 9.3 panel A).[3] This was a gross exaggeration of the true arrangement. A subsequent study by the same group, which used confocal microscopy,[4] correctly showed the presence within the ventricular walls of a complex three-dimensional meshwork of aggregated cardiomyocytes (Figure 9.3 panel B).[5]

The arrangement reflects the hierarchy of support for the individual cardiomyocytes provided by the mural fibro-collagenous matrix.[6] Thus, digestion of the individual cardiomyocytes within the ventricular walls shows that each cell is encased within an endomysial sheath (Figure 9.4 panel A). Units of individual cells are then encased in thicker perimysial units. It is the units aggregated in perimysial fashion that can be recognized histologically (Figure 9.4 panel B). The clefts between the entities produced by the perimysial aggregation provide the channels for access of the cardiac vasculature and nerves. In the ventricles, it is the clefts that permit the aggregated units to slide against one another during ventricular systole, thus providing the required answer to the conundrum of systolic mural thickening.[3] The overall myocardial masses are then encased within the epimysial component of the matrix (Figure 9.5).

As already indicated, the manner of aggregation of the cardiomyocytes within the atrial walls produces the preferential pathways for internodal conduction. At the same time, their contraction underscores atrial emptying. Within the ventricles, the cardiomyocytes are activated from the apex towards the base, with the impulse also spreading from endocardium to epicardium via the ramifications of the ventricular bundle branches. The ventricular walls, nonetheless, must also contract in coordinated fashion so as to ensure systolic emptying. In order to achieve this haemodynamic effect, the manner of aggregation is much more complicated than seen in the atrial walls.

Aggregation of the Cardiomyocytes Within the Atrial Walls

The arrangement of the atrial cardiomyocytes has previously been described on the basis of the existence of discrete muscle bundles within the walls.[7,8] The cardiomyocytes making up the bundles, furthermore, have been described as "fibres". As with the alleged ventricular laminar entities, both descriptions are incorrect. The working unit of the myocardial walls is the cardiomyocyte.[1] And, to

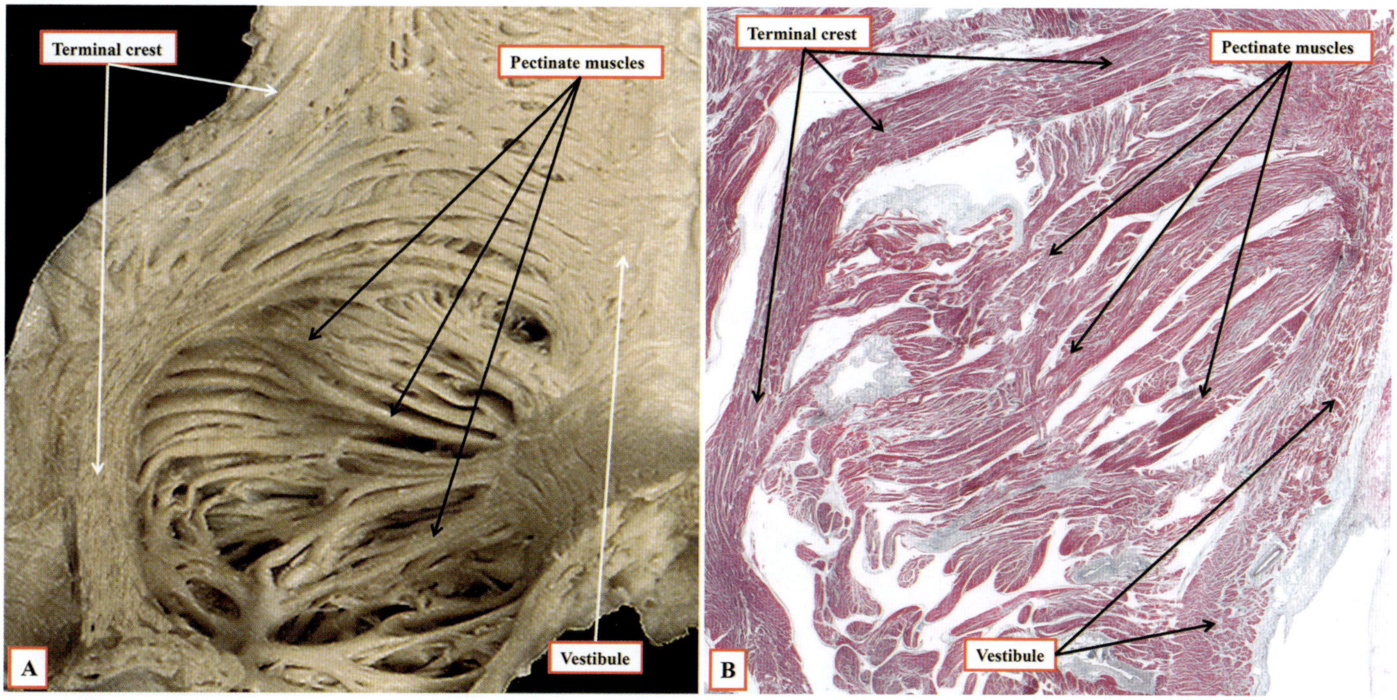

Figure 9.2. Panel A shows the internal surface of the right atrial appendage, having removed the endocardial lining. The major muscle bundle of the terminal crest can be seen, with the pectinate muscles originating at right angles and extending towards the vestibule of the tricuspid valve. Panel B shows a comparable histological section from a different heart, showing how the aggregation of the cardiomyocytes produces the obvious "grain" observed in the dissected specimen.

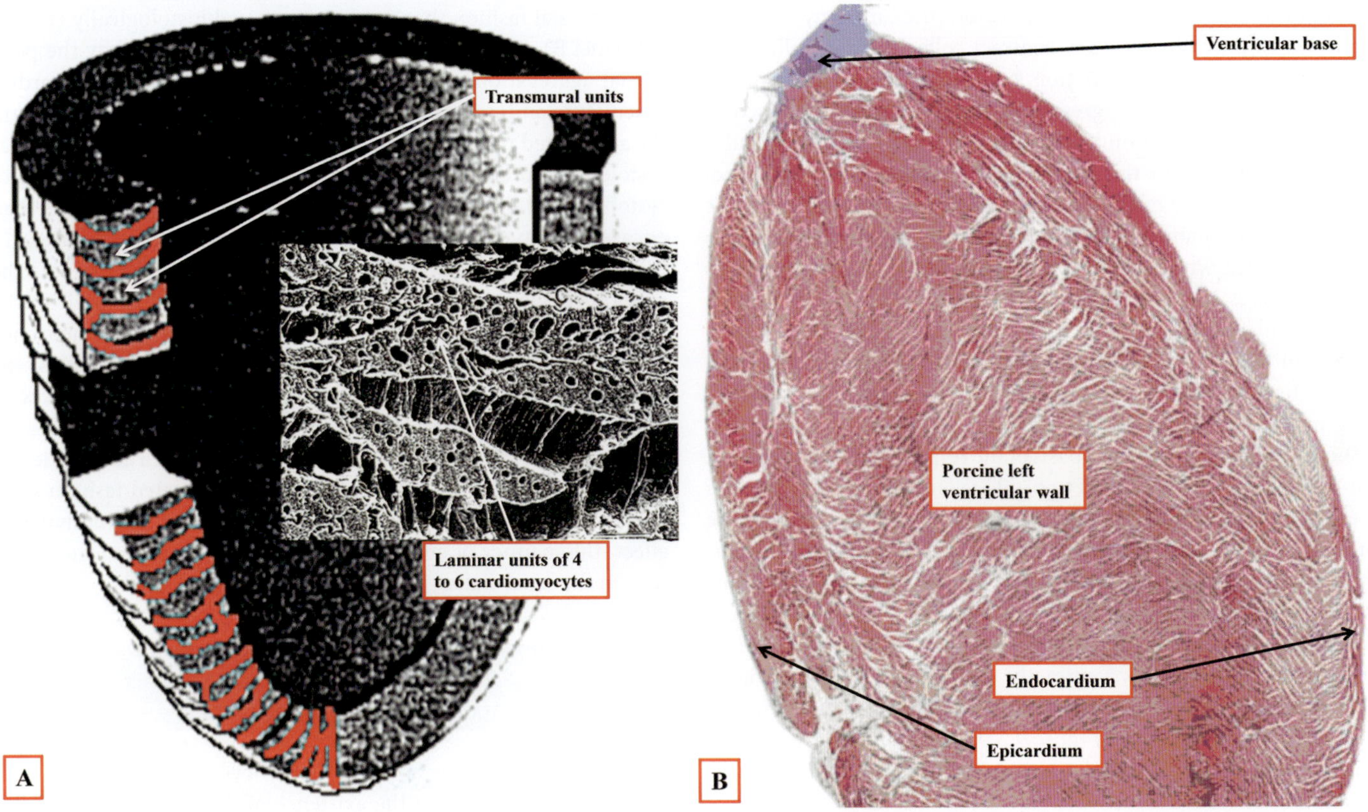

Figure 9.3. Panel A shows a modified version of the drawing produced by Legrice and colleagues to illustrate their concept of the presence of laminar aggregations of individual cardiomyocytes, with emphasis placed on shelves separating the units.[3] They had envisaged the presence of sheets made up of four to six cardiomyocytes, but illustrated the sheets, as can be seen, as extending in full mural thickness. Panel B shows a section across the ventricular wall of the porcine heart, prepared by Professor Paul Lunkenheimer and reproduced with his permission. The cardiomyocytes are, indeed, aggregated together, but they do not form full-thickness sheets. The arrangement is better described as a three-dimensional mesh.

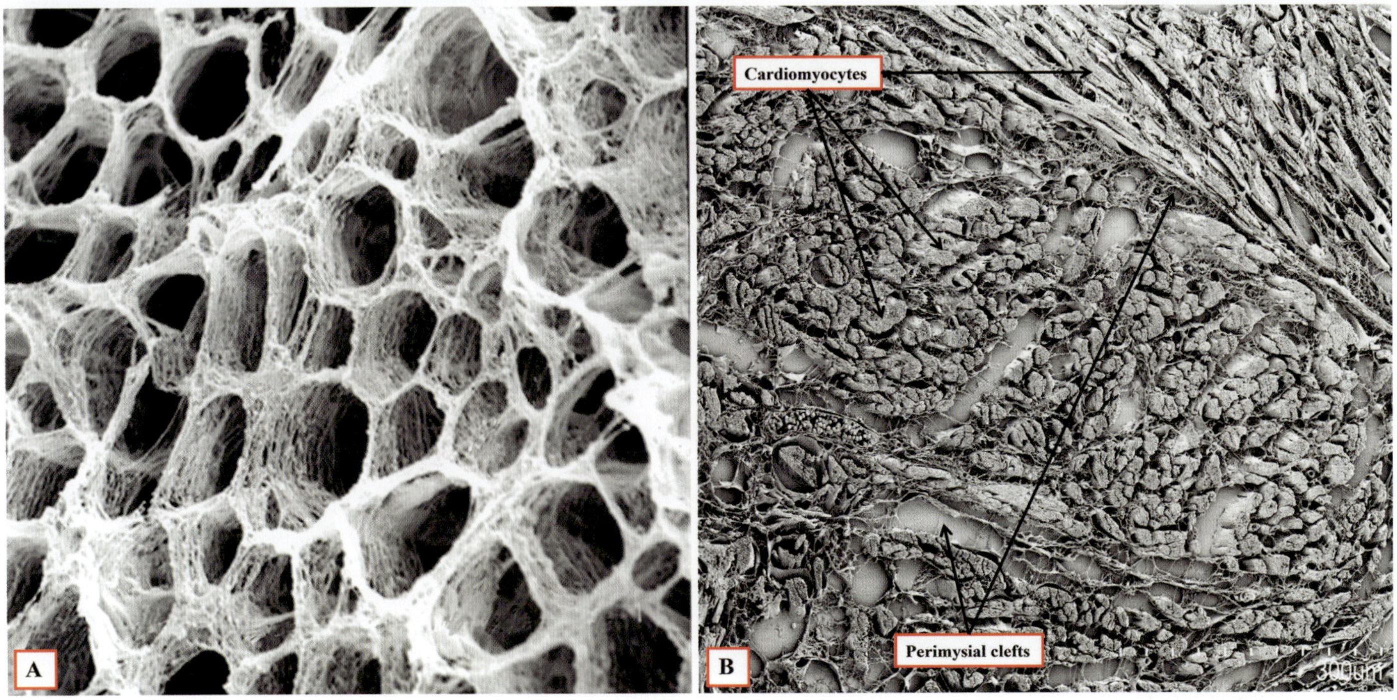

Figure 9.4. The images show scanning electron micrographs of human ventricular myocardium. In the image shown in panel A, the individual cardiomyocytes have been digested away to reveal the supporting endomysial scaffold within an aggregated unit. Panel B shows how the perimysial components of the fibrous scaffold aggregate together the individual cardiomyocytes. Note the marked change in alignment of cardiomyocytes in the body of the panel, as opposed to the aggregate in the top right-hand corner. Note also how the neurovascular elements extend within the perimysial clefts between adjacent aggregated entities.

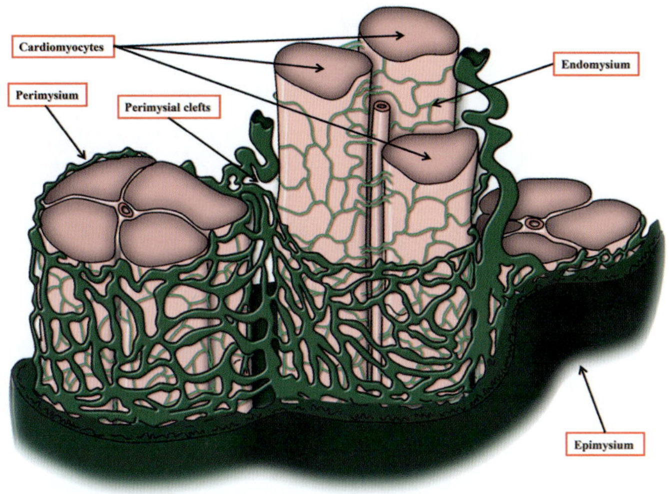

Figure 9.5. The drawing shows the hierarchy within the supporting fibrous matrix of the myocardial walls of the cardiac chambers, with its epimysial, perimysial, and endomysial components. The original drawing was made by Mrs Gemma Price and has been modified with her permission.

emphasize again, in the atrial walls it is the manner of aggregation of the individual cells that underscores conduction (Figure 9.6).

All cardiomyocytes have the capacity to conduct. Within the atrial walls, however, some of the cardiomyocytes are aggregated together so as to produce the nodes that generate, and then delay, the cardiac impulse (Figure 9.7). The anatomy of the conduction system is discussed in detail in Chapter 12. In brief, the sinus node can be recognized because its individual cardiomyocytes, which are smaller than the working cardiomyocytes, are supported by a particularly dense fibrous matrix. The nodal myocytes merge with the working atrial myocytes at the nodal margins (Figure 9.7 panel A). The atrioventricular node is a more complex structure, receiving inputs from the right and left atrial vestibules and the buttress of the atrial septum (Figure 9.7 panel B). It is recognized on the basis of its distinct cellular architecture, with the nodal cells themselves again being no larger than the working atrial cardiomyocytes. Almost all of the remaining walls of the right atrium are then made up of atrial cardiomyocytes aggregated together to produce contraction, but also to facilitate conduction between the sinus and atrioventricular nodes. Some of these cells are aggregated together as prominent bundles, such as the terminal crest and the pectinate muscles (Figure 9.2 panel A). In all these bundles, the speed of conduction is faster along the long axis of the aggregated cardiomyocytes than across their short axis (Figure 9.2 panel B). Such anisotropic conduction was long since shown to be sufficient to explain the arrhythmogenic propensity of these cardiomyocytes aggregated to provide preferential conduction.[9]

The walls of the left atrium are much thicker than those of the right. In consequence, the aggregation of the cardiomyocytes is more complex. The major function of the left atrial walls is to contract, so as to produce atrial systole. But the contraction must itself be orderly and hence depends on conduction of the cardiac impulse. Many of the cells are aggregated together in parallel fashion, therefore, so as to facilitate conduction from the sinus node into the left atrium. This is the pattern that is seen in Bachmann's bundle (Figure 9.6) and in the rims of the oval fossa. Much more variability in manner of aggregation is found in the roof of the left atrium (Figure 9.8), with particular mixing of the orientation of the aggregated entities at the pulmonary venoatrial junctions (Figure 9.9). The overall arrangement, nonetheless, remains one of individual cardiomyocytes aggregated together to produce a three-dimensional meshwork. At no places within the atrial walls are the cells ensheathed so as to permit the recognition of discrete anatomical subunits over and above the cardiomyocyte (Figures 9.1 panel B, 9.8). And, within the walls of the left atrium, there are no aggregations of cardiomyocytes to produce "nodes" (Figure 9.8), nor is there any evidence to support the notion that the cardiomyocytes of the pulmonary venous sleeves are "specialized" (Figure 9.9).[10,11] The manner of aggregation of the cardiomyocytes within the sleeves is also complex. Within the thickness of the walls, some of the cardiomyocytes are aggregated in circumferential fashion, but these are interconnected with other aggregates having a longitudinal orientation.[12] Such an arrangement may theoretically lead to anisotropic conduction between the cells, which in itself can act as a focal trigger or a substrate for micro re-entry.

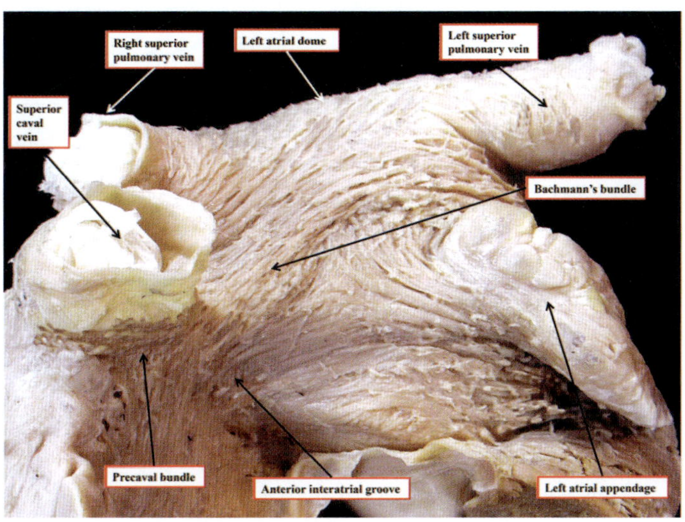

Figure 9.6. The dissection shows how the individual cardiomyocytes are aggregated together in parallel fashion within the walls of the atrial chambers so as to facilitate preferential conduction.

Aggregation of the Ventricular Cardiomyocytes

Simple stepwise dissection of the ventricular walls reveals an obviously helical arrangement of the aggregated cardiomyocytes (Figure 9.10). The change in the "grain" is known to reflect the alignment of the chains of individual cells when measured against the equator of the ventricular cone.[13] The spiral arrangement has been recognized since the 17th century. Thus, Richard Lower, by following the spiralling configuration of the aggregated cardiomyocytes, was able to dissect the ventricular mass so as to produce a band that started at the tricuspid valvar orifice and finished at the orifice of the mitral valve (Figure 9.11).[14]

In an important work published in the middle of the 19th century, Pettigrew provided a detailed account of the spiralling nature

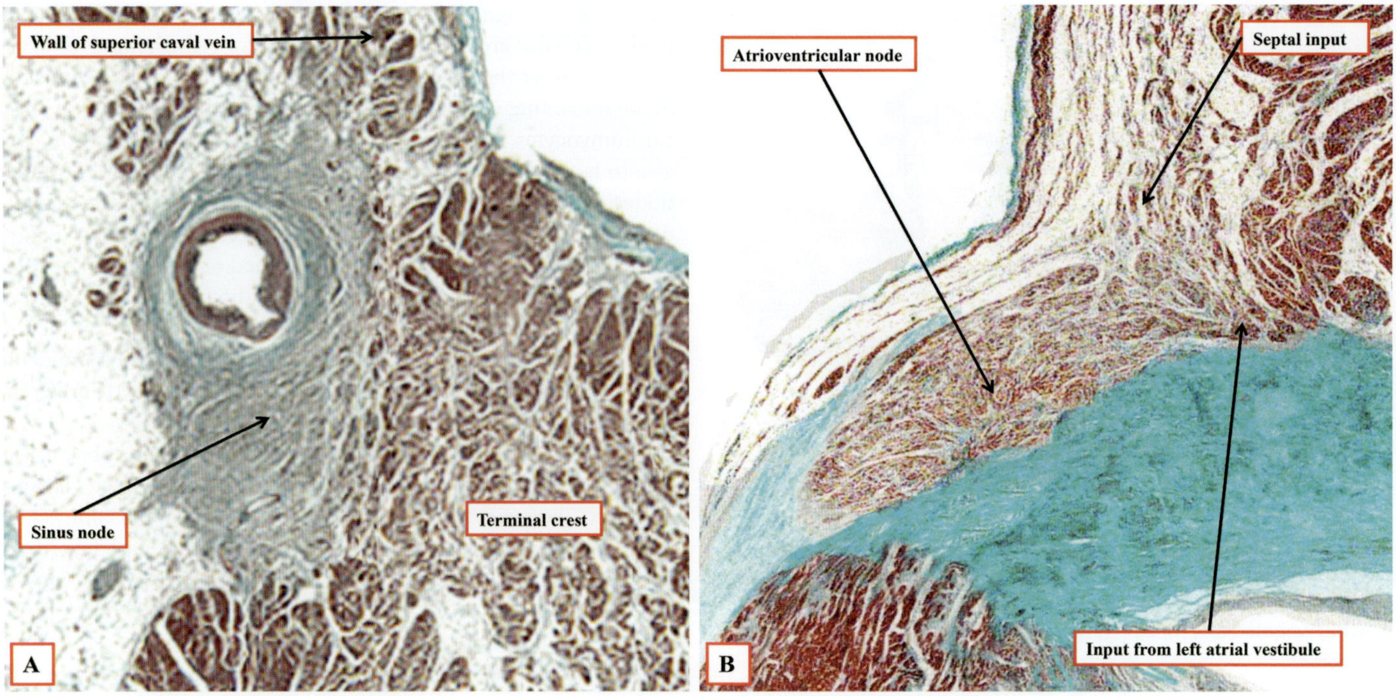

Figure 9.7. The histological sections show how, at discrete points within the walls of the atrial chambers and the atrial septum, it is possible to recognize the cardiomyocytes that are aggregated together within a special arrangement so as to produce the sinus (panel A) and atrioventricular (panel B) nodes. The nodal cardiomyocytes, however, although being histologically distinct, and traceable from section to section in serially sectioned datasets, are not insulated from the adjacent working atrial cardiomyocytes. Apart from the nodes and the paranodal area, the retroaortic node, and the ring tissues, the remainder of the atrial walls is made up exclusively of working atrial cardiomyocytes.

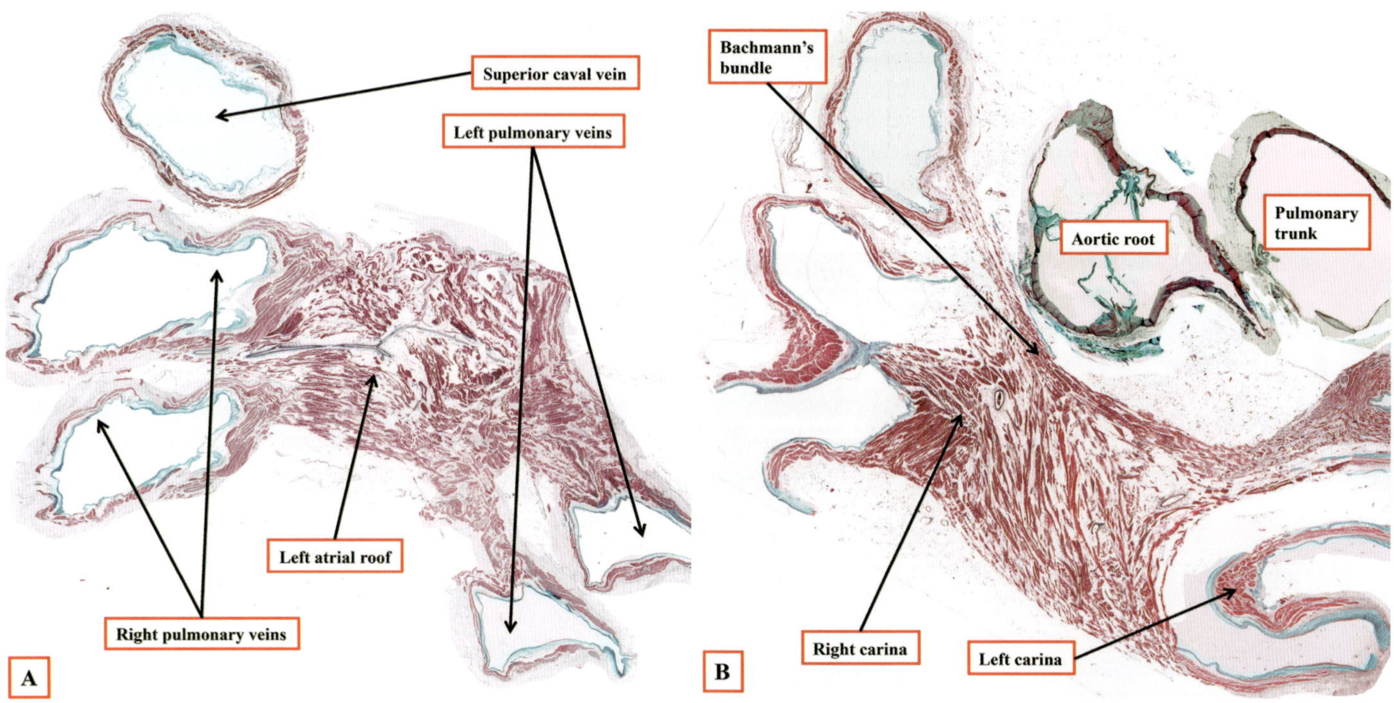

Figure 9.8. The images show two serial histological sections, stained using the trichrome technique, taken across the short axis of the atrial chambers at the site of the junction of the superior caval vein to the right atrium, and the pulmonary veins to the roof of the left atrium. The section shown in panel A is cranial to the one shown in panel B. The sections illustrate the manner of aggregation of the working atrial cardiomyocytes, which form a three-dimensional mesh, albeit with parallel aggregation of the cardiomyocytes in areas such as Bachmann's bundle. There are no anatomical boundaries that permit the identification of subunits within the three-dimensional mesh.

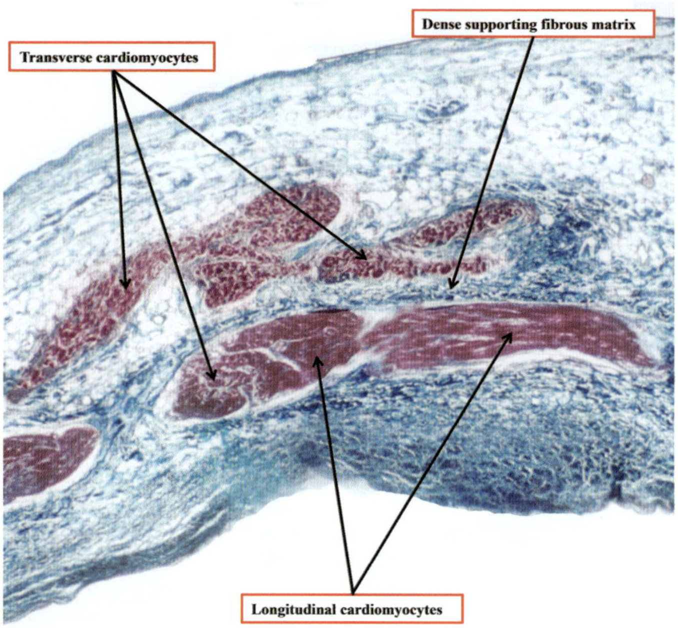

Figure 9.9. The image shows a histological section, stained using the trichrome technique, taken across the junction between one of the pulmonary veins and the dome of the left atrium. It shows how the pulmonary venous sleeves are made up of working atrial cardiomyocytes, albeit with markedly different angulation of the cardiomyocytes aggregated together in adjacent fashion. There is no evidence to support the notion that "Purkinje" cells are to be found within the venous sleeves.

of the cardiomyocytes.[15] Significantly, he noted the difference between skeletal and cardiac muscle, stating that the ventricular cardiomyocytes "as a rule, have neither origin nor insertion, i.e., they are continuous alike at the apex of the ventricles and at the base". His dissections demonstrated the changing helical angle that was subsequently measured by Streeter and colleagues.[13] In this regard, Pettigrew commented that the chains were "further distinguished by the almost total absence of cellular tissue as a connecting medium—the fibres being held together partly by splitting up and running into each other, and partly by the minute ramifications of the cardiac vessels and nerves". Those who followed Pettigrew, unfortunately, chose to ignore these explanations. By the end of the 19th century, anatomists had begun to analyse the ventricular cone on the basis of the morphology of the skeletal muscles, describing discrete components within its walls, and giving them titles such as the "bulbo-spiral muscle" and the "deep sinospiral muscle".[16] The alleged muscular entities, however, could not be demonstrated by dissection, as is the case for skeletal muscles, by following the fibrous sheaths that might enclose them. This is not surprising since, apart from the sheaths that insulate the ventricular bundle branches from the working myocardium of the ventricular septum, no additional fibrous sheaths are to be found within the ventricular mass.

The concept of describing the ventricular mass in terms of discrete muscles was subsequently challenged in the middle of the 20th century, when it was pointed out that the ventricular cone could be dissected, or sculpted, at the whim of the prosector.[17] This emphasis, however, did not deter a resurgence of interest amongst cardiologists in unwrapping the ventricular cone so as to produce a continuous

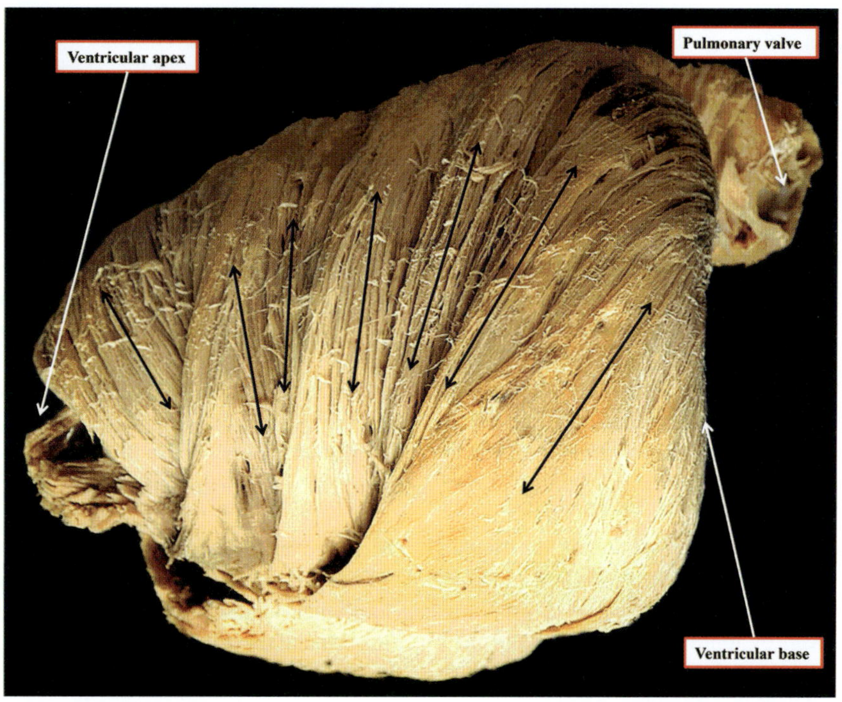

Figure 9.10. The ventricular cone of a porcine heart is shown from the left side. The cone has been dissected from the base to the apex by removing increasing increments of the wall. The process reveals the change in angulation of the aggregated chains of cardiomyocytes responsible for producing the obvious "grain". The orientation, shown by the double-headed black arrows, and known as the helical angle, changes from an epicardial spiral through a circumferential arrangement in the middle of the wall to a reciprocal endocardial spiral. The original dissection was made and photographed by Professor Paul Lunkenheimer. It has been relabelled with his permission.

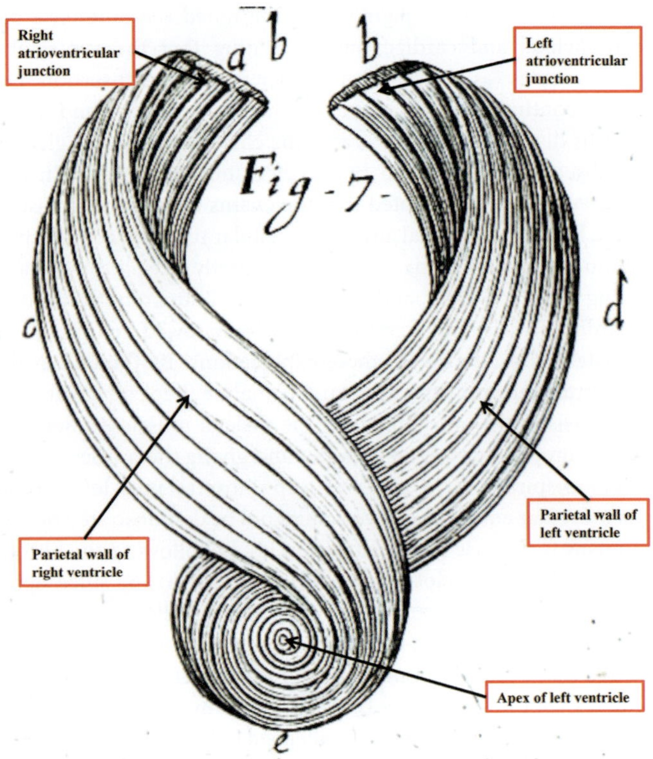

Figure 9.11. The drawing is taken from the work of Richard Lower, published in the 17th century.[13] It shows how Lower was able to produce a myocardial band that started at the right atrioventricular junction and finished at the left atrioventricular junction. Note the spiralling configuration shown by Lower at the apex of the left ventricle.

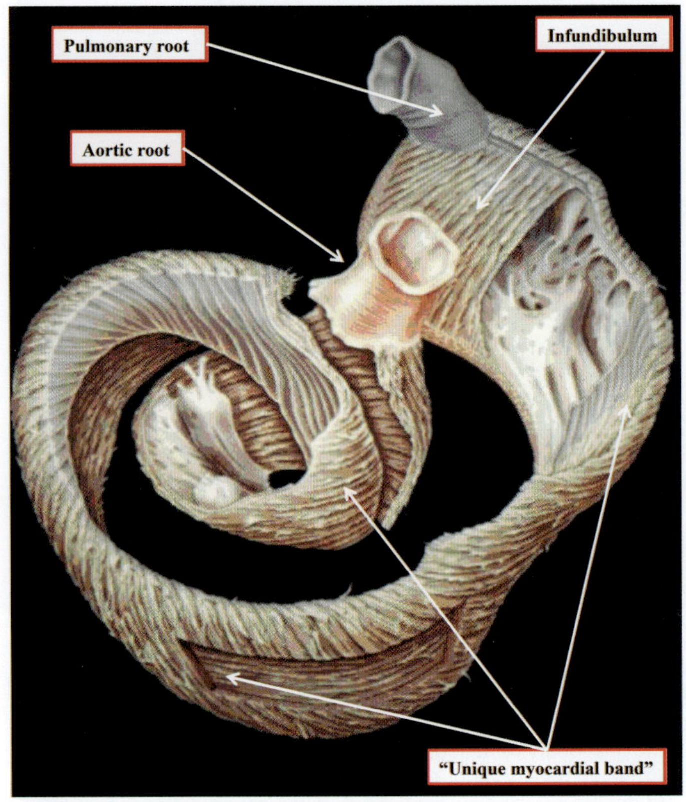

Figure 9.12. The drawing shows the fashion in which the ventricular mass can be sculpted to produce a helical band, which starts at the aortic root and ends at the pulmonary root. There are, however, no anatomical boundaries within the ventricular cone that can be followed by the prosector so as to reveal the end product. The drawing was made by Professor Paul Lunkenheimer and has been relabelled with his permission. The cut-away in the inferior wall shows the cardiomyocytes aggregated in circumferential fashion, showing that the concept of the "helical band" is fundamentally different from the change in helical angle of the aggregated cardiomyocytes. The change in angle is a real thing. The alleged band is an anatomical fiction.

helical strip. The prime mover of the concept of such unwrapping was Torrent-Guasp.[18] Like Lower, Torrent-Guasp showed that it was possible to unwrap the ventricular cone to produce a continuous myocardial band.[18] Although described as a "***helical band***", the concept should not be confused with the change in helical angle of the aggregated individual cardiomyocytes as seen in the changing depth of the ventricular walls. The change in helical angle is found throughout the walls of the left ventricle. The construct named by Torrent-Guasp as the helical band, however, started at the aortic root and ended at the pulmonary trunk (Figure 9.12). The concept, despite its lack of any anatomical foundation, was enthusiastically adopted by other cardiologists and surgeons during the latter decade of the 20th century and continued to be supported through the first decade of the new century.[19] Despite accounts pointing to the scientific deficiencies of the concept,[20] not least its incompatibility with the concept of laminar units underscoring mural thickening,[3,4] there are still those who press for the existence of the alleged helical band so as to explain the "wringing" motion observed during ventricular systole.[21]

The bands sculpted from the ventricular mass by Lower and Torrent-Guasp are not produced by following discrete anatomical boundaries within the cardiac walls. Histological sections taken through the ventricular mass, taken in orthogonal planes, show the lack of any such boundaries (Figures 9.3 panel B, 9.13). Dissections do reveal, nonetheless, obvious patterns in terms of the aggregation of the individual cardiomyocytes within the supporting fibrous matrix. Of these patterns, the most obvious is the helical configuration of the changing "grain" (Figure 9.10). To reiterate, the changing helical angle should not be conflated with the "helical band".

Removing the epicardial surface of the ventricular mass reveals that the most superficial cardiomyocytes on the anterior surface of the ventricular mass, as well as having a marked angle relative to the ventricular equator, also encase the cavities of both the right and left ventricles, with the aggregated chains crossing the anterior interventricular groove (Figure 9.14 panel A). The arrangement is subtly different on the diaphragmatic surface of the ventricular mass. There is a degree of cross-over of the aggregated chains at the ventricular base, but the superficial cardiomyocytes then become restricted to each ventricle (Figure 9.14 panel B).

The spiralling configuration of the aggregated units is most obvious when viewing the ventricular apex (Figure 9.15). Continuing dissection of the left ventricle shows that, as revealed by the change in the "grain", the middle part of the wall is made up of cardiomyocytes aggregated together in circumferential fashion (Figure 9.16 panel A). These circular arrays were suggested by German investigators to provide the driving force, or "Triebwerkzeug", for ventricular systole.[22] Still further dissection then reveals a third spiral array in the endocardial layers of the left ventricle, but one that is reciprocal to

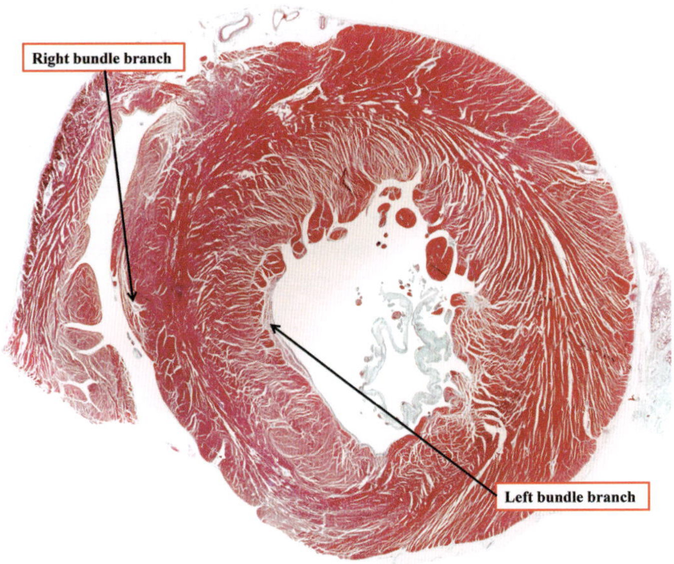

Figure 9.13. The panel shows a short axis histological section taken through the ventricular cone. There are no fibrous sheaths, other from those that enclose the ventricular bundle branches, that permit the myocardial masses to be interpreted as showing individual "muscles", as is the case for the skeletal musculature, nor boundaries that would permit the cone to be unwrapped to produce a continuous helical band. There are, nonetheless, obvious groupings that could slide relative to one another to underscore systolic mural thickening. Similar groupings can be seen in the section shown in Figure 9.3 panel B, in which the wall has been cut in longitudinal, rather than short axis, fashion.

the spiral array shown in the epicardial layers of the left ventricular wall (Figure 9.16 panel B). This, of course, does no more than mirror the findings produced by measurement of the change in the helical angle as revealed by histological sectioning.[13,23]

The changing alignment of the long axis of the aggregated cardiomyocytes within the walls of the left ventricle can also be demonstrated using diffusion tensor magnetic resonance (Figure 9.17).[24] The advantage of assessing the alignment of the chains of cardiomyocytes when using magnetic resonance is that the ventricular cone itself remains intact. This permits the angulations to be assessed as seen in short axis of the ventricular cone, confirming the gradual change in helical angulation across the thickness of the wall (Figure 9.18). The angulations, however, can be measured not only as seen tangential to the surface of the ventricular cone so as to produce the helical angle (Figure 9.18 panel A). It is also possible to demonstrate a transmural angulation of some of the aggregates (Figure 9.18 panel B).

The existence of intruding or extruding aggregates is important since, during the 20th century, those interpreting cardiodynamics usually followed the concept of Frank.[25] This presumed that all the spiralling cardiomyocytes were exclusively tangential, without any significant degree of transmural intrusion or extrusion. At the beginning of the 19th century, however, Brachet had suggested that a separate transmural set of cardiomyocytes was involved during the cardiac cycle so as to produce consecutive contractions, with the transmural cells actively producing ventricular dilation during diastole.[26] Subsequent histological observations, such as those of Streeter and colleagues,[13] failed to show any reciprocal tangential

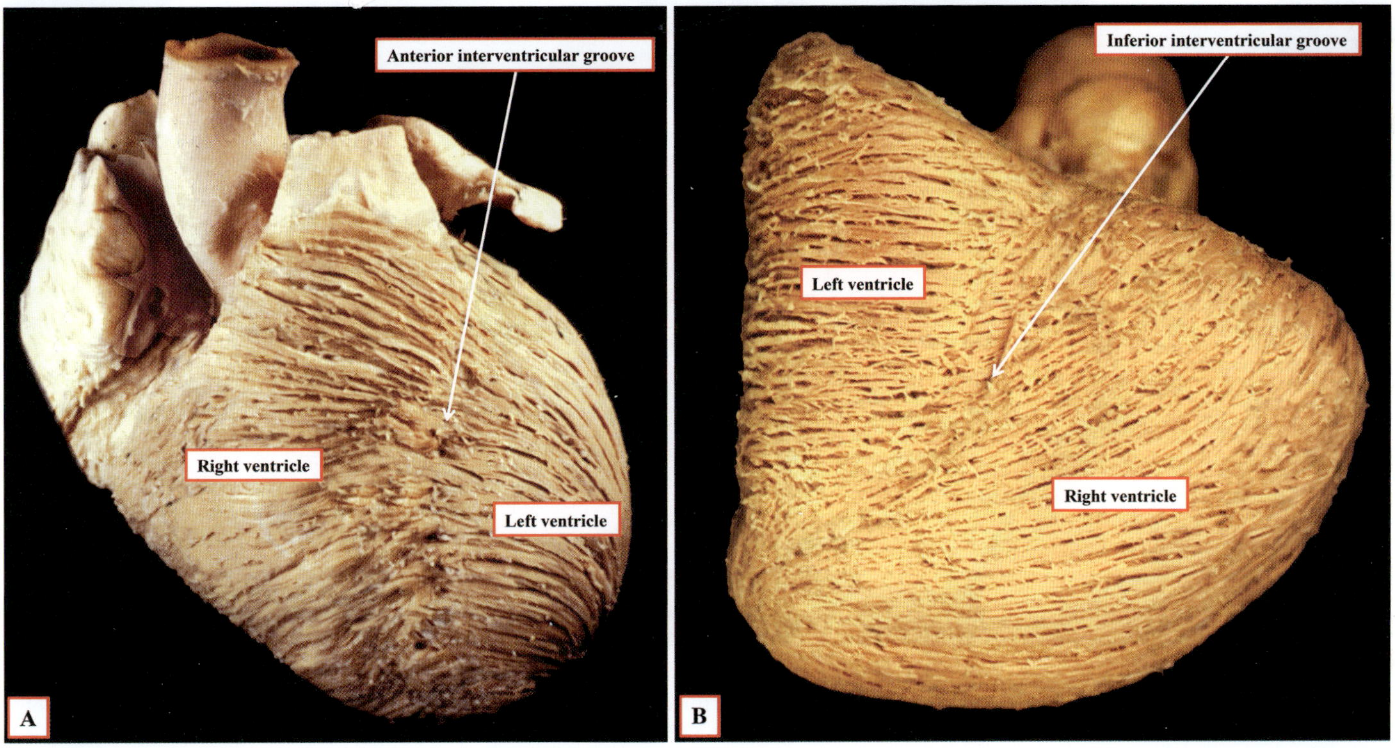

Figure 9.14. The images show how the overall alignment of the aggregated ventricular cardiomyocytes can be revealed by removing the epicardial surface of the ventricular cone. Panel A shows the anterior surface of the cone, with the superficial cardiomyocytes crossing the anterior interventricular groove so as to be part of the walls of both right and left ventricles. Panel B shows the diaphragmatic surface of the same heart. There is some cross-over of cardiomyocytes at the base, but towards the apex the cardiomyocytes are aggregated such that they belong to either the right or the left ventricular walls.

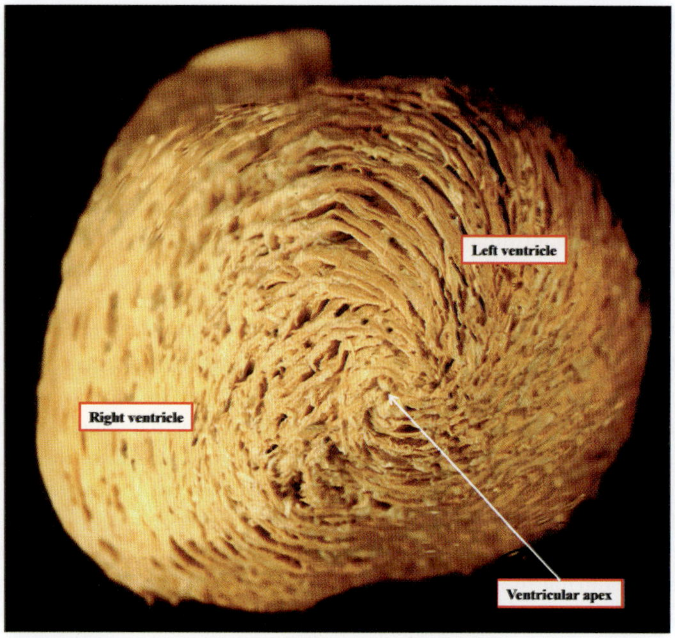

Figure 9.15. The image shows the apical view of the same heart as shown in Figure 9.14. The aggregation of the superficial cardiomyocytes has been revealed by stripping away the epicardial lining of the ventricular mass. The dissection shows the obvious spiralling of the cardiomyocytes at the apex.

and transmural chains as envisaged by Brachet. Experiments using transmural force probes, nonetheless, have now demonstrated that forces, over and above the regular unloading forces, are generated during ventricular systole. These forces were interpreted as tempering the effects of ventricular constriction so as to modulate focal deformation and thus prevent over-constriction. In aiding the process of ventricular unloading, they were described as being auxotonic.[26] And histological sections taken at the sites of such measured auxotonic forces do reveal the presence of cardiomyocytes aggregated together in intruding or extruding fashion. As shown in Figure 9.18 panel B, measurements taken from hearts interrogated using diffusion tensor magnetic resonance reveal the presence of such cardiomyocytes aggregated together in chains that extrude or intrude at significant angles. Such aggregates, when contracting, can be presumed principally to act in a dilatory fashion, thus serving to shape focal deformation of the walls. Their presence provides support for the concept of mural antagonism.[26] Examination of scanning electron microscopic images also reveals chains of cardiomyocytes adjacent to one another with markedly different angulations (Figure 9.4 panel B). The question remains as to how the chains of transmural cardiomyocytes are combined with the helical configuration of the tangential chains to produce an overall three-dimensional mural meshwork. Initial information in this regard has now been provided by interrogation of hearts processed using microcomputed tomography.[27] Even when using this technique, problems remain in

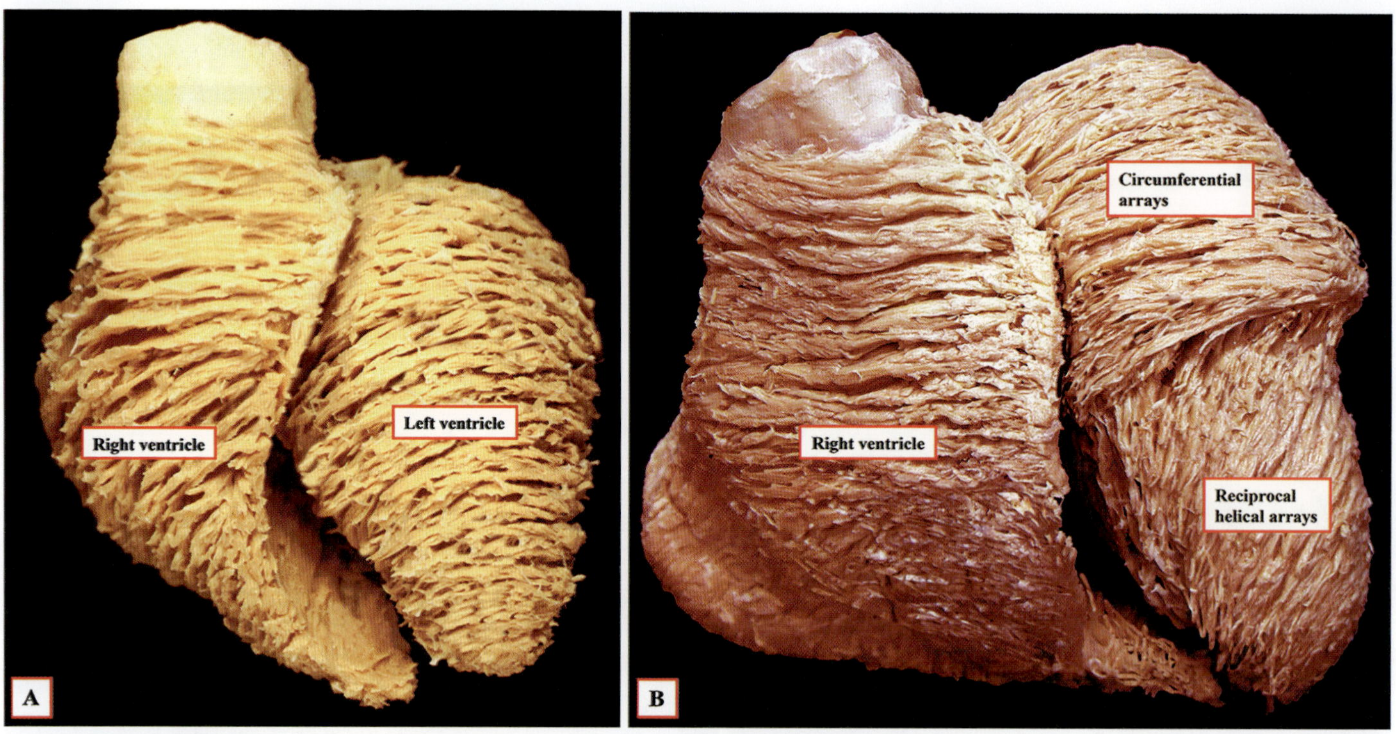

Figure 9.16. The heart shown in Figures 9.14 and 9.15 has been dissected further to produce these images by removing the superficial cardiomyocytes of the ventricular walls. Removing the superficial layer of the wall of the left ventricle, as shown in panel A, reveals the circumferential arrays of aggregated cardiomyocytes that make up the middle layer. It is these circumferential cardiomyocytes that were identified as producing the "driving force" for ventricular systolic ejection. Further dissection of the left ventricular wall, as shown in panel B, reveals the deeper layer of cardiomyocytes, which spiral in reciprocal fashion relative to the superficial cardiomyocytes shown in Figure 9.14.

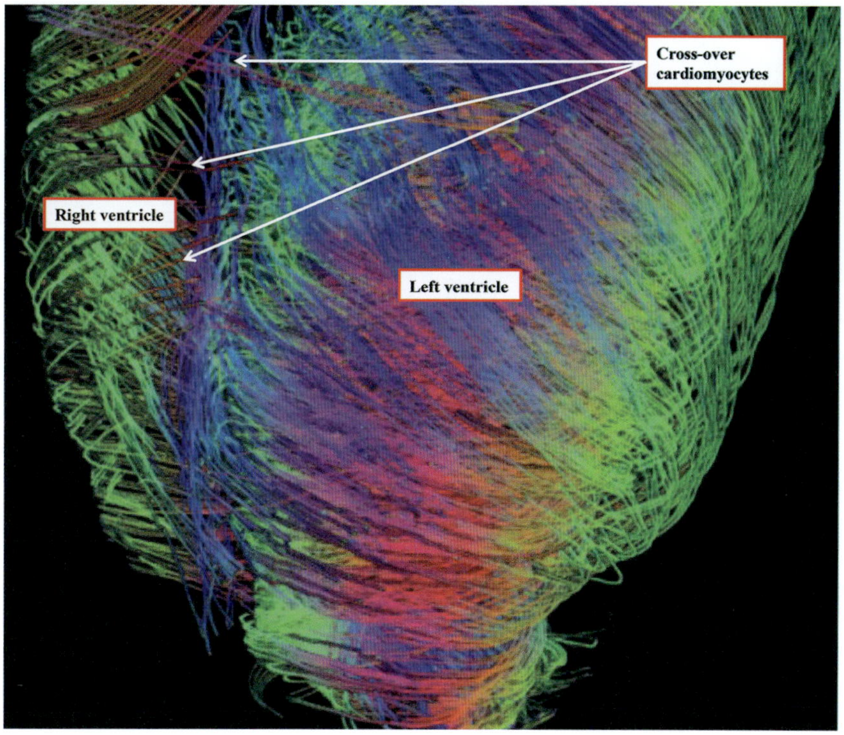

Figure 9.17. The image shows the porcine ventricular cone as imaged using diffusion tensor magnetic resonance. The technique shows the change in helical angle of the cardiomyocytes aggregated together in tangential fashion. Note also the superficial aggregates which cross over so as to belong to the walls of both ventricles. The original image was prepared by Dr Peter Agger, and has been relabelled with his permission.

distinguishing the extent of individual aggregated units within the overall three-dimensional mesh.[28] Nonetheless, by taking biopsies across the ventricular walls, it has proved possible to trace the chains of cardiomyocytes aggregated together within the perimysial component of the fibrous matrix, stopping the reconstruction when the chosen aggregate branches with its neighbours (Figure 9.19).

It is then possible to assess the angulation of the reconstructed entities in terms of both the helical and transmural angulation of their contained cardiomyocytes. The measurements show that as the helical angle changes, so, to a greater or lesser extent, the chains either intrude or extrude within the three-dimensional mesh (Figure 9.20).

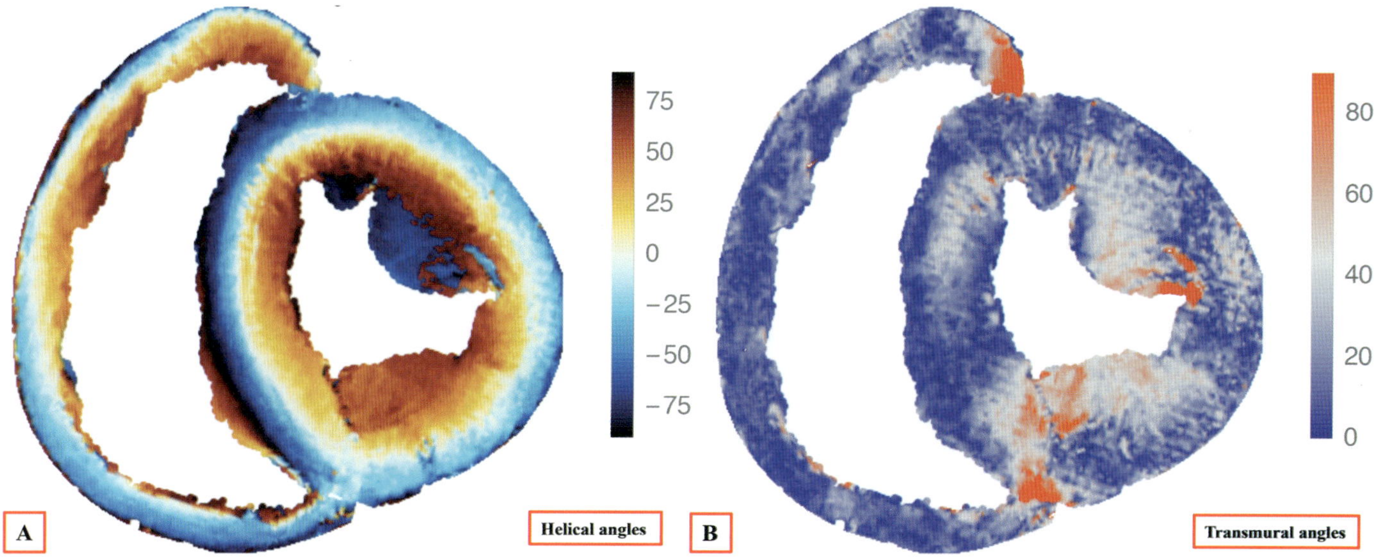

Figure 9.18. The images show short axis sections across the ventricular mass of the porcine heart subsequent to interrogation using diffusion tensor magnetic resonance. Panel A shows how the technique reveals the changing helical angle, as shown in the numbers, whilst panel B shows the change in transmural angulation of the aggregated cardiomyocytes, again as shown in the numbers. The original images were prepared by Dr Peter Agger and have been relabelled with his permission.

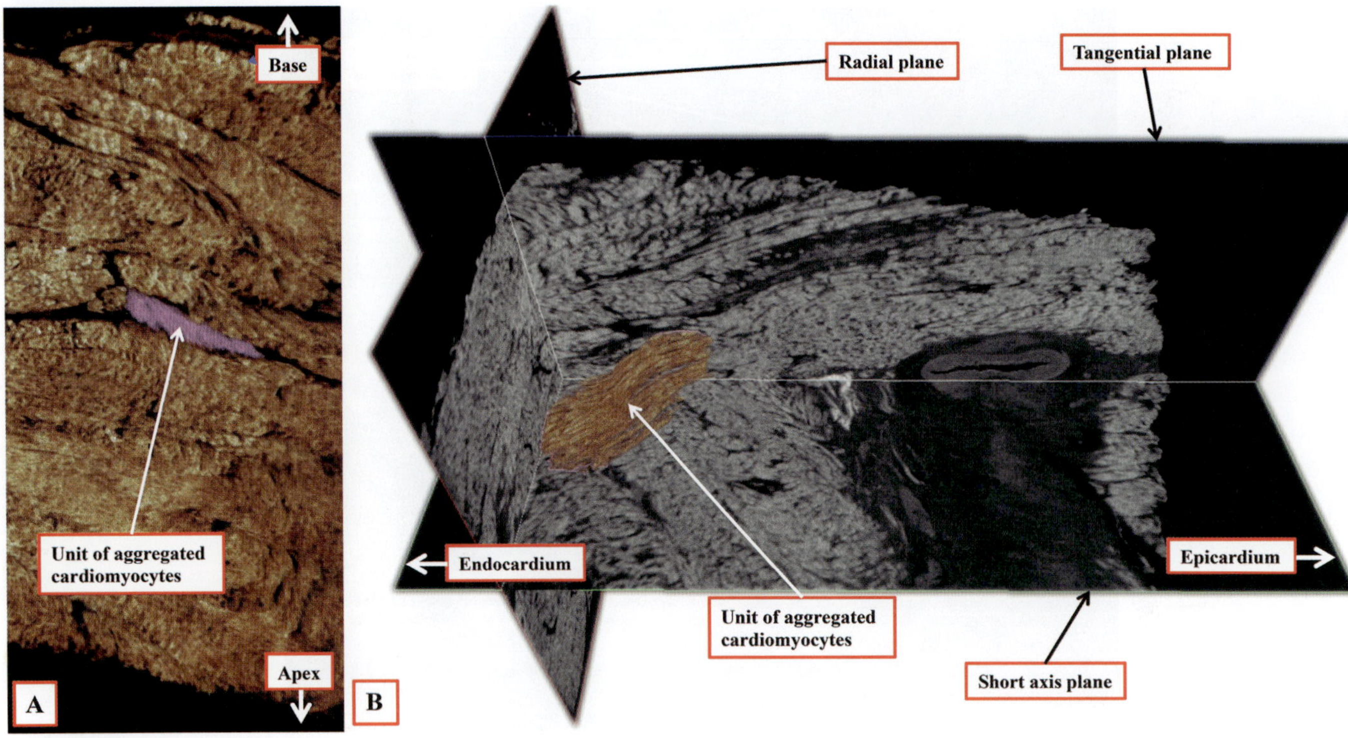

Figure 9.19. The images are taken from a biopsy of a human heart interrogated using microcomputed tomography. Panel A shows a section across the biopsy taken in the tangential plane. It is possible to identify a collection of cardiomyocytes within the three-dimensional mesh aggregated together by the endomysial component of fibrous matrix and separated by perimysial clefts from its neighbours. Panel B shows how it is possible, by using three-dimensional reconstructions, to track the angulation of the aggregated entity relative to the radial, tangential, and short axis planes of the ventricular cone. The reconstructed aggregate extends in transmural fashion within the thickness of the ventricular wall. The images were prepared initially by Dr Peter Agger and have been relabelled with his permission.

Within the biopsies, it also proved possible to identify aggregates within the mesh that extended with a marked transmural angulation relative to their neighbours (Figure 9.21). These transmural entities likely correspond with the cardiomyocytes identified as producing auxotonic forces.[26] Further information regarding the overall orientation of the aggregates within the three-dimensional architecture of the ventricular walls can be provided by detailed assessment of the datasets now produced using Synchrotron scanning of intact human

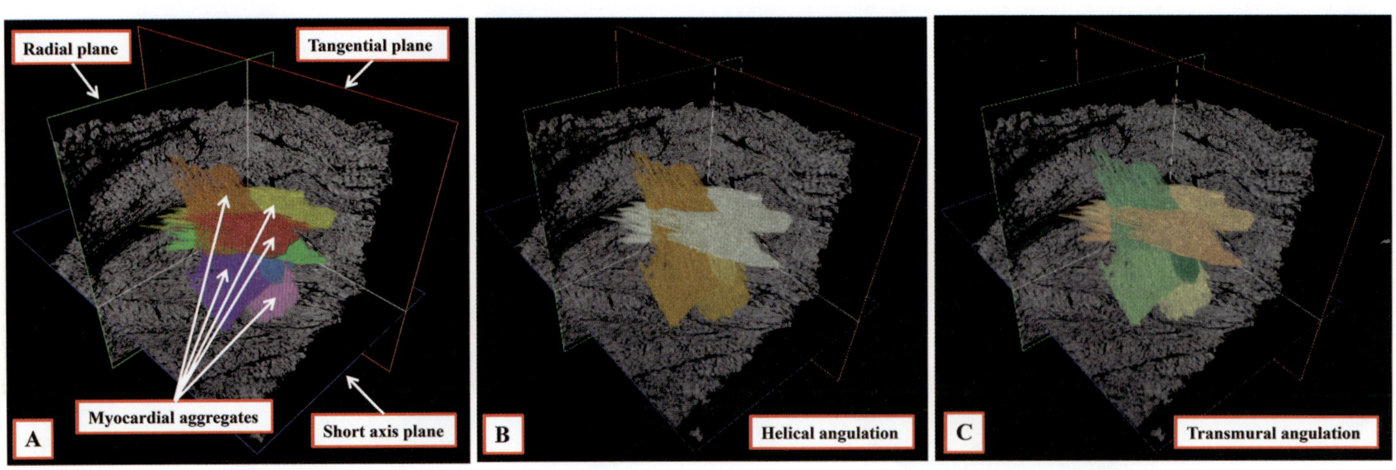

Figure 9.20. The images show how, using the biopsies interrogated using microcomputed tomography, it is possible to identify a group of aggregated cardiomyocytic units and then to measure the helical and transmural angulation of their contained cardiomyocytes. In panel A, the aggregated entities have been coloured in random fashion. Panel B shows the changing helical angulation, with the aggregated units shown in grey having zero angulation relative to the ventricular equator, and the ones shown in degrees of brown having increased spiralling angulation. Panel C shows the angulation of the cardiomyocytes of the same aggregates, but now relative to the short axis of the ventricular mass. Zero angulation, in other words a tangential arrangement, is shown in green. The aggregates shown in brown have increasing angles of intrusion or extrusion, with the darker shade of brown showing a transmural angulation of 45 degrees. The original images were prepared by Dr Peter Agger and have been relabelled with his permission.

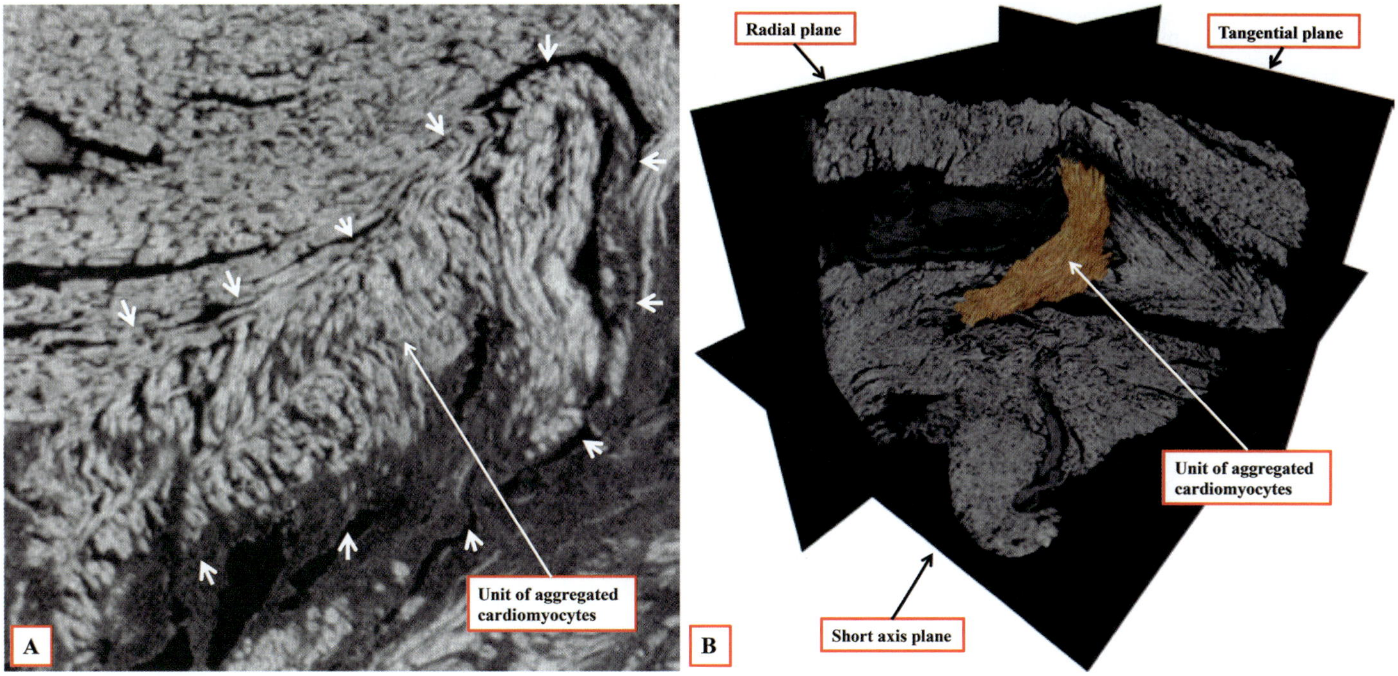

Figure 9.21. Panel A shows an aggregated group of cardiomyocytes from one of the biopsies of the human heart as shown in Figures 9.19 and 9.20. In this instance, as revealed by the reconstruction shown in panel B, the aggregated cardiomyocytes extend in markedly transmural fashion compared to their neighbouring components of the three-dimensional mesh. It is likely that transmural cardiomyocytes aggregated together in the fashion shown are responsible for the auxotonic forces identified during ventricular systolic contraction.[25] The images were prepared initially by Dr Peter Agger and have been relabelled with his permission.

hearts.[29] Such interrogation should finally demonstrate the overall three-dimensional arrangement of the ventricular mural architecture, resolving any remaining controversies relating to the alleged helical band or discrete laminar sheets.

REFERENCES

1. Stephenson RS, Agger P, Lunkenheimer PP, Zhao J, Smerup M, Niederer P, Anderson RH, Jarvis JC. The functional architecture of skeletal compared to cardiac musculature: myocyte orientation, lamellar unit morphology, and the helical ventricular myocardial band. *Clin Anat*. 2016;**29**:316–332. doi: 10.1002/ca.22661
2. Spotnitz HM, Spotnitz WD, Cottrell TS, Spiro D, Sonnenblick EH. Cellular basis for volume related wall thickness changes in the rat left ventricle. *J Mol Cell Cardiol*. 1974;**6**:317–331. doi: 10.1016/0022-2828(74)90074-1
3. Legrice IJ, Hunter PJ, Smaill BH. Laminar structure of the heart: a mathematical model. *Am J Physiol*. 1997;**272**:H2466–H2476. doi: 10.1152/ajpheart.1997.272.5.H2466
4. Pope AJ, Sands GB, Smaill BH, LeGrice IJ. Three-dimensional transmural organization of perimysial collagen in the heart. *Am J Physiol Heart Circ Physiol*. 2008;**295**:H1243–H1252. doi: 10.1152/ajpheart.00484.2008
5. Anderson RH, Niederer PF, Sanchez-Quintana D, Stephenson RS, Agger P, et al. How are the cardiomyocytes aggregated together within the walls of the left ventricular cone? *J Anat*. 2019;**235**:697–705. doi: 10.1111/joa.13027
6. Borg TK, Caulfield JB. The collagen matrix of the heart. Fed Proc. 1981;**40**:2037–2041. PMID: 7227559
7. Papez JW. Heart musculature of the atria. *Am J Anat* 1920;**27**:255–277. doi: 10.1002/aja.1000270302
8. Wang K, Ho SY, Gibson DG, Anderson RH. Architecture of atrial musculature in humans. *Br Heart J*. 1995;**73**:559–565. doi: 10.1136/hrt.73.6.559
9. Spach MS, Miller WT, 3rd, Dolber PC, Kootsey JM, Sommer JR, Mosher CE, Jr. The functional role of structural complexities in the propagation of depolarization in the atrium of the dog. Cardiac conduction disturbances due to discontinuities of effective axial resistivity. *Circ Res*. 1982;**50**:175–191. doi: 10.1161/01.res.50.2.175
10. Anderson RH, Mohun TJ, Sanchez-Quintana D, Mori S, Spicer DE, Cheung JW, Lerman BB. The anatomic substrates for outflow tract arrhythmias. *Heart Rhythm*. 2019;**16**:290–297. doi: 10.1016/j.hrthm.2018.08.014
11. Perez-Lugones A, McMahon JT, Ratliff NB, Saliba WI, Schweikert RA, Marrouche NF, Saad EB, Navia JL, McCarthy PM, Tchou P, et al. Evidence of specialized conduction cells in human pulmonary veins of patients with atrial fibrillation. *J Cardiovasc Electrophysiol*. 2003;**14**:803–809. doi: 10.1046/j.1540-8167.2003.03075.x
12. Sanchez-Quintana D, Lopez-Minguez JR, Pizarro G, Murillo M, Cabrera JA. Triggers and anatomical substrates in the genesis and perpetuation of atrial fibrillation. *Curr Cardiol Rev*. 2012;**8**:310–326. doi: 10.2174/157340312803760721
13. Streeter DD, Jr., Spotnitz HM, Patel DP, Ross J, Jr., Sonnenblick EH. Fiber orientation in the canine left ventricle during diastole and systole. *Circ Res*. 1969;**24**:339–347. doi: 10.1161/01.res.24.3.339
14. Lower R. Tractatus de Corde. In: Gunther RT (ed.) *Early Science in Oxford, Volume 9*. Oxford: Oxford; 1669, 1932.

15. Pettigrew JB. On the arrangement of the muscular fibres in the ventricles of the vertebrate heart, with physiological remarks. *Phil Trans R Soc*. 1864;**154**:445–500.
16. Mall FP. On the muscular architecture of the ventricles of the human heart. *Am J Anat*. 1911;**11**:211–266. doi: 10.1002/aja.1000110302
17. Lev M, Simkins CS. Architecture of the human ventricular myocardium; technic for study using a modification of the Mall–MacCallum method. *Lab Invest*. 1956;**5**:396–409. PMID: 13358198
18. Torrent Guasp F. *Anatomia Funcional del Corazon: La Actividad Ventricular Diastólica y Sistólica*. Madrid: Paz Montalvo; 1957.
19. Torrent-Guasp F, Kocica MJ, Corno AF, Komeda M, Carreras-Costa F, Flotats A, Cosin-Aguillar J, Wen H. Towards new understanding of the heart structure and function. *Eur J Cardio-thorac Surg*. 2005;**27**:191–201. doi: 10.1016/j.ejcts.2004.11.026
20. MacIver DH, Partridge JB, Agger P, Stephenson RS, Boukens BJD, Omann C, Jarvis JC, Zhang H. The end of the unique myocardial band: Part II. Clinical and functional considerations. *Eur J Cardio-thorac Surg*. 2018;**53**:120–128. doi: 10.1093/ejcts/ezx335
21. Antunez-Montes OY, Kocica MJ, Olavarria AS, Corno AF, Millan RA, Rosales CI, Sanchez Aparicio HE. Helical structure of the ventricular myocardium. A narrative review of cardiac mechanics. *Echocardiography*. 2023;**40**:161–173. doi: 10.1111/echo.15515
22. Feneis H. Das gefüge des herzmuskels bei systole und diastole. *Gegenbauers Morphol Jb*. 1944;**944/5**:S371–S406. doi: 10.1002/ar.a.20326
23. Greenbaum RA, Ho SY, Gibson DG, Becker AE, Anderson RH. Left ventricular fibre architecture in man. *Br Heart J*. 1981;**45**:248–263. doi: 10.1136/hrt.45.3.248
24. Schmid P, Jaermann T, Boesiger P, Niederer PF, Lunkenheimer PP, Cryer CW, Anderson RH. Ventricular myocardial architecture as visualised in postmortem swine hearts using magnetic resonance diffusion tensor imaging. *Eur J Cardio-thorac Surg*. 2005;**27**:468–472. doi: 10.1016/j.ejcts.2004.11.036
25. Frank O. Isometrie und isotonie des herzmuskels. *Z Biol*. 1901;**41**:14–34.
26. Brachet JL. *Sur la Cause du Mouvement de Dilatation du Coeur*. Paris: Faculté de Médecine de Paris; 1813.
27. Agger P, Stephenson RS. Assessing myocardial architecture: the challenges and controversies. *J Cardiovasc Dev Dis*. 2020;**7**:47. doi: 10.3390/jcdd7040047
28. Stephenson RS, Agger P, Omann C, Sanchez-Quintana D, Jarvis JC, Anderson RH. Resolving the true ventricular mural architecture. J Cardiovasc Dev Dis. 2018;**5**:34. doi: 10.3390/jcdd5020034
29. Brunet J, Cook AC, Walsh CL, Cranley J, Tafforeau P, Engel K, Arthurs O, Berruyer C, Burke O'Leary E, Bellier A, et al. Multidimensional analysis of the adult human heart in health and disease using hierarchical phase-contrast tomography. *Radiology*. 2024;**312**:e232731. doi: 10.1148/radiol.232731

10

The Intrapericardial and Extrapericardial Arterial Pathways

The arterial pathways are important anatomical entities adjacent to the main structure of the heart. When analysing the congenitally malformed heart, one of the parts addressed when using the process of segmental analysis is the arterial segment.[1,2] This part has intrapericardial and extrapericardial components. The difference between the two parts has received scant attention from anatomists and pathologists. The need to enter the pericardial cavity in order to approach the intrapericardial components, however, has obvious implications for the surgeon, and for the modern-day interventionist, who needs to be well aware of the location of the pericardial reflections separating the parts. Furthermore, the intrapericardial components of the arterial trunks, united within their sleeve of serous pericardium, serve as the major pathway for the sympathetic component of the autonomic nervous system to enter the heart. The extrapericardial parts of the pathways may be deemed the province of the vascular rather than cardiac specialist. But diagnosis of coarctation, or the finding of a persistently patent arterial duct, or the potential implications of a retro-oesophageal right subclavian artery are very much within the realm of the cardiologist. The major nerve trunks extending across the fibrous pericardial sac also have important relationships to the branches of the extrapericardial arterial pathways.

The Intrapericardial Arterial Pathways

The parts of the aorta and pulmonary trunk contained within the pericardial cavity are short. Each vessel originates at its junction with the sinuses of its arterial root (Figure 10.1). In the normal heart, the intrapericardial components show the first evidence of the spiralling configuration that is the essence of the usual ventriculo-arterial connections (Figure 10.2).[1,2]

Within the pericardial cavity, the two arterial trunks are enclosed together within the sleeve of serous pericardium that initially clothed the arterial pole of the developing ventricular outflow tract (Figure 10.3 panel A). They transition to their extrapericardial parts as they exit through the cranial attachments of the fibrous pericardium, with the visceral and parietal layers of the serous pericardium reflecting back on themselves at these levels (Figure 10.3 panel B). When first formed, the walls of the intrapericardial outflow tract were exclusively myocardial. The ingrowth of non-myocardial tissues from the heart-forming fields eventually produces not only the walls of the intrapericardial trunks themselves, but also the arterial walls of the aortic and pulmonary valvar sinuses. The precise mechanisms and timing of these processes have still to be clarified.[3]

The intrapericardial component of the ***aorta*** is right-sided and posterior as it emerges from the aortic root at the sinutubular junction (Figure 10.1). The junction itself is well formed within the aortic pathway (Figure 10.4), but is less obvious in the pulmonary root. The coronary arteries usually arise within the arterial walls of the valvar sinuses adjacent to the pulmonary root. Origin just distal to the sinutubular junction, however, is not uncommon (Figure 10.4).[4] In the adult heart, origin more than 1 cm distal to the junction is considered to represent a congenital malformation. If associated with an intramural course, and particularly when the heart itself is congenitally malformed, such high origin can represent a risk for sudden cardiac death.[5,6] The intrapericardial component of the ***pulmonary trunk*** is often described as the "main pulmonary artery". It is properly described as the pulmonary trunk. It has comparable length to the intrapericardial aorta, but its long axis is almost perpendicular to the aortic channel (Figure 10.2).

At the margins of the pericardial cavity, the trunk divides into the right and left pulmonary arteries, which are themselves extrapericardial (Figure 10.5). During embryonic and fetal life and during the first 2 or 3 days of postnatal life the pulmonary trunk continues extrapericardially as the arterial duct (Figure 10.3 panel B). With normal closure of the duct, the extrapericardial component of the channel becomes the arterial ligament. The pericardial reflections provide the distinguishing feature between persistent patency of the duct as opposed to presence of an aortopulmonary window. The persistently patent duct and the ligament in postnatal life are exclusively extrapericardial, whereas the window is a congenital communication between the intrapericardial arterial trunks.[7]

The Extrapericardial Arterial Pathways

Having passed through the pericardial reflections, the extrapericardial components of the arterial pathways make up the superior part of the mediastinum, with the heart itself enclosed

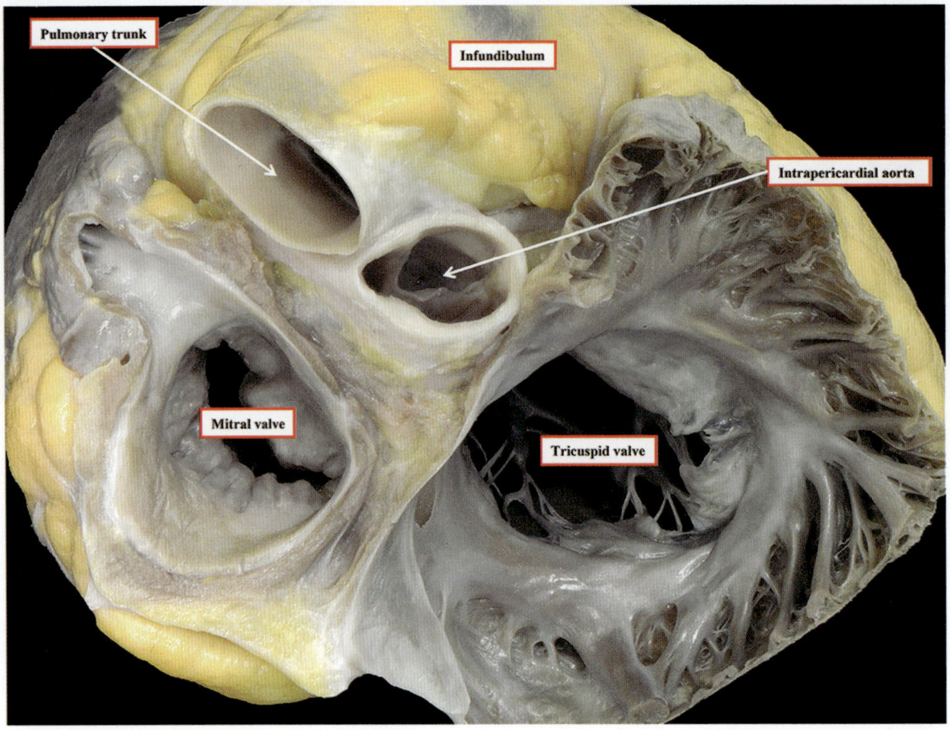

Figure 10.1. The image shows the base of the ventricular mass as viewed from the atrial aspect, having removed the walls of the atrial chambers and transected the intrapericardial arterial trunks just distal to the sinutubular junctions. The pulmonary trunk takes its origin from the infundibulum of the morphologically right ventricle in anterior and left-sided position. It is possible to recognize the beginning of the spiral relationship between the pulmonary trunk and the intrapericardial component of the aorta.

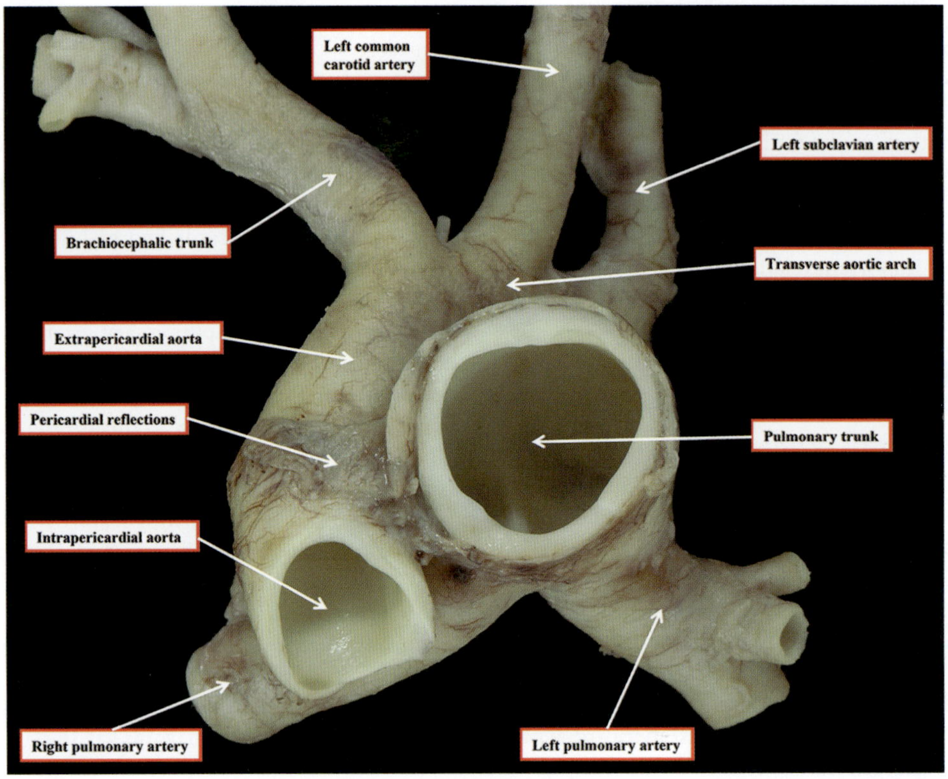

Figure 10.2. This image shows the arterial pathways viewed from the ventricular aspect, having transected the intrapericardial trunks just distal to the sinutubular junctions. It is possible to recognize the location of the pericardial reflections on the aorta, separating its intrapericardial and extrapericardial components. The pulmonary trunk can also be seen to be wrapped in its serous pericardial sleeve. The axes of the aortic and pulmonary pathways are almost at a right angle to each other, with the pathways spiralling as they extend into the middle part of the mediastinum.

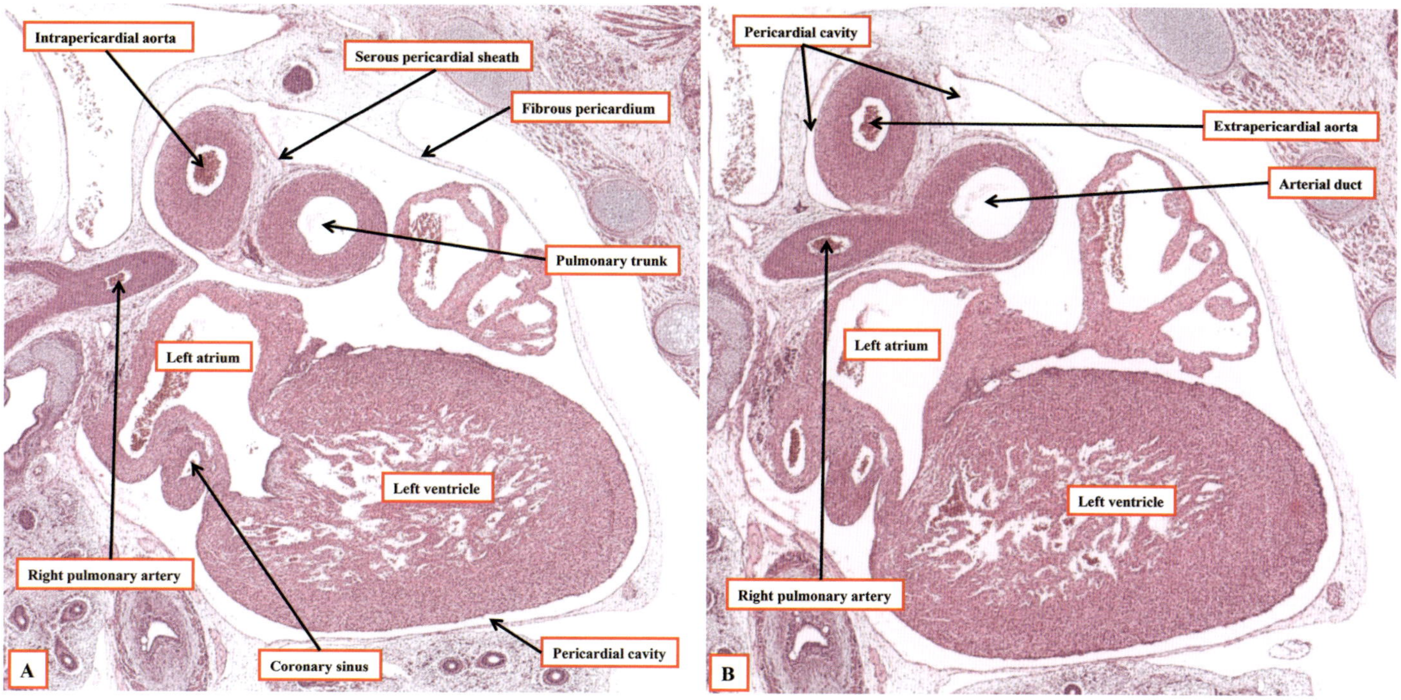

Figure 10.3. The images are serial histological sections of a human embryo at Carnegie stage 23 stained with haematoxylin and eosin. The sections are taken from the e-histology viewer of the HDBR Atlas, available for free interrogation. The heart is sectioned in the frontal plane. Panel A shows how the intrapericardial arterial trunks are enclosed together within the sleeve of serous pericardium. Careful interrogation shows the presence of autonomic nerves within the sleeve. Panel B shows how the pulmonary trunk has branched at the margins of the pericardial cavity into its right and left branches, with only the right pulmonary artery seen in this section. The trunk, during embryonic and foetal life, continues extrapericardially as the arterial duct. The aorta is cut at its transition from its intrapericardial to its extrapericardial component.

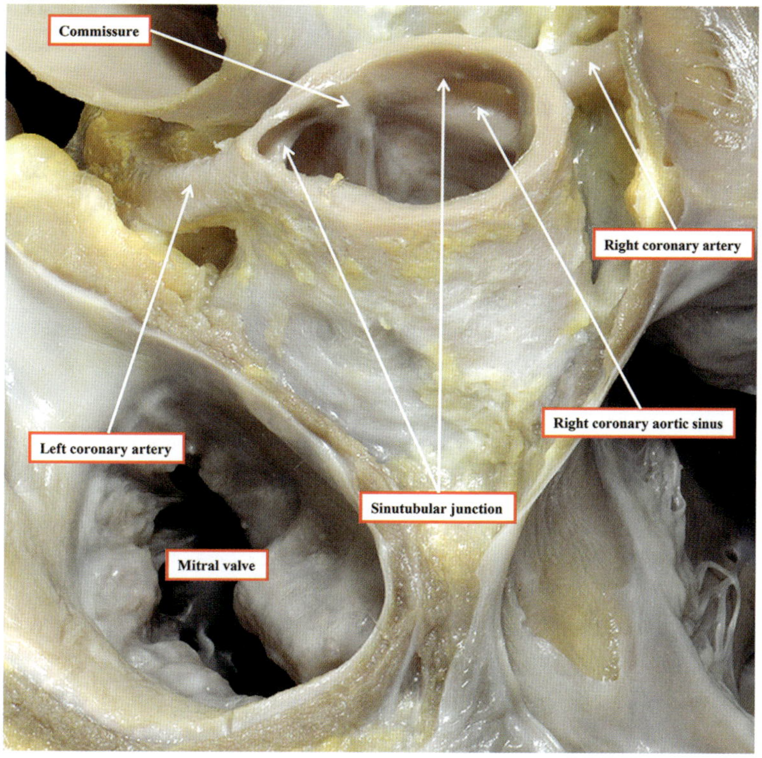

Figure 10.4. In this heart, the intrapericardial component of the aorta has been transected distal to the sinutubular junction. The junction itself can be visualized as an obvious boundary between the tubular component of the aorta and the sinuses of the aortic root. The boundary is not as well marked in the pulmonary root. Note that, in this heart, the main stem of the left coronary artery is arising distally relative to the sinutubular junction. This is considered a normal variant. In the normal adult heart, origin more than 1 cm distal to the junction is deemed to be a congenital malformation, potentially carrying the risk of sudden cardiac death when associated with an intramural course.

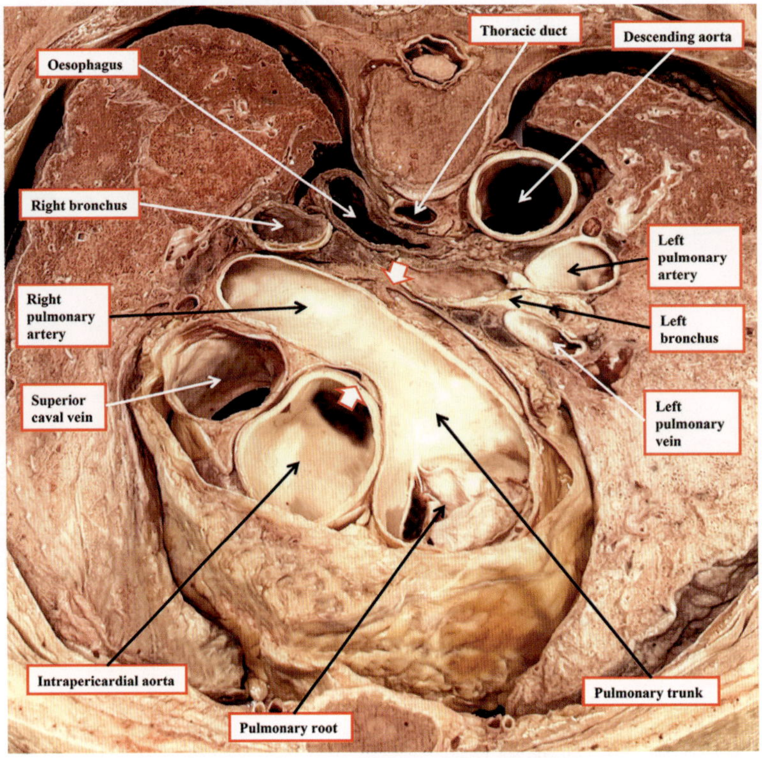

Figure 10.5. The image shows a short axis of the mediastinum taken at the level of the intrapericardial arterial trunks. The white arrows with red borders show the reflections of the pericardium at the site of bifurcation of the pulmonary trunk. The pulmonary trunk itself is exclusively within the pericardial cavity, but its right and left branches are extrapericardial. Only the extrapericardial right pulmonary artery is seen in this section.

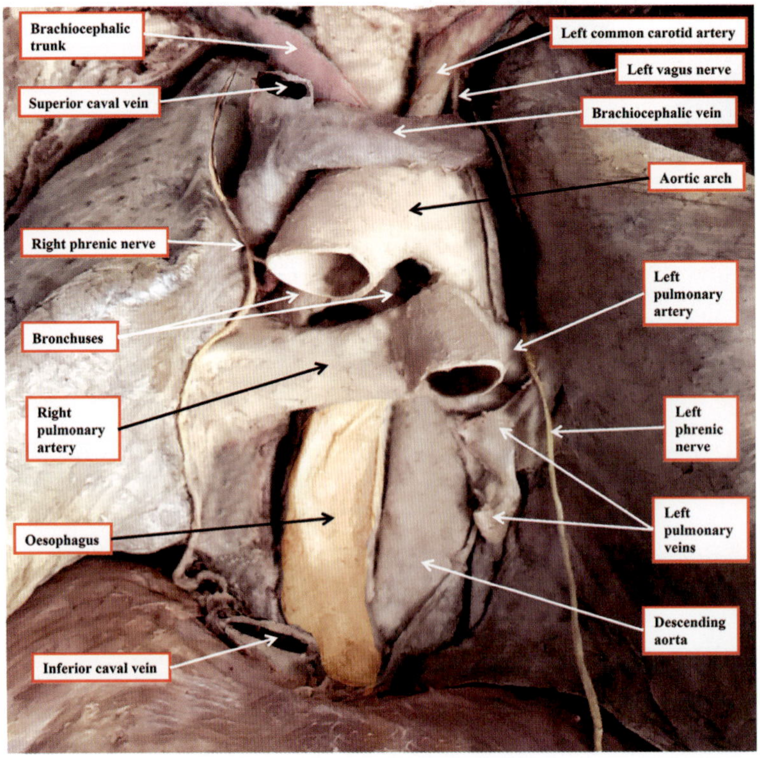

Figure 10.6. The image shows the view of the mediastinum, having removed the heart and its fibrous pericardial sac. The extrapericardial components of the arterial pathways occupy the superior part of the mediastinum, with the aortic arch crossing over the right pulmonary artery and then the left bronchus. It is the crossing of the left bronchus that is the criterion for definition of a left aortic arch. The right and left pulmonary arteries on each side enter the pulmonary hilums, along with the bronchuses and the pulmonary veins. Note the location of the phrenic nerves, which extend laterally across the fibrous pericardial sac.

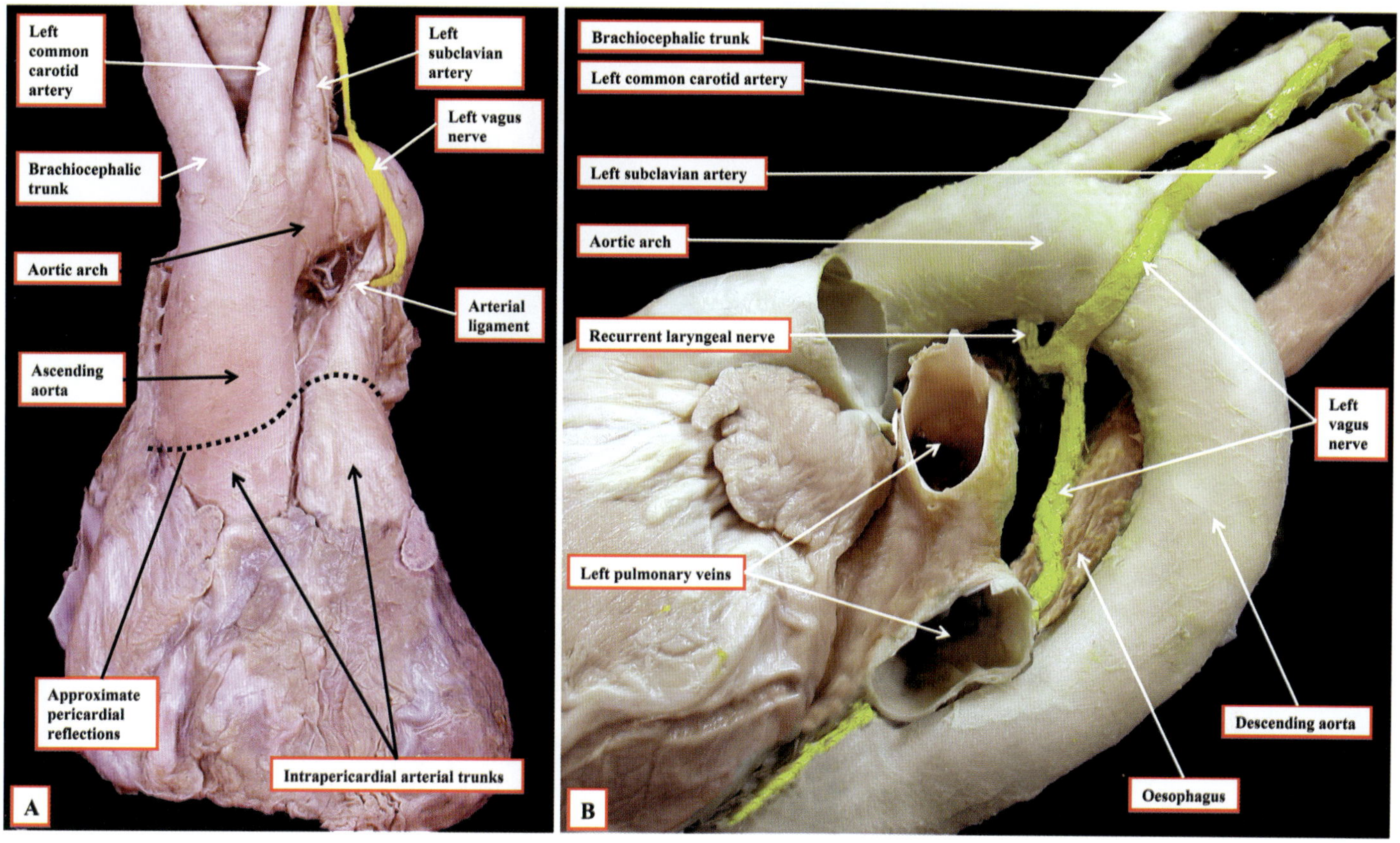

Figure 10.7. Panel A shows the heart removed from its pericardial cradle along with the arterial pathways. The approximate site of the pericardial reflections has been marked. The extrapericardial ascending aorta becomes the aortic arch, which extends posteriorly and leftward to cross the left bronchus. It is the crossing of the left bronchus that makes the arch left sided. The frontal view shows the origin from the arch of the brachiocephalic trunk, followed by the left common carotid and left subclavian arteries. In this specimen, the vagus nerve has been retained and coloured yellow. Further dissection of the heart, and viewing it from the left side, as shown in panel B, reveals how the recurrent laryngeal nerve passes underneath the arch before ascending to supply the larynx. As seen in panel A, the origin of the recurrent nerve is closely related to the arterial ligament. The left vagus nerve itself continues caudally on the surface of the oesophagus.

within its pericardial fibrous sac occupying the inferior part (Figure 10.6). The extrapericardial component of the aorta ascends, having exited the pericardial cavity, turning leftward as the ***aortic arch*** when it has crossed the right pulmonary artery. The arch itself then crosses the left bronchus as it becomes the descending aorta. It is the crossing of the left, rather than the right, bronchus that serves as the defining feature of a left aortic arch. A divided arch, with components which cross both bronchuses, is found rarely as the double aortic arch.[8] The presence of a right, as opposed to a left, arch was found to occur in less than 1% of otherwise normal individuals in an extensive meta-analysis.[9]

The aortic arch, in most instances, gives rise to the brachiocephalic trunk and then to the left common carotid and left subclavian arteries, with the brachiocephalic trunk itself usually dividing into the ***right common carotid*** and ***subclavian arteries*** (Figure 10.7). Having given off the left subclavian artery, the arch turns caudally to become the ***descending aorta*** (Figure 10.7 panel B). The ***left vagus nerve*** gives off its ***recurrent laryngeal branch*** in this area, with the laryngeal branch turning cranially around the aorta itself. The origin of the recurrent branch is closely related to the site of the ***arterial ligament*** (Figure 10.7 panel A).

During the first few days of postnatal life, of course, the ***arterial duct*** remains patent (Figure 10.8). This arrangement, seen immediately after birth, reveals the presence of the ***isthmus***. This is the segment of the aortic arch between the origin of the left subclavian artery and the union between the arterial duct and the descending aorta. It is this part of the arch that is most usually hypoplastic in the setting of aortic coarctation, although when found later in adolescence or adulthood, as may still be the case, the coarctation lesion itself is usually a fibrous shelf formed at the site of insertion of the arterial ligament into the aorta.[10] In the normal arrangement it is the left subclavian artery that is the last branch from the aortic arch. Assessment of the overall population, nonetheless, reveals rare instances in which it is the ***right subclavian artery*** that is the last branch of the arch, with the artery itself taking a retro-oesophageal course. Such an arrangement, which can also underscore problems with swallowing, was found in 0.7% of individuals included in the meta-analysis.[9] The analysis showed several other variants of

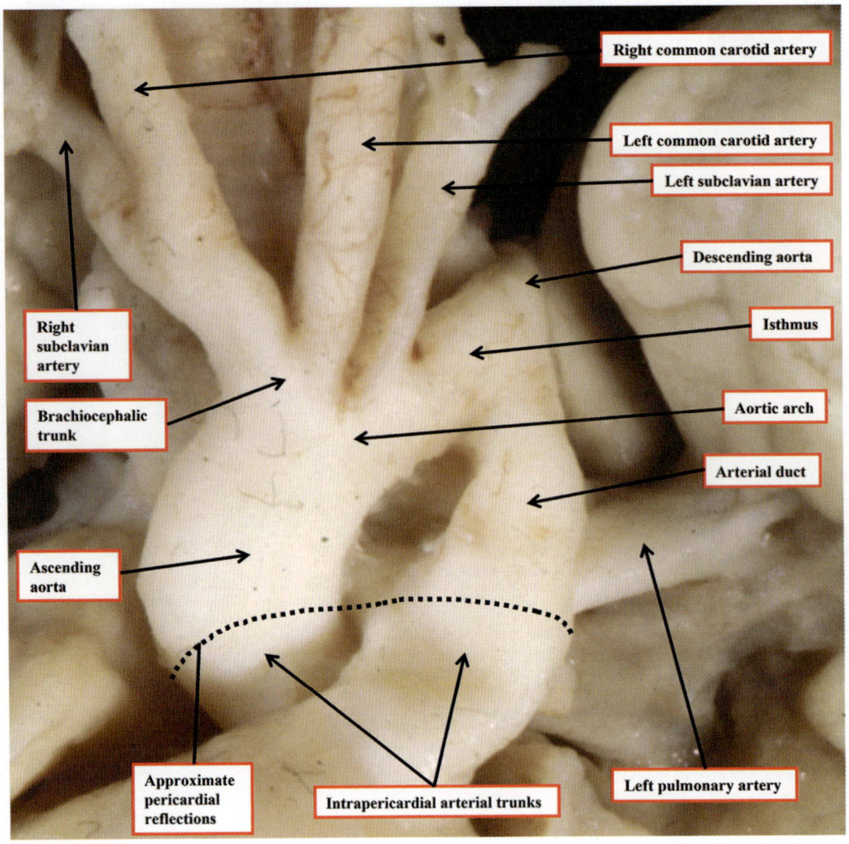

Figure 10.8. This image shows the arrangement of the extrapericardial pathways in the first days following birth. At this stage of neonatal life, the arterial duct remains patent and is the major pathway from the pulmonary trunk to the descending aorta. The segment of the aortic arch between the origin of the left subclavian artery and the union between the duct and the descending aorta is known as the isthmus. In this heart, the brachiocephalic trunk gives rise to not only the right common carotid and subclavian arteries, but also the left common carotid artery. This is the commonest variant in terms of branching in overall human populations. Although often described as the "bovine" variant, the arrangement bears no resemblance to the arrangements seen in oxen and other cattle.[11]

branching, with the second commonest pattern being the so-called "***bovine***" arrangement. In this variant, the brachiocephalic trunk gives rise to not only the right common carotid and subclavian arteries, but also the left common carotid artery (Figure 10.8). The adjective "bovine" is incorrect to describe the pattern, since cattle do not show this pattern.[11] Even though inappropriate, the name is unlikely to disappear. It is similarly unlikely that the term "innominate" will disappear as an alternative for the brachiocephalic trunk, although it is not clear why any structure should be considered to be "unnamed".

The ***pulmonary arteries***, having taken their origin extrapericardially from the pulmonary trunk, extend laterally to occupy the right and left pulmonary hilums, accompanied by the branches of the trachea and the right and left pulmonary veins. The vagus and phrenic nerves have important relationships to the pulmonary hilums, with the ***phrenic nerves*** coursing anteriorly across the pericardial sac and the vagus nerves turning posteriorly to approach the ***oesophagus***, having given off their recurrent laryngeal branches (Figure 10.9). In the usual situation, the left recurrent laryngeal nerve turns cranially around the aortic arch (Figure 10.7 panel B). The right nerve, in contrast, recurs around the right subclavian artery (Figure 10.9). Should the aortic arch be right-sided, as can happen in otherwise normal individuals,[9] it is the right recurrent laryngeal nerve that turns beneath the aortic arch, with the left nerve recurring around the left subclavian artery. There is a further recurrent neural pathway related to both subclavian arteries. This is the ***subclavian loop***, or the ansa subclavia. This part of the sympathetic nervous system supplies the iris. When diseased or damaged iatrogenically, it underscores ***Horner's syndrome***.[12]

On the right side, the ***azygos vein*** is an additional important component of the pulmonary hilum. Bringing back venous blood from the abdomen, this unpaired vessel opens into the superior caval vein in its extrapericardial course (Figure 10.10). The right phrenic nerve descends in front of the azygos vein, with the right vagus nerve turning posteriorly relative to the junction between the azygos and superior caval veins. On occasion, when the inferior caval vein is interrupted or diseased, the azygos vein can be the main venous tributary bringing back the abdominal venous return to the heart (see Chapter 4). When the caval vein is interrupted, however, the hepatic veins continue to drain the portal venous system to the right atrium.[13] The ***bronchuses***, the branches of the trachea, are the final components of the pulmonary hilums. In this regard, there is a significant morphological difference between the right and left bronchuses.

The morphologically left bronchus is significantly longer than its morphologically right partner, reflecting the fact that it is

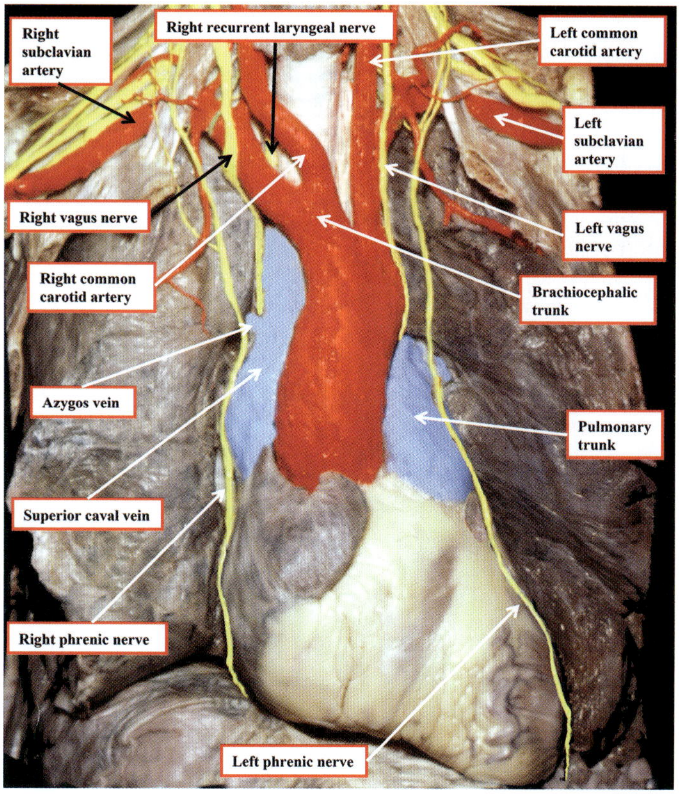

Figure 10.9. The heart has been dissected and coloured to show the relationship of the vagus and phrenic nerves to the extrapericardial pathways and the heart itself, albeit that the heart is usually enclosed within its fibrous pericardial sac. Note that the laryngeal nerve on the right side recurs around the right subclavian artery, whereas on the left side it turns around the aortic arch (see Figure 10.7). When the arch is rarely right-sided, it is the left nerve that will recur around the subclavian artery.

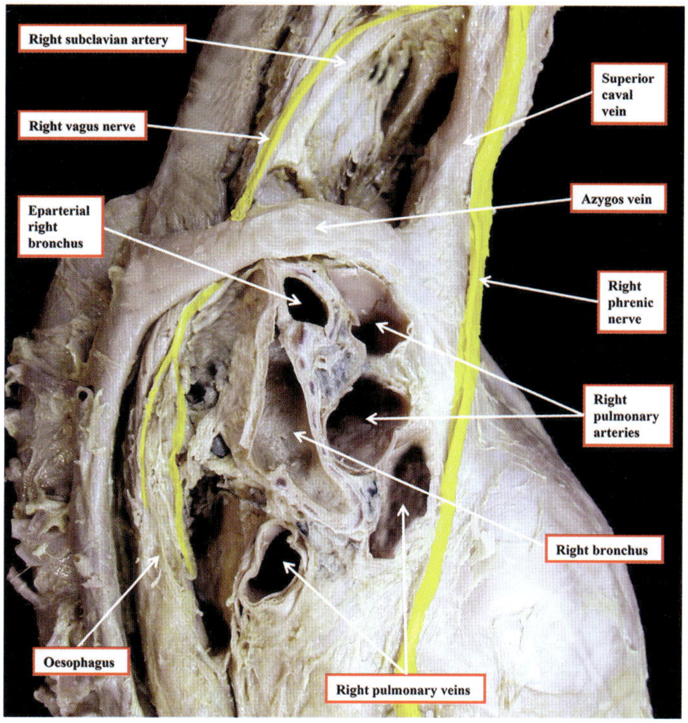

Figure 10.10. The right pulmonary hilum has been dissected to show its component parts, with the right vagus and phrenic nerves coloured yellow. Note their relationship to the azygos vein, which itself empties into the extrapericardial component of the superior caval vein.

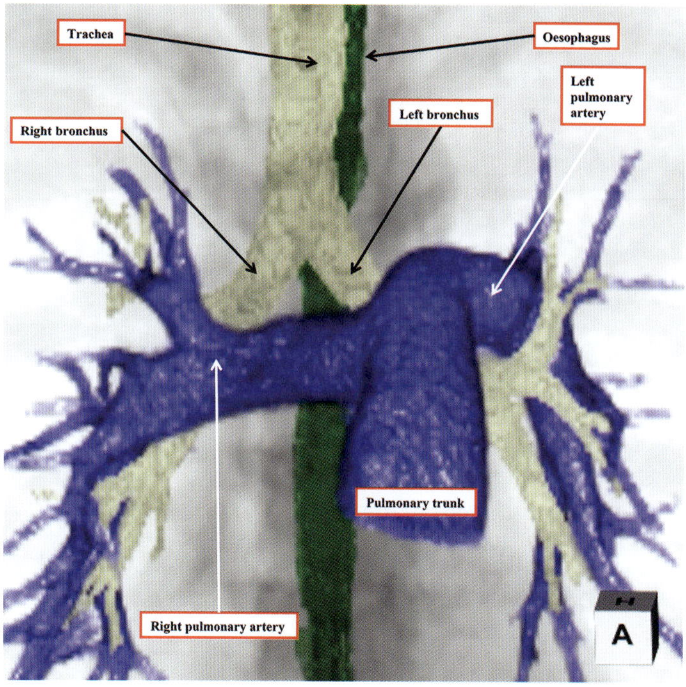

Figure 10.11. The image shows a reconstruction of the tracheobronchial tree from a computed tomographic dataset prepared from a normal adult individual. The morphologically left bronchus is significantly longer than the morphologically right bronchus. In addition, the right bronchus gives off its first branch before it is crossed by the branch of the right pulmonary artery supplying the middle and lower lobes of the right lung, making the first bronchial branch eparterial, or above the artery, as opposed to the left bronchus, which is hyparterial, not giving off its first branch before it has been crossed by the left pulmonary artery.

crossed by the aortic arch when the arch itself is left-sided (Figure 10.11). The right bronchus also gives off its first branch before it is crossed by the branches of the pulmonary artery, making the bronchus eparterial (Figure 10.10). The first branch of the morphologically left bronchus, in contrast, is hyparterial. It takes its origin only after the bronchus has been crossed by the left pulmonary artery. These arrangements serve to distinguish between the morphologically right and left bronchuses in the setting of so-called ***visceral heterotaxy***, where the thoracic organs, along with the bronchial tree, can show evidence of isomerism rather than being lateralized.[14]

REFERENCES

1. Van Praagh R. Terminology of congenital heart disease. Glossary and commentary. *Circulation*. 1977;**56**:139–143. doi: 10.1161/01.cir.56.2.139
2. Anderson RH, Becker AE, Freedom RM, Macartney FJ, Quero-Jimenez M, Shinebourne EA, Wilkinson JL, Tynan M. Sequential segmental analysis of congenital heart disease. *Pediatr Cardiol*. 1984;**5**:281–287. doi: 10.1007/BF02424973
3. Anderson RH, Lamers WH, Hikspoors J, Mohun TJ, Bamforth SD, Chaudhry B, Eley L, Kerwin J, Crosier M, Henderson DJ. Development of the arterial roots and ventricular outflow tracts. *J Anat*. 2024;**244**:497–513. doi: 10.1111/joa.13973
4. Muriago M, Sheppard MN, Ho SY, Anderson RH. Location of the coronary arterial orifices in the normal

heart. *Clin Anat*. 1997;**10**:297–302. doi: 10.1002/(SICI)1098-2353(1997)10:5<297::AID-CA1>3.0.CO;2-O
5. Frescura C, Basso C, Thiene G, Corrado D, Pennelli T, Angelini A, Daliento L. Anomalous origin of coronary arteries and risk of sudden death: a study based on an autopsy population of congenital heart disease. *Hum Pathol*. 1998;**29**:689–695. doi: 10.1016/s0046-8177(98)90277-5
6. Li J, Tulloh RM, Cook A, Schneider M, Ho SY, Anderson RH. Coronary arterial origins in transposition of the great arteries: factors that affect outcome. A morphological and clinical study. *Heart*. 2000;**83**:320–325. doi: 10.1136/heart.83.3.320
7. Ho SY, Gerlis LM, Anderson C, Devine WA, Smith AV. The morphology of aortopulmonary windows with regard to their classification and morphogenesis. *Cardiol Young*. 1994;**4**:146–155. doi: 10.1017/S1047951100002092
8. Weinberg PM. Aortic arch anomalies. *J Cardiovasc Magn Reson*. 2006;**8**:633–643. doi: 10.1080/10976640600713756
9. Popieluszko P, Henry BM, Sanna B, Hsieh WC, Saganiak K, Pękala PA, Walocha JA, Tomaszewski KA. A systematic review and meta-analysis of variations in branching patterns of the adult aortic arch. *J Vasc Surg*. 2018;**68**:298–306.e210. doi: 10.1016/j.jvs.2017.06.097
10. Dijkema EJ, Leiner T, Grotenhuis HB. Diagnosis, imaging and clinical management of aortic coarctation. *Heart*. 2017;**103**:1148–1155. doi: 10.1136/heartjnl-2017-311173
11. Layton KF, Kallmes DF, Cloft HJ, Lindell EP, Cox VS. Bovine aortic arch variant in humans: clarification of a common misnomer. *AJNR Am J Neuroradiol*. 2006;**27**:1541–1542. PMID: 16908576
12. Walton KA, Buono LM. Horner syndrome. *Curr Opin Ophthalmol*. 2003;**14**:357–363. doi: 10.1097/00055735-200312000-00007
13. Piciucchi S, Barone D, Sanna S, Dubini A, Goodman LR, Oboldi D, Bertocco M, Ciccotosto C, Gavelli G, Carloni A, Poletti V. The azygos vein pathway: an overview from anatomical variations to pathological changes. *Insights Imaging*. 2014;**5**:619–628. doi: 10.1007/s13244-014-0351-3
14. Loomba RS, Pelech AN, Shah PH, Anderson RH. Determining bronchial morphology for the purposes of segregating so-called heterotaxy. *Cardiol Young*. 2016;**26**:725–737. doi: 10.1017/S1047951115001195

11

The Coronary Vasculature

The heart, which drives the overall circulation, requires its own vascular supply. This is provided by the coronary arteries which take their origin from the aortic root. The blood is then returned to the heart through the coronary veins. There is a third component of the coronary vasculature. This is the lymphatic drainage from the heart, which has been least well investigated and least well understood.[1] The role of the lymphatic component is now becoming increasingly appreciated, thanks to the ability to recognize the lymphatic channels using clinical imagery, at least within the body if not yet the heart. The advent of HiP-CT technology also permits the recognition of the location of the lymphatic channels within the heart.

The Coronary Arterial Circulation

The major coronary arteries are the first branches of the aorta, emerging from the sinuses of the aortic root that are adjacent to the subpulmonary infundibulum (Figure 11.1).[2] There are three sinuses within the aortic root, but only two major coronary arteries. The aortic sinus that is not adjacent to the infundibulum does not usually give rise to a coronary artery. This permits the sinuses themselves to be named as being ***non-coronary***, ***right coronary***, and ***left coronary*** (Figure 11.2).

Very rarely, even in otherwise normal individuals, the sinus that is not adjacent to the infundibulum can give rise to a coronary artery.[3] In those circumstances, it would be inappropriate to label the sinus as being non-coronary. It can then be described as being ***non-adjacent***. In other circumstances, all the coronary arteries arise from the same sinus of the aortic root, leaving not only the non-adjacent but one of the adjacent sinuses without a coronary artery. Such arrangements are more frequent when the heart is congenitally malformed, but origin of a coronary artery from an inappropriate sinus, particularly when the artery in question takes an intramural

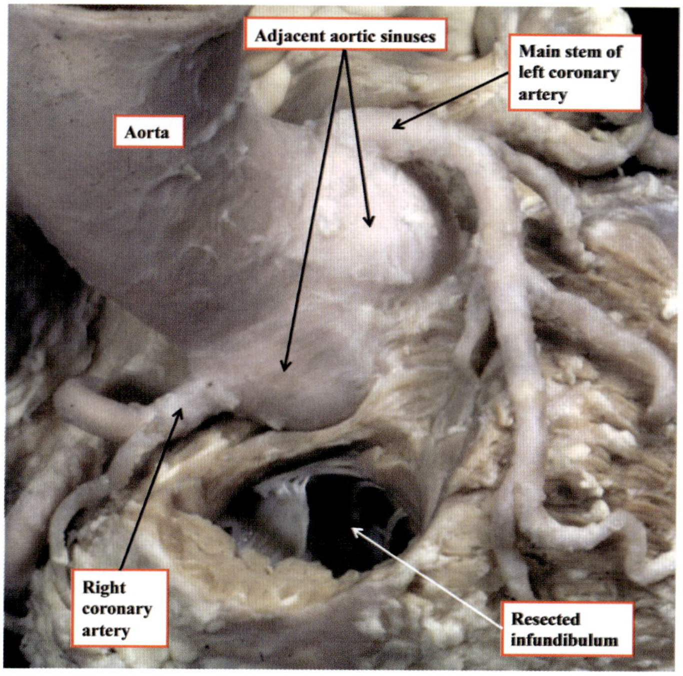

Figure 11.1. The pulmonary root and its supporting infundibulum have been removed to show the anterior surface of the aortic root. The right and left coronary arteries take their origin from the aortic valvar sinuses adjacent to the pulmonary root.

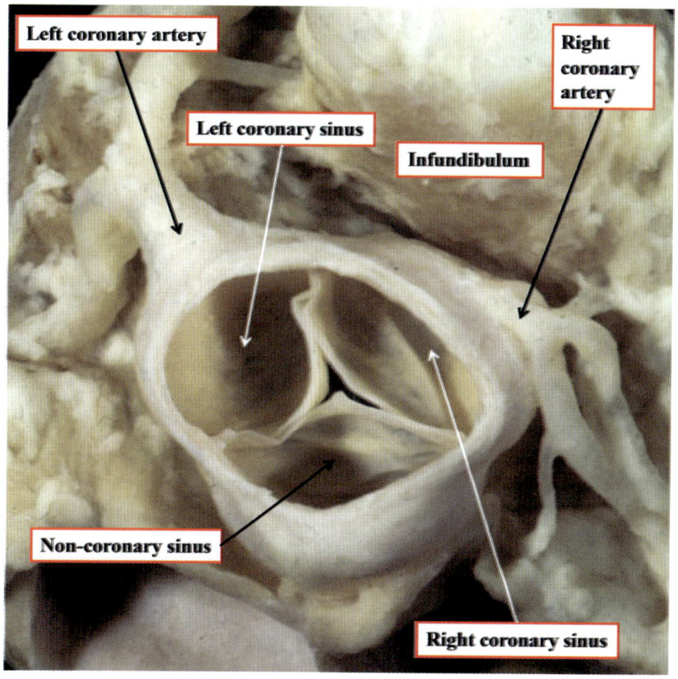

Figure 11.2. The subpulmonary infundibulum has been reflected anterior and the intrapericardial aorta removed at the level of the sinutubular junction. It can be seen that the right and left coronary arteries take their origin from the sinuses of the aortic root adjacent to the infundibulum. The third sinus does not usually give rise to a coronary artery and hence can be described as the non-coronary sinus. In rare instances, however, a coronary artery may arise from the third sinus and can be described as being non-adjacent.

course between the aorta and pulmonary artery, is increasingly recognized as a cause of sudden cardiac death. It is convenient to have a means of describing the aortic valvar sinuses, therefore, that is independent of either the location of the aortic root in space or the origin of the coronary arteries. This is provided by considering one sinus, as described above, as being non-adjacent relative to the pulmonary root. The other sinuses can then be described as viewed by the observer standing in the non-adjacent sinus and looking towards the pulmonary root (Figure 11.3). One of the sinuses is then to the right hand of the observer and is conventionally known as ***sinus 1***. The other sinus is to the left hand and is known as ***sinus 2***.[4] It is, of course, also possible to describe the sinuses according to the attitudinal location. Nonetheless, when comparing the origins of the coronary arteries in congenitally malformed hearts with paired arterial roots, it helps to have a system that continues to work irrespective of the rotation or tilt of the roots. The convention of distinguishing the sinuses according to their adjacency to the pulmonary root was designed to cater for the need to make such comparisons, particularly in the setting of discordant ventriculo-arterial connections.[4]

The vessels arising directly from the aortic root are the ***right*** and ***left coronary arteries***. The left coronary artery usually originates within the middle third and the right coronary artery within the posterior third of their respective sinuses, though with marked variability (Figure 11.4 panel A).[5] Preprocedural identification of arteries originating immediately adjacent to a commissure helps to plan the appropriate modified surgical or transcatheter approach in those individuals considered for valvar-sparing root replacements or implantation of a bioprosthetic aortic valve.[6] On occasion, either the right or the left coronary artery can be found taking its origin well above the sinutubular junction (Figure 11.4 panel B).[7] As with origin of the arteries relative to the valvar commissures, a potential

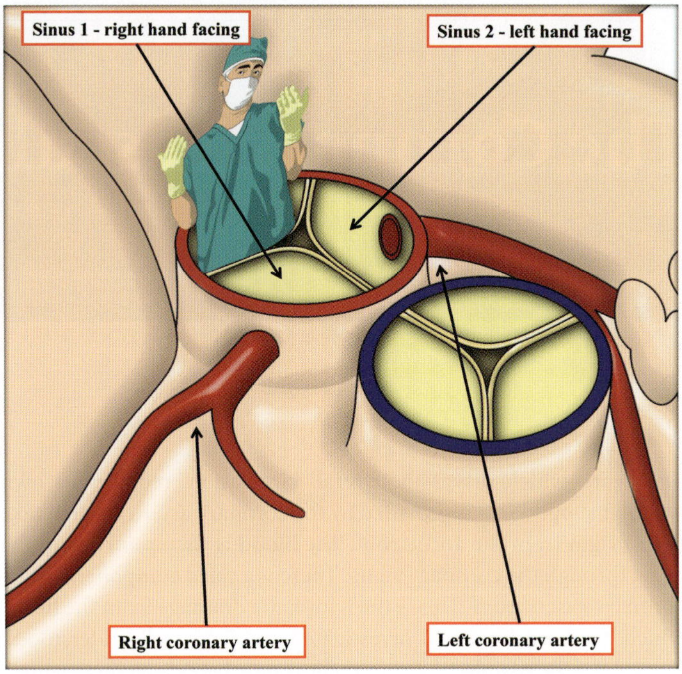

Figure 11.3. The drawing shows the concept used for identifying the sinuses of the aortic root that is independent of the origin of the coronary arteries. The observer, shown in the drawing as a surgeon, positions himself or herself in the non-adjacent aortic valvar sinus. In hearts with trisinuate aortic roots, the adjacent sinuses are then always to either the right hand or the left hand of the observer. By convention, the sinus to the right hand is numbered 1. In the normal heart, this sinus gives rise to the right coronary artery. The sinus to the left hand is numbered 2, and usually it gives rise to the left coronary artery. The original drawing was made by Mrs Gemma Price and has been modified with her permission.

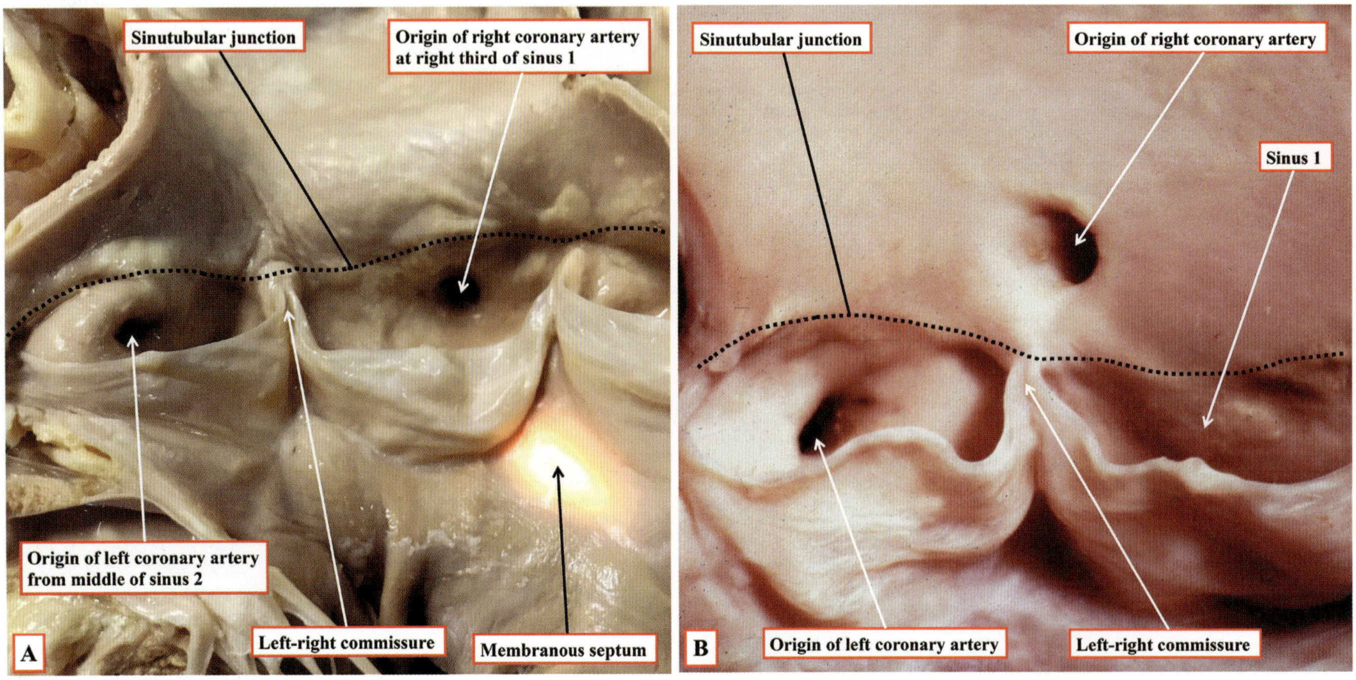

Figure 11.4. The image in panel A illustrates the opened aortic root viewed from behind, with the membranous septum transilluminated from the right side. The arrangement shown for the coronary arteries is the usual pattern. Both coronary arteries arise within the sinuses of the root adjacent to the pulmonary trunk. The orifice of the left coronary artery is more-or-less in the middle of the sinus, whereas the orifice of the right coronary artery is located towards the commissure between sinus 1 and the non-coronary aortic sinus. In the arrangement illustrated in panel B, again showing the opened aortic root from behind, the left coronary artery takes its anticipated origin from sinus 2, but the right coronary artery originates at least 1 cm above the sinutubular junction. This is high take-off of the right coronary artery, but in this case there was no intramurality of the artery.

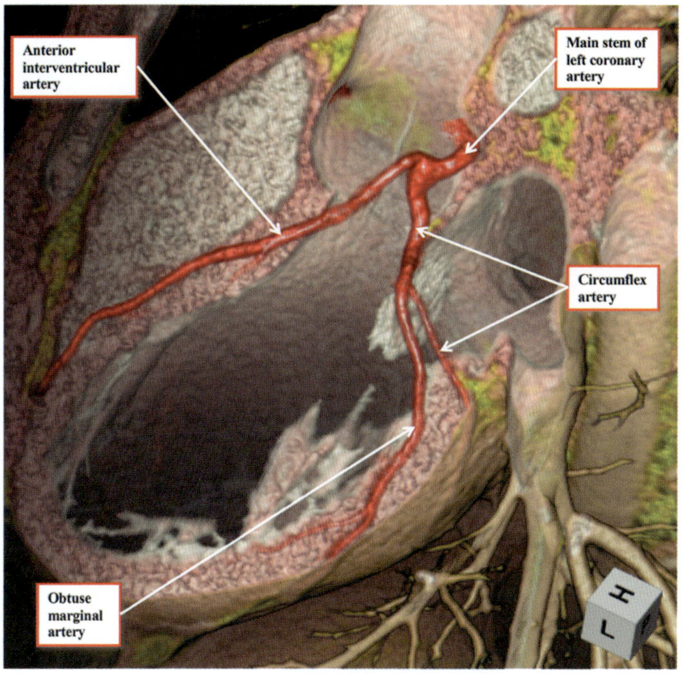

Figure 11.5. The clinical computed tomogram, shown in left lateral projection, has been segmented to show the branches of the left coronary artery. The left artery itself has a very short main stem before it divides into its anterior interventricular and circumflex branches. The circumflex artery then gives rise to a major obtuse marginal branch, diminishing in size as it enters the left atrioventricular groove.

significance of high origin is the relationship of the feature to sudden cardiac death. This, in turn, requires a uniform definition for "high origin". In a review of the literature providing details of nearly 13,000 reports, the criterion proposed for high origin was a distance greater than 1 cm above the sinutubular junction in adult hearts, or greater than one-fifth the depth of the supporting valvar sinus in those yet to reach adulthood.[8] When using these values, high take-off was exceedingly rare, at no more than 0.2% within the general population, with only one-tenth of these reported cases associated with sudden cardiac death. This suggests that the extent of intramurality is likely to be the key feature in determining the pathogenicity of the finding.

Irrespective of its precise origin from the aortic root, the ***left coronary artery*** has a very short course. This is because it divides rapidly into the anterior interventricular and circumflex arteries (Figure 11.5). This means that, although only two coronary arteries arise from the aortic root, the overall coronary arterial circulation can be assessed in terms of three major vessels, namely the ***right***, ***anterior interventricular***, and ***circumflex arteries***. The anterior interventricular artery is usually described by cardiologists as the left anterior descending coronary artery.

The right coronary and the circumflex arteries occupy the atrioventricular grooves (Figure 11.6), whereas the anterior interventricular artery is positioned within the anterior interventricular groove (Figure 11.7). It is these locations that underscore the patterns of the branches of these three major coronary arteries.

There is then a fourth major coronary artery, which occupies the inferior interventricular groove (Figure 11.8). It follows that this

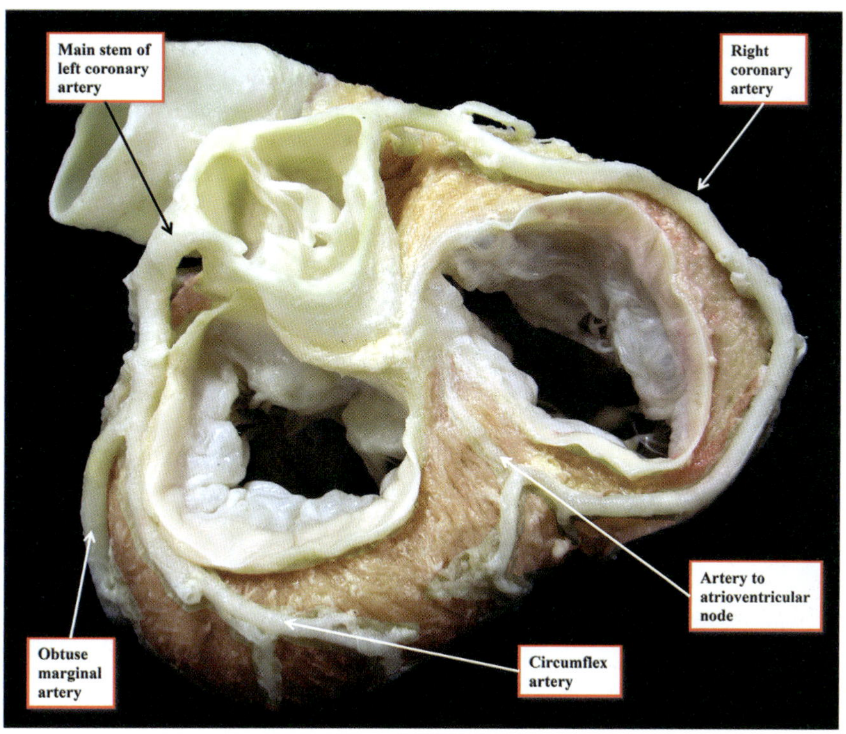

Figure 11.6. The heart has been dissected to show how the circumflex and right coronary arteries occupy the atrioventricular grooves. The circumflex artery gives rise to a major obtuse marginal branch prior to entering the left atrioventricular groove. The right coronary artery, in contrast, gives rise to the artery of the atrioventricular node at the crux, continuing to supply part of the diaphragmatic wall of the left ventricle. This is right coronary arterial dominance. The right coronary artery also gives rise to the inferior interventricular artery, which is not well seen in this dissection.

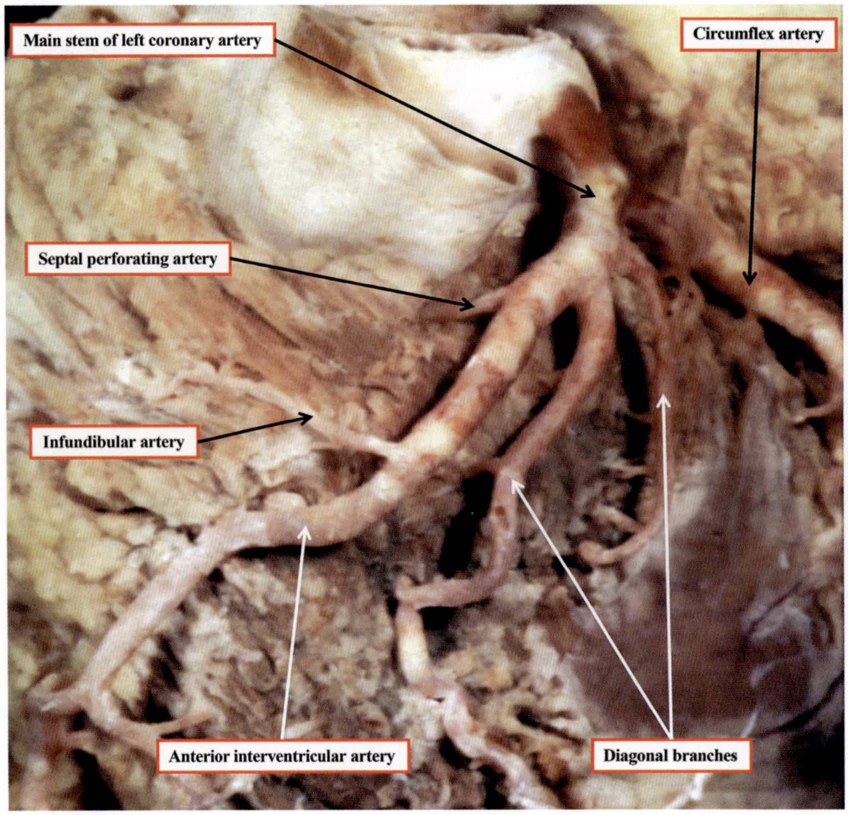

Figure 11.7. The location of the anterior interventricular artery in the anterior interventricular groove permits it to provide perforating branches directly into the crest of the ventricular septum, along with diagonal branches to supply the anterior wall of the left ventricle, and an infundibular branch to supply the subpulmonary infundibulum.

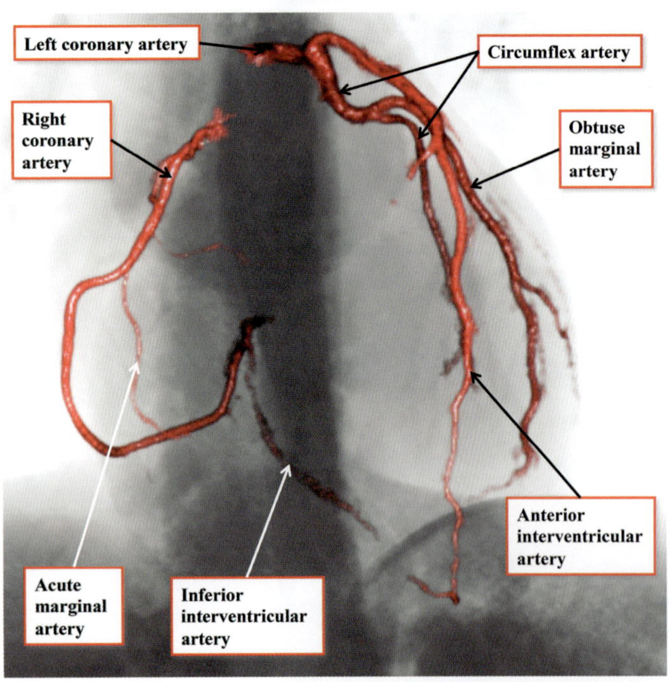

Figure 11.8. This is the same computed tomogram as was shown in Figure 11.5, but in this image shown in frontal projection. The artery that for many years was described as the posterior descending artery can be seen to supply the diaphragmatic surface of the ventricular mass. In this patient, the artery does descend as it moves towards the apex of the ventricular mass, but it is better described as being inferior rather than posterior.

vessel, which irrigates the diaphragmatic surface of the heart, is the ***inferior interventricular artery***. Generations of both anatomists and cardiologists have incorrectly named this artery as being posterior and descending. The very fact that the artery branches to supply the diaphragmatic surface of the ventricular mass indicates that it is inferior, as well as being posterior. It is not always the case, furthermore, that the artery descends as it runs its course towards the apex of the ventricular cone. More significantly, it has long been accepted that occlusion of the artery produces inferior myocardial ischaemia or infarction. The advent of three-dimensional reconstructions of computed tomographic datasets now leaves little doubt that the artery is inferior and interventricular (Figure 11.8). This artery, together with the collateral vessels that develop in the context of chronic total occlusions, may play a role in the retrograde approach for revascularization.[9]

It is the origin of the inferior interventricular artery, furthermore, which underscores the concept of ***coronary arterial dominance***. In about four-fifths of individuals, it is the right coronary artery that gives rise to the inferior interventricular artery. In these individuals, the right coronary artery then usually continues beyond the crux to supply the diaphragmatic surface of the left ventricle, thus producing ***right coronary arterial dominance*** (Figure 11.9).

At the crux, when dominant, the right coronary artery also gives rise to the artery that supplies the atrioventricular node. In about one-tenth of individuals, it is the circumflex artery that gives rise to the interventricular artery, with the artery often continuing beyond the crux to supply the inferior wall of the right ventricle. This arrangement is described as ***left coronary arterial dominance*** (Figure 11.10).

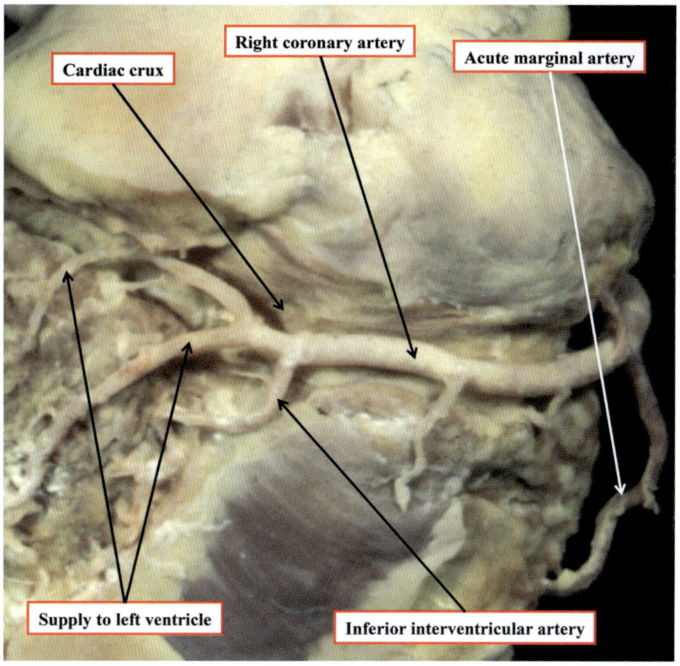

Figure 11.9. The heart has been turned to show its inferior surface. The right coronary artery gives rise to the inferior interventricular artery at the crux and continues to supply the diaphragmatic surface of the left ventricle. This is another example of right coronary arterial dominance.

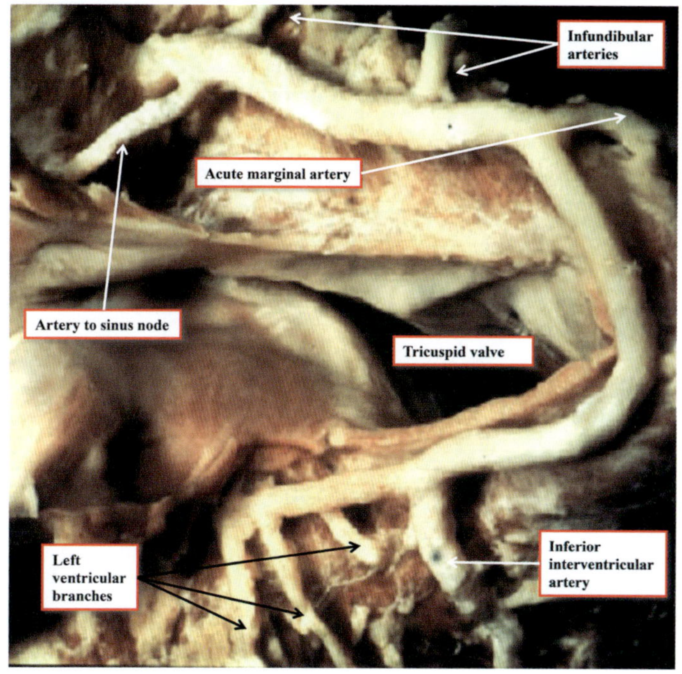

Figure 11.11. The right atrioventricular groove has been dissected to show the usual arrangement of the right coronary artery. In this example, as in three-fifths of individuals, its first branch is the artery to the sinus node.

In this setting, the artery to the atrioventricular node arises from the circumflex artery. In the remaining one-tenth of individuals, both the right and circumflex arteries provide branches to the inferior walls of the ventricular cone at the crux. This produces a balanced pattern to the circulation.

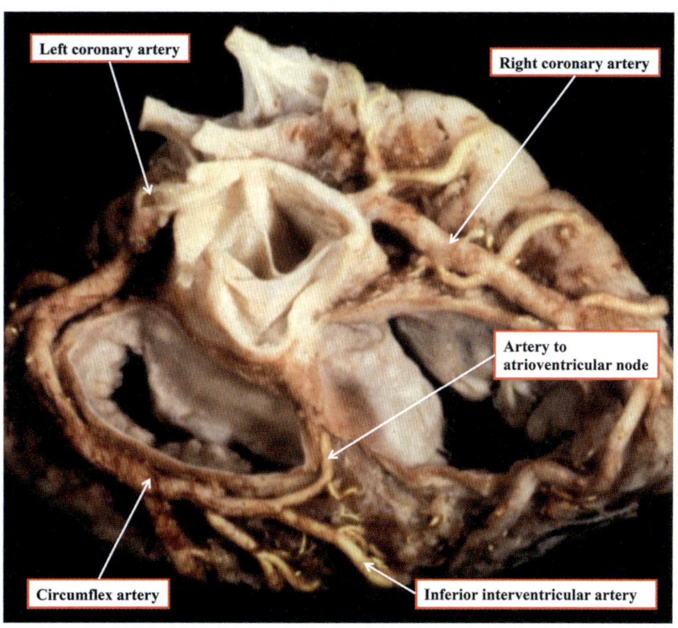

Figure 11.10. The heart has been dissected to show the atrioventricular grooves. The circumflex artery gives rise to the artery to the atrioventricular node and the inferior interventricular artery. This is an example of left coronary arterial dominance. Note that the circumflex artery is much more closely related to the left atrioventricular junction than when the right coronary artery is dominant.

The ***right coronary artery*** enters the right atrioventricular groove directly above the supraventricular crest of the right ventricle. It then encircles the parts of the right atrioventricular junction from which hinge the antero-superior and -inferior leaflets of the tricuspid valve (Figure 11.11).

In approximately three-fifths of individuals, the first branch of the right coronary artery supplies the ***sinus node*** (Figure 11.12 panel A). At the acute margin of the junction, the right coronary artery gives rise to the ***acute marginal artery***. As already explained, in four-fifths of individuals, having entered the inferior right atrioventricular junction, the right coronary artery gives rise to the inferior interventricular artery, usually then continuing to supply parts of the inferior wall of the left ventricle in the arrangement known as right dominance (Figure 11.9). Again, as emphasized, it is the dominant coronary artery that supplies the artery to the atrioventricular node (***atrioventricular nodal artery***). Thus, when the left coronary artery is dominant, the nodal artery arises from the circumflex artery at the crux.[10] In addition to the supply provided by the artery to the atrioventricular node, which ascends within the inferior pyramidal space, the node can be supplied by the septal branches of the left anterior interventricular artery.[10–12]

The main stem of the left coronary artery exits from the aortic root to enter the space directly behind the subpulmonary infundibulum, with the tubular left atrial appendage forming the roof of the space (Figure 11.13). This area of the ventricular base beneath the artery is the ***left ventricular summit***. It receives this name because, when viewed attitudinally, it is the most superior part of the myocardium making up the ventricular cone.[13] The wall extending inferiorly and posteriorly from the area of the summit is the ventricular component of the mural atrioventricular junction. The main stem of the ***left coronary artery*** branches within the area of the summit into the ***anterior interventricular*** and ***circumflex*** arteries, often giving

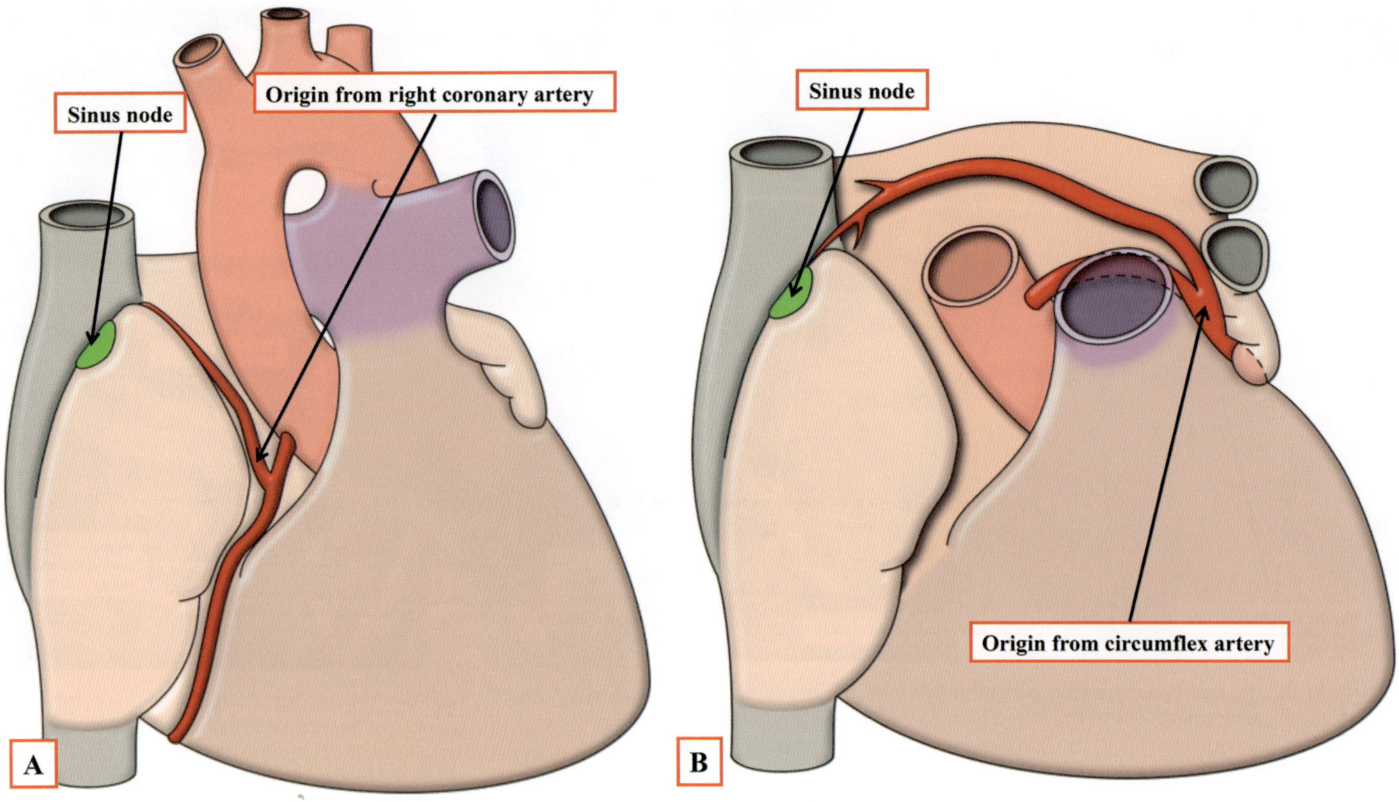

Figure 11.12. The drawings show the arrangement of the sinus node artery when it arises, as in the case of three-fifths of the population, from the right coronary artery (panel A), and in the remaining two-fifths from the circumflex artery (panel B). As shown in these drawings, the artery in either instance is usually the first branch of the parent artery. In some circumstances, however, the artery can arise more distally. When arising from the right coronary artery it then crosses the right atrial appendage, whereas when arising from the circumflex artery it crosses the dome of the left atrium from behind. The original drawings were made by Mrs Gemma Price and have been modified with her permission.

off a third ***intermediate*** branch (Figure 11.13).[14] The ***left anterior interventricular*** artery, also frequently described as being ***anterior descending***, has an oblique course as it extends towards the cardiac apex through the anterior interventricular groove (Figures 11.5, 11.8). It gives rise to diagonal branches that supply blood to the left ventricular myocardium, and important septal perforating branches that supply blood to the muscular ventricular septum. These perforating branches also supply the branches of the atrioventricular conduction axis. The right bundle branch is supplied only by the septal perforating arteries. The left bundle branch, in contrast, is supplied by both septal perforating arteries and the atrioventricular nodal artery. Thus, left bundle branch block in the setting of acute myocardial infarction does not automatically suggest isolated occlusion of the left anterior interventricular artery. Occlusion of the first septal perforating branch of the left anterior interventricular artery is known to produce right bundle branch block.[15]

The ***circumflex artery*** runs its course within the left atrioventricular groove, extending to various degrees to supply the diaphragmatic surface of the heart. In two-fifths of individuals, it gives rise, as its first branch, to the artery supplying the sinus node (Figure 11.12 panel B). Its more constant branches are the ***obtuse marginal artery***, additional ***marginal branches***, and sometimes an ***infero-lateral branch***. When dominant, as is the case in around one-tenth of individuals, the artery gives rise to the inferior interventricular artery, usually then continuing to supply the diaphragmatic wall of the right ventricle (Figure 11.10). And, to emphasize again, in this setting the dominant circumflex artery will also give rise to the artery supplying the atrioventricular node. The ***intermediate artery*** (Figure 11.13) is found when there is trifurcation of the main stem of the left coronary artery. The intermediate artery then has a distribution similar to that of a diagonal branch of the anterior interventricular artery, or the obtuse marginal artery.[16]

Many congenital coronary arterial anomalies have been described, reflecting their abnormal embryonic development.[2] As already discussed, anomalous origin from an unexpected aortic valvar sinus is now recognized as a frequent cause of sudden cardiac death, particularly when the artery takes an intramural course across a commissure of the aortic root (Figure 11.14). A more severe congenital variant is found when one of the coronary arteries takes origin from the pulmonary trunk or one of its branches.[17]

The Coronary Venous System

The cardiac venous system is divided into the ***greater*** and ***lesser components***. The greater system, made up of the veins located in the outer layer of the myocardium, drains in its greater part to the coronary sinus (Figure 11.15). The ***anterior cardiac veins*** and the lesser venous vasculature, with the latter forming the ***Thebesian system***,[18] in contrast drain directly into the cavities of the atrial chambers.

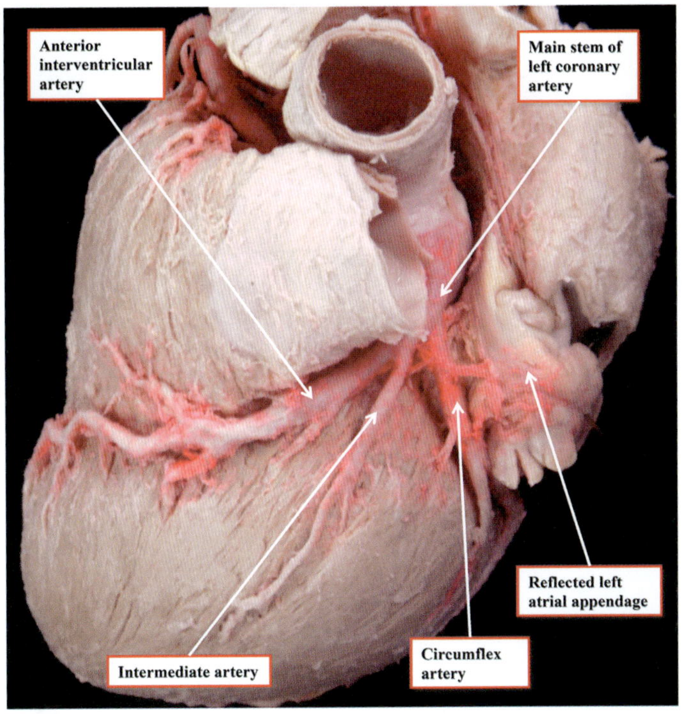

Figure 11.13. The heart is photographed from the left lateral side, having reflected the left atrial appendage. This shows how the main stem of the left coronary artery enters the space between the left appendage and the subpulmonary infundibulum. It rests on the area of the ventricular cone known as the left ventricular summit. In this heart, the left coronary artery trifurcates, giving rise to an intermediate branch, which replaces the obtuse marginal branch of the circumflex artery.

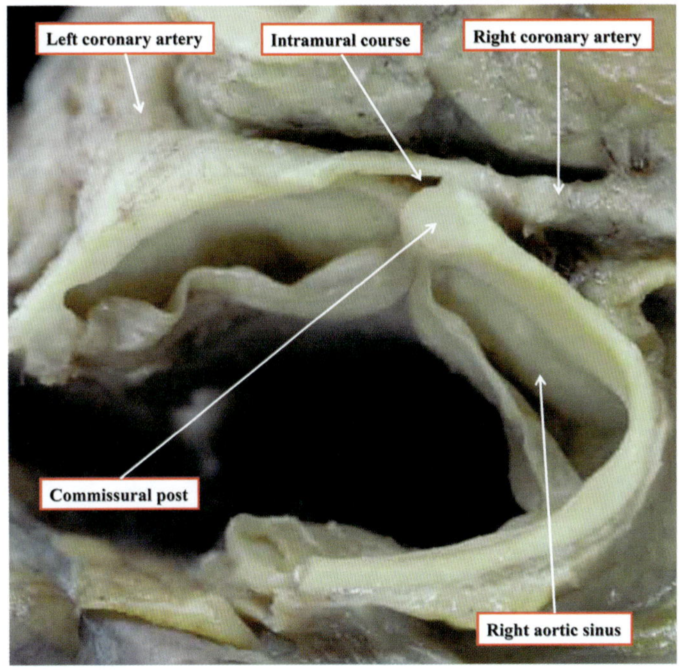

Figure 11.14. In this heart, the right coronary artery takes an intramural course, crossing the commissure between the sinuses which are adjacent to the pulmonary trunk. In consequence, the left-sided sinus of the aortic root gives rise to both the right and left coronary arteries. Such an intramural arrangement, with origin from an unexpected aortic valvar sinus, can be a harbinger of sudden cardiac death.

The ***coronary sinus*** is formed at the union of the great cardiac vein and the oblique vein of the left atrium. It then runs, with its own walls, within the left atrioventricular groove, opening into the cavity of the right atrium (Figures 11.15, 11.16, 11.17). Its major tributary is the great cardiac vein, which accompanies the anterior interventricular artery as it ascends within the anterior interventricular groove. The ***great cardiac vein*** enters the inferior atrioventricular groove at the left ventricular summit, where it receives the ***obtuse marginal vein***. Within the inferior atrioventricular groove, it receives the ***inferior left ventricular vein*** before it is joined by the ***oblique vein*** to form the coronary sinus. The oblique vein is also known as the ***vein of Marshall***. It is a remnant of the left superior caval vein, with the coronary sinus itself being the persisting component of the left sinus horn seen during early embryonic development (see Chapter 2).

On this basis, the junction between the oblique vein and the great cardiac vein can be used to provide the best marker for the distal boundary of the coronary sinus. It is usual, nonetheless, to find a prominent valve at the junction, which is known as the ***valve of Vieussens*** (Figure 11.16). Others take the site of the valve of Vieussens as marking the boundary of the coronary sinus. An additional remnant of the left superior caval vein, continuous with the oblique vein, can be seen as the ***ligament of Marshall***.[19] The ligament, at its junction with the oblique vein, co-locates with the autonomic nerves feeding left atrial ganglionated plexuses.[20] It was often

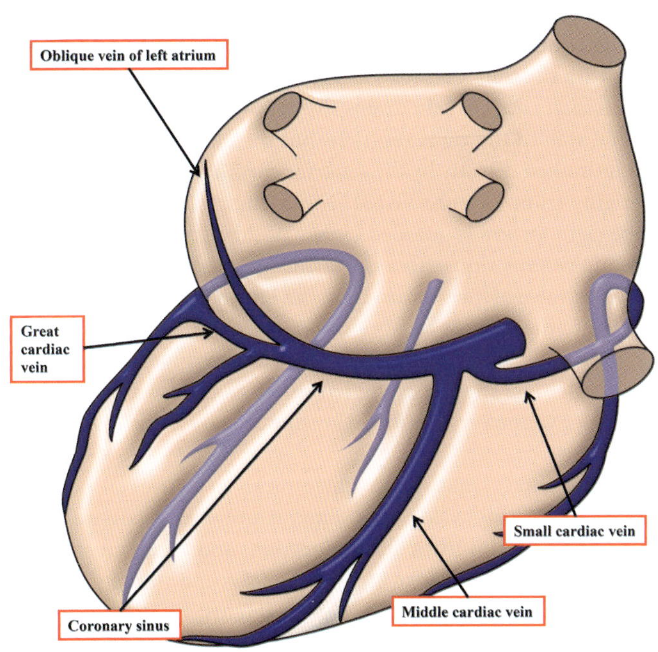

Figure 11.15. The drawing, showing the heart as seen from behind, illustrates the pattern of the greater cardiac venous system, with the cardiac veins being tributaries of the coronary sinus. The original drawing was made by Mrs Gemma Price and has been modified with her permission.

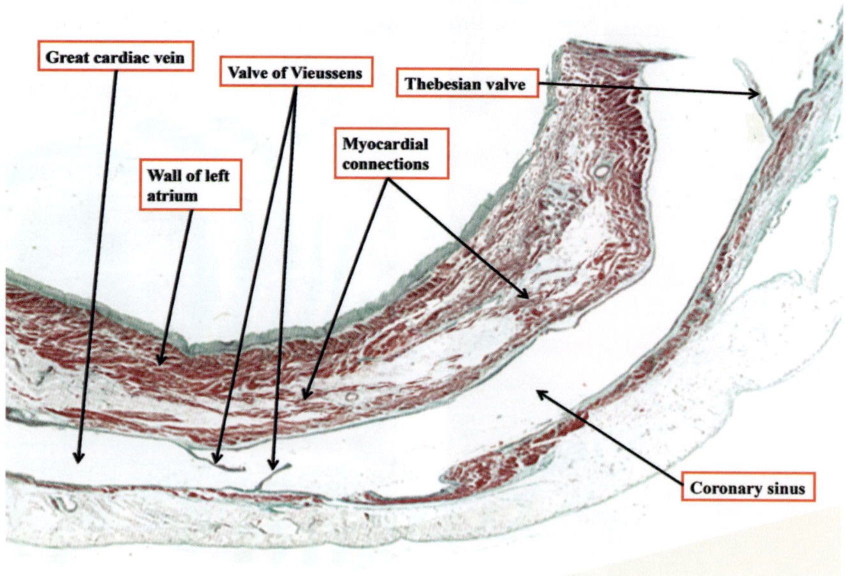

Figure 11.16. The histological section shows the course of the coronary sinus through the left atrioventricular groove. Note the location of the valve of Vieussens at the junction between the great cardiac vein and the coronary sinus. Note also the presence of a second valve, the Thebesian valve, which guards the entrance of the sinus to the right atrium. Note in addition the myocardial strands that pass between the walls of the coronary sinus and the left atrium.

claimed that the myocardial wall of the coronary sinus was shared with the vestibular wall of the left atrium. In fact, the two walls are discrete and separate, although myocardial strands extend between the two layers (Figure 11.16).[21] The middle and small cardiac veins join the coronary sinus at the cardiac crux (Figure 11.17). The ***middle vein*** accompanies the inferior interventricular artery, whilst the small cardiac vein occupies the right atrioventricular groove along with the right coronary artery.

The ***small cardiac vein*** drains the majority of the blood from the parietal wall of the right ventricle, but the blood from the anterior wall is drained directly by the ***anterior cardiac veins*** to the cavity of the right atrium (Figure 11.18). The opening of the coronary sinus to the right atrium is guarded by one of the persisting valves of the systemic venous sinus. This is the ***Thebesian valve*** (Figure 11.16). The other valve of the venous sinus, the ***Eustachian valve***, guards the opening of the inferior caval vein.

On occasion, the Thebesian valve can be imperforate (Figure 11.19 panel A). The persisting left superior caval vein then drains the greater venous system to the brachiocephalic vein (Figure 11.19 panel B).

The coronary sinus is an anatomical structure of particular interest to electrophysiologists. First, it provides access to epicardial accessory atrioventricular connections and to the substrates for both atrial and ventricular arrhythmias. Second, the myocardium that wraps around the coronary sinus (Figure 11.16) can itself be a source of atrial arrhythmias.[22,23] At its distal extent, the left atrial ridge is a reliable endocardial target for radiofrequency ablation of the vein of Marshall.[24] Inside the atrium, a prominent ridge lies between the orifices of the left pulmonary veins and the ostium of the appendage. Epicardially, the ridge is a fold containing the remnant of the oblique vein or ligament of Marshall with its accompanying autonomic nerves and can be the source of atrial arrhythmia. It can be approached and ablated through the distal coronary sinus.[25] In

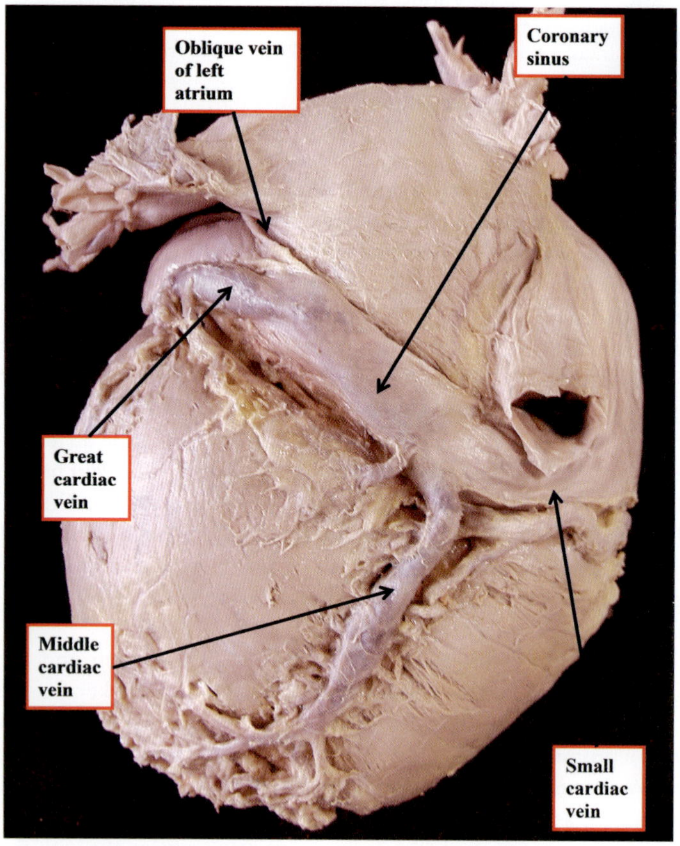

Figure 11.17. The diaphragmatic surface of the heart has been dissected to show the tributaries of the coronary sinus. The sinus itself has as its distal boundary the junction between the great cardiac vein and the oblique vein of the left atrium, which is ligamentous in this specimen as it extends between the left pulmonary veins and the left atrial appendage. This is the ligament of Marshall.

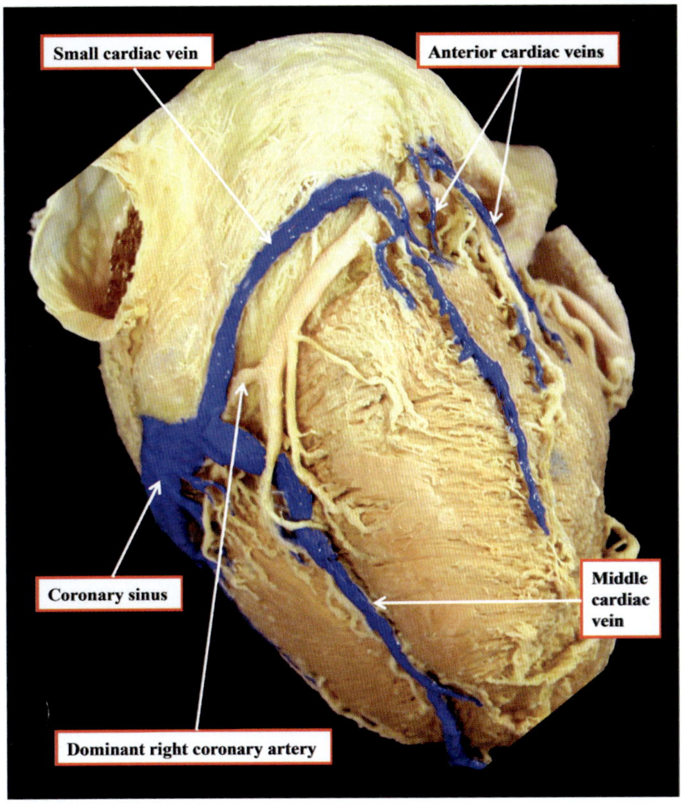

Figure 11.18. The inferior and anterior walls of the right ventricle have been dissected to show the location of the middle and small cardiac veins, along with the anterior cardiac veins. The veins themselves have been coloured blue.

a randomized comparison, however, empirical isolation of the coronary sinus using either endocardiac or epicardial lesions as an adjunct to isolation of the pulmonary veins, even when combined with a roofline ablation, was not associated with improved freedom from atrial arrhythmias.[26]

In addition to the venous tributaries that drain directly to the coronary sinus, and the anterior cardiac veins, there are multiple small veins that, like the anterior veins, drain directly to the cavities of the right and left atrial chambers. These are the ***Thebesian veins***, which together make up the lesser cardiac venous system.[27] The small venous channels are found throughout the myocardium. They drain to a subendocardial system of vessels, which, in turn, connects the intramural coronary arterial system with all four chambers of the heart. The Thebesian vessels themselves, which are highly variable in length and number, have no specific orientation and hence appear to be randomly arranged.[28] The overall small venous system can itself be subcategorized into ***venosinusoidal***, ***venoluminal***, ***arteriosinusoidal***, and ***arterioluminal*** components. Unlike the veins of the greater system, the walls of the Thebesian vessels are formed exclusively by endothelial cells, themselves continuous with the endothelial linings of the cardiac chambers. The venous orifices empty directly into all four cardiac chambers. It can be argued that the vessels are not strictly veins, since the arteriosinusoidal and arterioluminal vessels connect directly with branches of the coronary arteries. As such, therefore, it is suggested that the vessels should be considered as arteriovenous anastomoses.[28,29] The lesser system is responsible for a significant part of the myocardial drainage. It drains most of the right appendage and much of the muscular ventricular septum. The right side of the heart relies to a significant extent on the

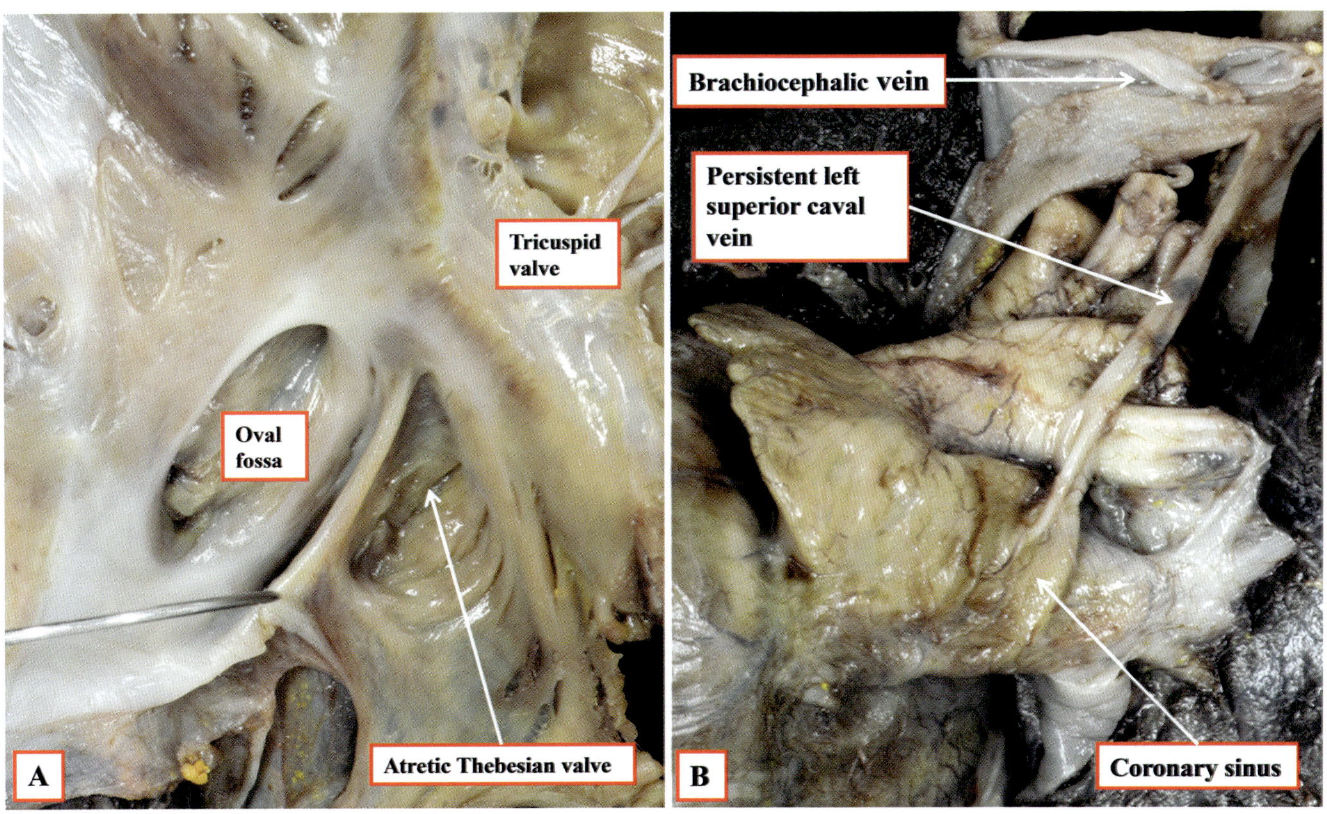

Figure 11.19. In this heart, as shown in panel A, the mouth of the coronary sinus is blocked by an imperforate Thebesian valve. In this setting, the venous drainage from the greater cardiac venous system then returns to the heart through the persistently patent left superior caval vein, as shown in panel B.

smaller system for its venous drainage, but the number of Thebesian veins is significantly reduced on the left.[28,29]

The Cardiac Lymphatic System

Far less is known in regard to the arrangement of the cardiac lymphatics when compared to knowledge of the coronary arteries and veins.[1] Responsible for maintaining homeostasis by receiving proteins and excess fluid from the interstitial tissues and returning them to the venous system, lymphatic channels are found within the heart, just as in all the other bodily components. It is unusual, however, to find the topic of the lymphatics discussed in textbooks of cardiology. This is surprising, since over one hundred years ago three lymphatic plexuses had been identified by injecting dye into the hearts of living mammals.[30] The plexuses were located subendocardially, within the myocardium, and subepicardially. These findings had been confirmed by the end of the next decade, with further experiments in mammalian hearts showing that the flow of the cardiac lymph flow originated in the subendocardial area, from whence it was collected in valveless channels, which passed through the myocardium to drain in the epicardial plexuses. It was then drained by major lymphatic trunks into the regional cardiac lymph nodes.[1] The epicardial plexuses largely occupy the interventricular grooves, with the major cardiac lymph node located between the origins of the intrapericardial arterial roots. This node, along with posterior mediastinal nodes, then drains to the thoracic duct, which in turn drains to the brachiocephalic vein. Other nodes related to the intrapericardial arterial trunks, at least in the dog, drain via a right lymphatic channel directly to the superior caval vein.[31]

REFERENCES

1. Loukas M, Abel N, Tubbs RS, Grabska J, Birungi J, Anderson RH. The cardiac lymphatic system. *Clin Anat.* 2011;**24**:684–691. doi: 10.1002/ca.21104
2. Loukas M, Groat C, Khangura R, Owens DG, Anderson RH. The normal and abnormal anatomy of the coronary arteries. *Clin Anat.* 2009;**22**:114–128. doi: 10.1002/ca.20761
3. Garg A, Ogilvie BC, McLeod AA. Images in cardiology. Anomalous origin of the left coronary artery from the non-coronary sinus of Valsalva. *Heart.* 2000;**84**:136. doi: 10.1136/heart.84.2.136
4. Gittenberger-de Groot AC, Koenraadt WMC, Bartelings MM, Bokenkamp R, DeRuiter MC, Hazekamp MG, Bogers A, Quaegebeur JM, Schalij MJ, Vliegen HW, et al. Coding of coronary arterial origin and branching in congenital heart disease: the modified Leiden Convention. *J Thorac Cardiovasc Surg.* 2018;**156**:2260–2269. doi: 10.1016/j.jtcvs.2018.08.009
5. Toh H, Mori S, Tretter JT, Izawa Y, Shimoyama S, Suzuki M, Takahashi Y, Tsuda D, Toba T, Fujiwara S, et al. Living anatomy of the ventricular myocardial crescents supporting the coronary aortic sinuses. *Semin Thorac Cardiovasc Surg.* 2020;**32**:230–241. doi: 10.1053/j.semtcvs.2020.01.001
6. Redondo A, Baladron Zorita C, Tchetche D, Santos-Martinez S, Delgado-Arana JR, Barrero A, Gutierrez H, Serrador Frutos A, Ybarra Falcon C, Gomez MG, et al. Commissural versus coronary optimized alignment during transcatheter aortic valve replacement. *JACC Cardiovasc Interv.* 2022;**15**:135–146. doi: 10.1016/j.jcin.2021.10.005
7. Muriago M, Sheppard MN, Ho SY, Anderson RH. Location of the coronary arterial orifices in the normal heart. *Clin Anat.* 1997;**10**:297–302. doi: 10.1002/(SICI)1098-2353(1997)10:5<297::AID-CA1>3.0.CO;2-O
8. Loukas M, Andall RG, Khan AZ, Patel K, Muresian H, Spicer DE, Tubbs RS. The clinical anatomy of high take-off coronary arteries. *Clin Anat.* 2016;**29**:408–419. doi: 10.1002/ca.22664
9. Arnold R, Gervasoni R, Leclercq F. Chronic total occlusions: current approaches, evidence and outcomes. *J Clin Med.* 2025;**14**:4695. doi: 10.3390/jcm14134695
10. Kuniewicz M, Ostrowski P, Bonczar M, Kwiecinska M, Mozdzen K, Murawska A, Dziedzic M, Zytkowski A, Goncerz G, Walocha J, et al. The anatomy of the atrioventricular nodal artery: a meta-analysis with implications for cardiothoracic surgery and ablation procedures. *Clin Anat.* 2023;**36**:951–957. doi: 10.1002/ca.24072
11. Esrailian AJ, Mori S, Sato T, Izawa Y, Shivkumar K. Understanding cardiac anatomy and imaging to improve safety of procedures: the atrioventricular node artery. *JACC Case Rep.* 2025;**30**:102753. doi: 10.1016/j.jaccas.2024.102753
12. Saremi F, Abolhoda A, Ashikyan O, Milliken JC, Narula J, Gurudevan SV, Kaushal K, Raney A. Arterial supply to sinuatrial and atrioventricular nodes: imaging with multidetector CT. *Radiology.* 2008;**246**:99–107; discussion 108–109. doi: 10.1148/radiol.2461070030
13. McAlpine W.A. *Heart and Coronary Arteries: An Anatomical Atlas for Clinical Diagnosis, Radiological Investigation, and Surgical Treatment.* New York: Springer; 1975.
14. Angelini P. Normal and anomalous coronary arteries: definitions and classification. *Am Heart J.* 1989;**117**:418–434. doi: 10.1016/0002-8703(89)90789-8
15. Strauss DG, Loring Z, Selvester RH, Gerstenblith G, Tomaselli G, Weiss RG, Wagner GS, Wu KC. Right, but not left, bundle branch block is associated with large anteroseptal scar. *J Am Coll Cardiol.* 2013;**62**:959–967. doi: 10.1016/j.jacc.2013.04.060
16. Baz RO, Refi D, Scheau C, Savulescu-Fiedler I, Baz RA, Niscoveanu C. Coronary artery anomalies: a computed tomography angiography pictorial review. *J Clin Med.* 2024;**13**:3920. doi: 10.3390/jcm13133920
17. Fuenzalida JJV, Becerra-Rodriguez ES, Quivira Munoz AS, Baez Flores B, Escalona Manzo C, Orellana-Donoso M, Nova-Baeza P, Suazo-Santibanez A, Bruna-Mejias A, Sanchis-Gimeno J, et al. Anatomical variants of the origin of the coronary arteries: a systematic review and meta-analysis of prevalence. *Diagnostics (Basel).* 2024;**14**:1458. doi: 10.3390/diagnostics14131458
18. Zehan IG, Eotvos CA, Moldovan MP, Andrei MG, Schiop-Tentea CP, Lazar RD, Sarb AD, Coseriu G, Avram T, Serban A, et al. Angiographic anatomy of the left coronary veins: beyond conventional cardiac resynchronization therapy. *Curr Cardiol Rep.* 2025;**27**:58. doi: 10.1007/s11886-025-02204-z
19. Cabrera JA, Ho SY, Climent V, Sanchez-Quintana D. The architecture of the left lateral atrial wall: a particular anatomic region with implications for ablation of atrial fibrillation. *Eur Heart J.* 2008;**29**:356–362. doi: 10.1093/eurheartj/ehm606
20. Pauza DH, Skripka V, Pauziene N, Stropus R. Morphology, distribution, and variability of the epicardiac neural ganglionated subplexuses in the human heart. *Anat Rec.* 2000;**259**:353–382. doi: 10.1002/1097-0185(20000801)259:4<353::AID-AR10>3.0.CO;2-R

21. Chauvin M, Shah DC, Haissaguerre M, Marcellin L, Brechenmacher C. The anatomic basis of connections between the coronary sinus musculature and the left atrium in humans. *Circulation*. 2000;**101**:647–652. doi: 10.1161/01.cir.101.6.647
22. Katritsis DG. The coronary sinus: passive bystander or source of arrhythmia? *Heart Rhythm*. 2004;**1**:113–116. doi: 10.1016/j.hrthm.2004.02.005
23. Morita H, Zipes DP, Morita ST, Wu J. The role of coronary sinus musculature in the induction of atrial fibrillation. *Heart Rhythm*. 2012;**9**:581–589. doi: 10.1016/j.hrthm.2011.11.041
24. Macedo PG, Kapa S, Mears JA, Fratianni A, Asirvatham SJ. Correlative anatomy for the electrophysiologist: ablation for atrial fibrillation. Part I: Pulmonary vein ostia, superior vena cava, vein of Marshall. *J Cardiovasc Electrophysiol*. 2010;**21**:721–730. doi: 10.1111/j.1540-8167.2010.01728.x
25. Katritsis D, Ioannidis JP, Anagnostopoulos CE, Sarris GE, Giazitzoglou E, Korovesis S, Camm AJ. Identification and catheter ablation of extracardiac and intracardiac components of ligament of Marshall tissue for treatment of paroxysmal atrial fibrillation. *J Cardiovasc Electrophysiol*. 2001;**12**:750–758.
26. Ariyaratnam JP, Middeldorp ME, Brooks AG, Thomas G, Kadhim K, Mahajan R, Pathak RK, Young GD, Kalman JM, Sanders P. Coronary sinus isolation for high-burden atrial fibrillation: a randomized clinical trial. *JACC Clin Electrophysiol*. 2025;**11**:1–9. doi: 10.1016/j.jacep.2024.09.017
27. Loukas M, Bilinsky S, Bilinsky E, el-Sedfy A, Anderson RH. Cardiac veins: a review of the literature. *Clin Anat*. 2009;**22**:129–145. doi: 10.1002/ca.20745
28. von Ludinghausen M. The venous drainage of the human myocardium. *Adv Anat Embryol Cell Biol*. 2003;**168**:I–VIII, 1–104. doi: 10.1007/978-3-642-55623-4
29. von Ludinghausen M. Clinical anatomy of cardiac veins, Vv. cardiacae. *Surg Radiol Anat*. 1987;**9**:159–168. doi: 10.1007/BF02086601
30. Aagaard OC. *Les Vaisseaux Lymphatique du Coeur Chez l'Homme et Chez Quelques Mammifères*. Copenhagen: Levin & Munksgaard; 1924.
31. Ullal SR. Cardiac lymph and lymphatics. Experimental observations and clinical significance. *Ann R Coll Surg Engl*. 1972;**51**:282–298. PMID: 4646747

12

The Conduction System

All the cardiomyocytes making up the walls of the cardiac chambers have the capacity to conduct. If diseased or abnormal, they also have the capacity to give rise to, or become part of a circuit for, cardiac arrhythmias. A specific subset of cardiomyocytes is now recognized as providing the so-called "conduction system". When assessed grossly, there is no way of distinguishing these cells from the so-called working cardiomyocytes, with the latter cells making up the greater part of the chamber walls. This has led to multiple controversies as to which cardiomyocytes should, or should not, be considered to belong to the "system".[1] The arguments have largely related to the pathways for interatrial conduction, although other disagreements have focused on the nature of the cardiomyocytes found within the pulmonary venous sleeves. In both instances, the disputes usually relate to whether any of the cells can be recognized as being "specialized" based on histological examination. Subsequent to the initial debate regarding the pathways for internodal conduction, a series of criterions had been proposed to permit recognition, when using the light microscope, of the "specialized" cardiomyocytes. Now known as the Aschoff–Monkeberg criterions, the rules dictated that the cardiomyocytes, in the first instance, should be histologically discrete when assessed relative to adjacent working cardiomyocytes. The second proposed criterion reflected the ability to follow the cardiomyocytes from section to section in serially sectioned histological datasets. The final criterion, which was specific to the definition of specialized tracts as opposed to both sinus and atrioventricular nodes, was that the cardiomyocytes should be insulated from their working neighbours. For this purpose, the exemplar for a specialized tract was taken to be the atrioventricular conduction axis as described by Tawara.[2] Thus far, no evidence has been provided to question the validity of these criterions.[1] When assessed on this basis, the specialized components responsible for generating and disseminating the cardiac impulses in the normal heart can be considered in terms of the sinus node, along with the atrioventricular conduction axis (Figure 12.1). With the advent of techniques such as transcriptomics, which permit the assessment of the genetic make-up of individual cells, and laser histological capture, which permits recognition of such cells in histological sections, it may well prove possible to identify histologically indistinct cardiomyocytes that possess particular features that influence conduction. At the present time, it is the Aschoff–Monkeberg criterions that serve to distinguish between the specialized and the working cardiomyocytes.

Sinus Node

Initially described by Keith and Flack during the first decade of the 20th century,[3] the sinus node is usually located laterally within the terminal crest, with the groove corresponding to the crest marking the junction between the appendage and the systemic venous sinus of the right atrium (Figures 12.2, 12.3 panel A). On occasion, the node can straddle the crest of the right atrial appendage

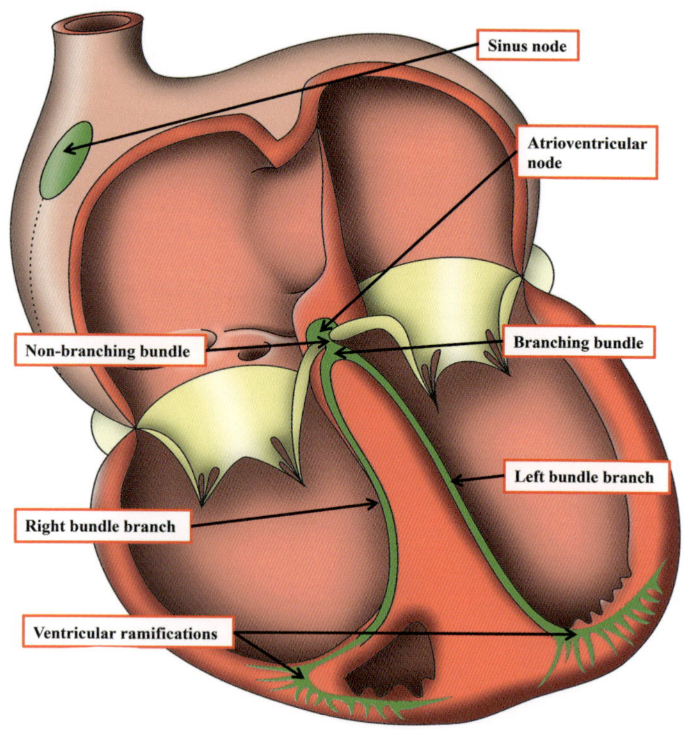

Figure 12.1. Locations of the so-called conduction system of the heart. The cardiac impulse is generated by the sinus node. It is then disseminated through the working atrial cardiomyocytes, until delayed at the atrioventricular node. The non-branching bundle, or the bundle of His, is the only myocardial connection across the plane of insulation provided at the atrioventricular junctions. The conduction axis then branches on the crest of the muscular ventricular septum, with the right and left bundle branches insulated until they ramify within the ventricular apical trabeculations. The right bundle branch crosses the ventricular cavity with the moderator band. The original drawing was made by Mrs Gemma Price and has been modified with her permission.

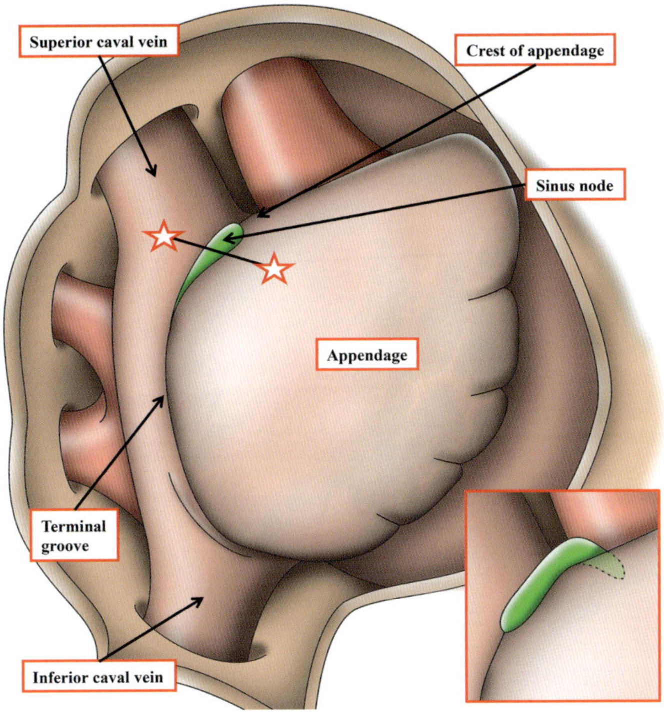

Figure 12.2. The drawing shows the usual location of the sinus node. The inset shows the "horseshoe" arrangement, found in up to one-tenth of individuals. The line between the two stars shows the plane of section taken to reveal the histology of the node, as shown in Figure 12.3 panel A. The histology of the horseshoe variant is shown in Figure 12.3 panel B. The original drawing was made by Mrs Gemma Price and has been modified with her permission.

in horseshoe fashion (Figures 12.2 inset, 12.3 panel B).[4] With its cardiomyocytes supported in a dense fibrous matrix, the node lies directly subepicardially (Figure 12.3). Its margins are irregular. The supporting fibrous matrix does not insulate the contained cardiomyocytes from the adjacent working myocardium.[5] Instead, its histologically specialized cardiomyocytes merge at its margins with the muscular sleeve of the superior caval vein, and with the working myocardium of the terminal crest (Figure 12.3 panel A). It possesses an extensive tail, which extends subepicardially, to varied individual extent, running within the crest along the terminal groove towards the orifice of the inferior caval vein.

Cardiac electrical activity starts by the spontaneous excitation of the nodal cells, which are smaller than the adjacent working cardiomyocytes (Figure 12.4 panel B). Its automaticity is dependent on phase 4 of spontaneous diastolic repolarization. This generates rhythmic action potentials, with the speed of their production determining the heart rate through various currents, including the I_f current.[6] The heart rate is further modulated by the rich innervation of the node provided by postganglionic adrenergic and cholinergic nerve terminals.[7] Once generated, the sinus impulse is transmitted to the working atrial cardiomyocytes via the multiple pathways formed at the nodal margins.[8] The process of excitation then depolarizes the working cardiomyocytes, providing a wave within the atrial walls which moves towards the atrioventricular node via pathways made up of well-aligned working atrial cells.[9]

The suggestion had been made that some of the cardiomyocytes providing these pathways were histologically specialized. No evidence has yet been provided to support this speculation. The proposal, nonetheless, spawned the meeting at which the

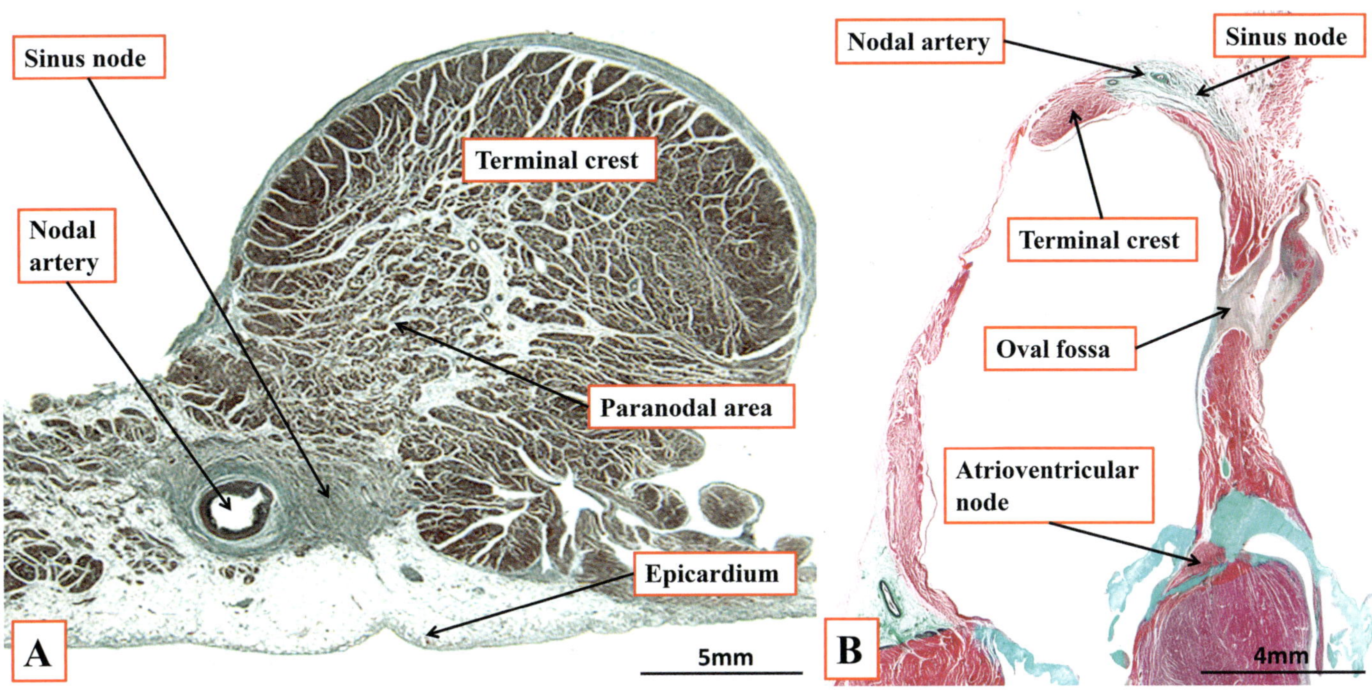

Figure 12.3. The histological sections, stained using the trichrome technique, show how it is possible to distinguish, when using the Aschoff–Monkeberg criterions, the cardiomyocytes making up the sinus node from those aggregated together as working cells within the atrial walls. Panel A shows the usual arrangement, with the plane of section as shown in Figure 12.2. Panel B shows the horseshoe variant, with the section shown in four-chamber orientation. Note also the presence of the paranodal area within the terminal crest as shown in panel A.

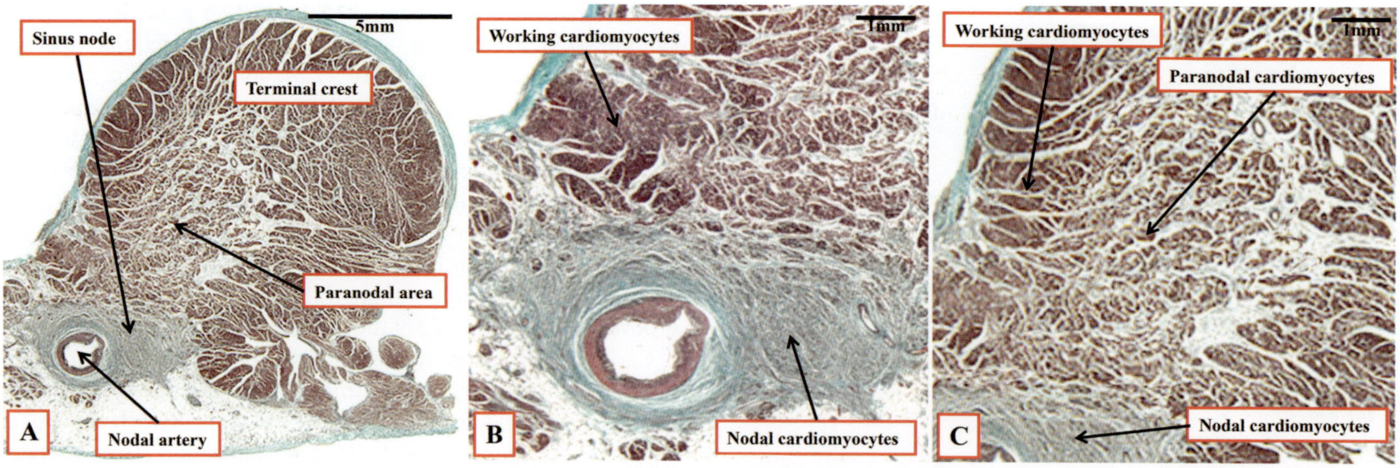

Figure 12.4. The images show how the Aschoff–Monkeberg criterions can be used to distinguish between the specialized cardiomyocytes making up the sinus node itself, as shown in panels A and B, the working cardiomyocytes of the terminal crest, as shown in panel B, and the cardiomyocytes making up the paranodal area, as shown in panel C. The paranodal cardiomyocytes are intermediate in character between the nodal and the working cardiomyocytes. The precise function of the paranodal area has yet to be established.

Aschoff–Monkeberg criterions emerged, with the intent of quelling such subsequent speculation. Despite the production of the histological criterions, the suggestion has again been made that the pathways were "specialized". The major proponent for revitalization of the concept of specialized internodal tracts, however, paid scant recognition to the arrangement of the atrioventricular conduction axis as the paradigm of a conducting tract. In particular, he ignored the third rule of Aschoff and Monkeberg, namely that any atrial tracts should be insulated by fibrous tissues from the adjacent working cardiomyocytes.[10] As shown in Figure 12.3 panel B, even at low magnifications it is possible histologically to recognize the sinus and atrioventricular nodes. Examination of serially sectioned datasets then shows that there are no insulated pathways within the atrial walls providing discrete tracts between the nodes. It is the aggregation of the working cardiomyocytes in parallel fashion that provides the substrate for preferential conduction through the atrial walls, particularly within the ***terminal crest*** and its continuation into the cavotricuspid isthmus (Figure 12.5).[11] A similar aggregation of working cardiomyocytes underscores the spread of conduction from the right to the left atrium through Bachmann's bundle.[12]

Although there are no insulated tracts extending through the atrial walls, it is possible to recognize a second area of cells within the terminal crest that does satisfy the Aschoff–Monkeberg criterions for histological specialization (Figure 12.4 panel B). This is the ***paranodal area***, which was shown by simulation studies to play a role in spreading the action potential from the sinus node to the atrial walls. As yet, its overall function remains to be established.[13] A notable feature of the sinus node is its organization around the prominent ***nodal artery***, which is the largest of the atrial arteries. The artery is a branch of the right coronary artery in just over half the population, and of the circumflex artery in the remainder. When taking proximal origin from its parent artery, the nodal artery ascends through the anterior interatrial groove to reach the node. It can then course in front of, or behind, the cavoatrial junction so as to enter the node, although in some individuals it branches to form a circle around the junction. When arising laterally from the right coronary artery, the nodal artery crosses the wall of the right atrial appendage to supply the node. This variant should be recognized during surgical procedures involving incisions into the wall of the appendage made parallel to the right atrioventricular groove. In a minority of individuals, the artery can arise distally from the circumflex artery and then supply the node, having ascended the posterior wall of the left atrium. This variant potentially poses a danger to surgeons dissecting the superior interatrial groove so as to gain access to the cavity of the left atrium.

The Atrioventricular Conduction Axis

Having traversed the pathways provided by the working atrial cardiomyocytes (Figure 12.5 panel A), the impulse generated by the sinus node arrives at the ***atrioventricular node*** (Figure 12.5 panel B). The function of the atrioventricular node is to delay the impulse so that the ventricular chambers are able to fill with blood during atrial systole. The node also functions as a filter to protect the ventricular myocardium from fast atrial rates, as well as providing a backup pacemaker in case of sinus nodal dysfunction.[14,15] It is located towards the apex of the ***triangle of Koch***, being uniformly located at the apex of the inferior pyramidal space, with the walls of the space enclosed by the ***pyramid of Koch***. The apex of both the triangle and the pyramid is directed superiorly when considered in an attitudinally appropriate fashion (Figure 12.6 panel A). The triangle, as viewed from the right atrium, is one face of the walls enclosing the inferior pyramidal space (Figure 12.6 panel B). The diverging inferior walls of the ventricles form the ventricular surface of the space. Its posterior atrial surface is the antero-inferior buttress of the atrial septum, with its parietal right and left walls formed by the atrial vestibules. Running through the space in almost all individuals is the ***artery to the atrioventricular node***.[16] To summarize, the walls enclose the inferior pyramidal space, with the triangle of Koch representing its right atrial wall.[17]

The node itself is the atrial component of the atrioventricular conduction axis. In the normal heart, the axis is the only pathway providing electrical continuity between the atrial and ventricular

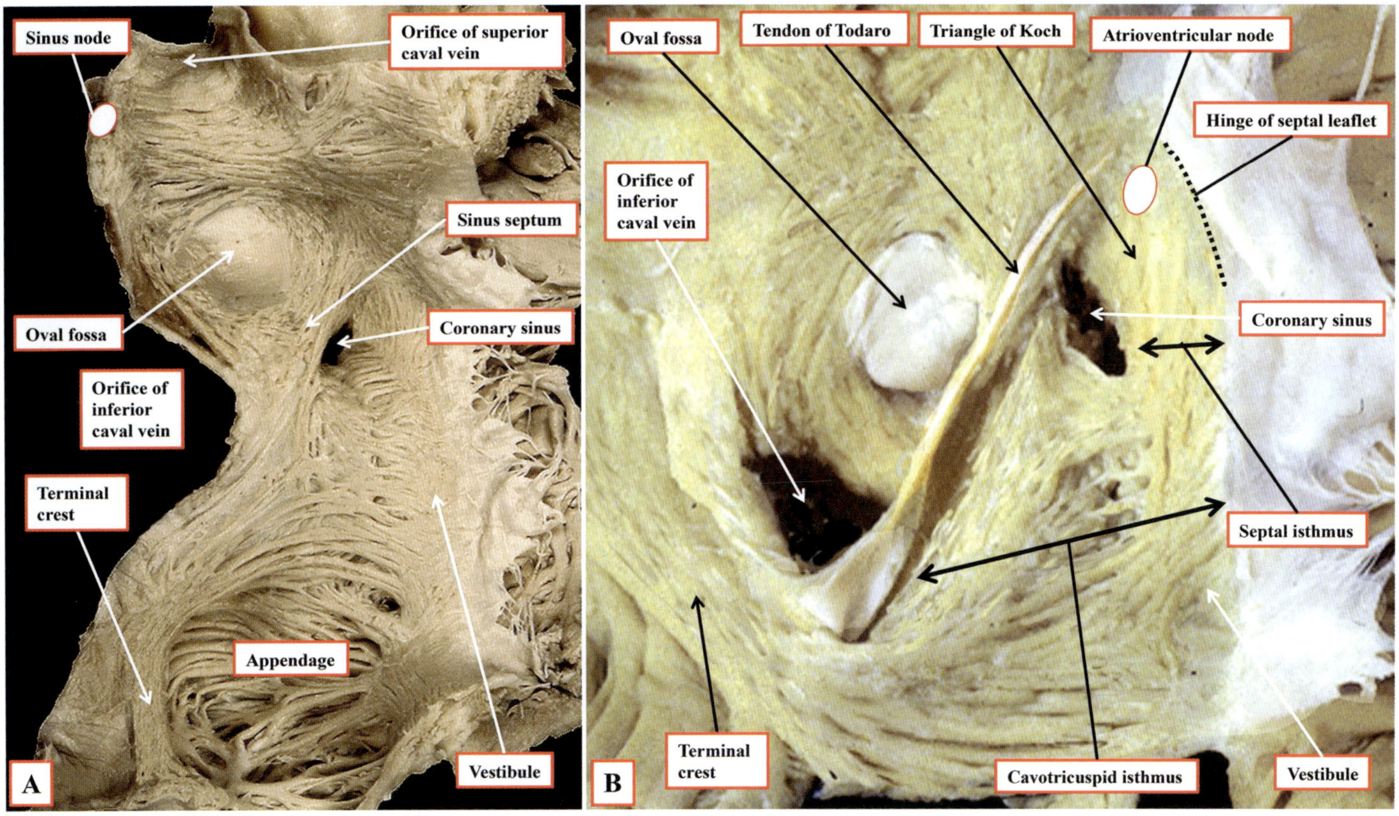

Figure 12.5. The manner of aggregation of the working atrial cardiomyocytes within the atrial walls has been revealed by stripping away the endocardial surface of the right atrium. Panel A shows an overview, revealing multiple areas where the parallel aggregation of the working cells favours preferential conduction through the atrial walls from the sinus node. Panel B is a close-up of a different heart, showing the extension of the terminal crest into the cavotricuspid isthmus. The dissection also shows the location of the triangle of Koch, which provides the landmark to the atrioventricular node.

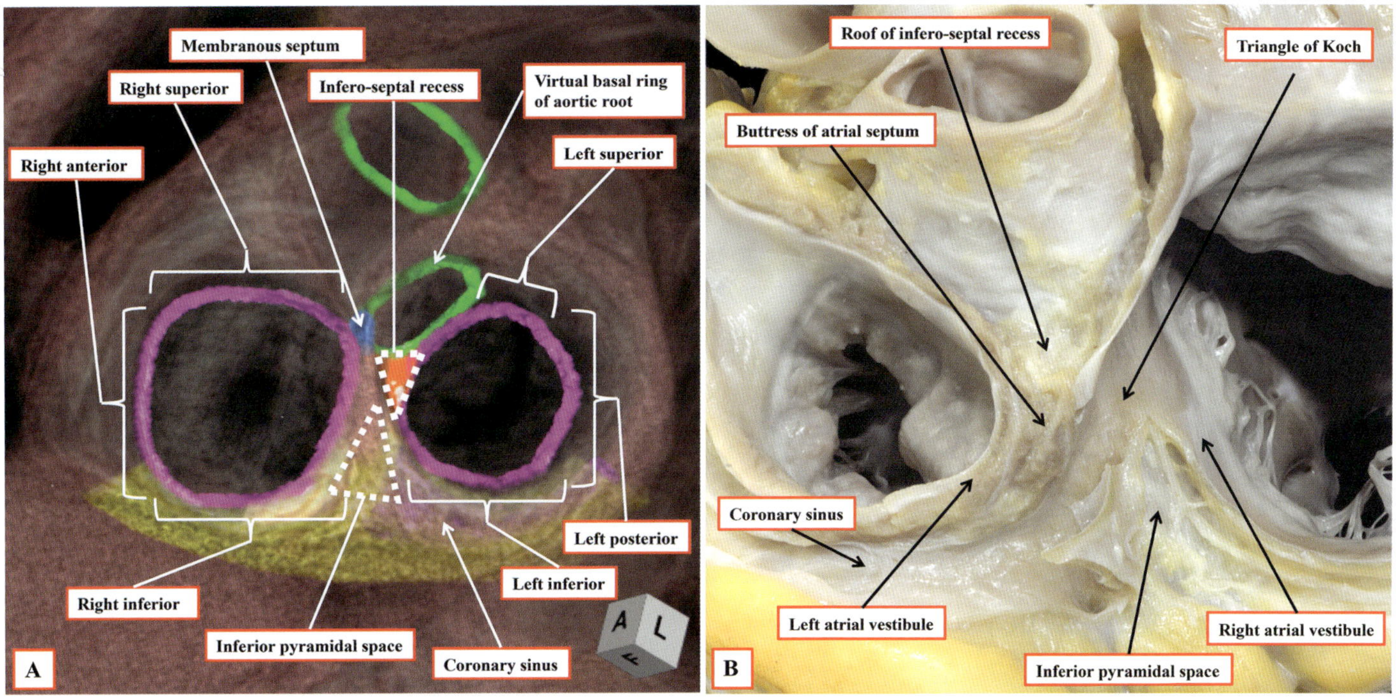

Figure 12.6. Panel A shows a segmented virtual dissection of a computed clinical dataset revealing the features of the atrioventricular junctions as viewed from the cardiac apex looking towards the base. Panel B is a dissection of a heart shown from the atrial aspect looking towards the apex. Panel A shows the overlap of the apexes of inferior pyramidal space and the infero-septal recess, whereas panel B shows how the inferior pyramidal space is a continuation of the inferior atrioventricular groove.

myocardial masses.[2] This is made possible because the atrial vestibules are insulated from the crests of the ventricular walls throughout the right and left atrioventricular junctions. Much was made in the past of atrioventricular "*annuluses*" providing the insulation. As was described in Chapter 6, this is a gross exaggeration. Throughout the right atrioventricular junction, and in large parts of the left atrioventricular junction, it is the fibroadipose tissues of the junctions that serve to separate the atrial and ventricular walls. This is also the case in the area of the pyramid of Koch, where the fibroadipose tissues of the ***inferior pyramidal space***, itself a continuation of the inferior atrioventricular groove (Figure 12.6 panel A), separate the atrial walls from the underlying diverging walls of the ventricular chambers (Figure 12.6 panel B). As was emphasized in Chapter 6, appreciation of this arrangement has necessitated the recognition that areas previously considered to be "*septal*" are properly described as being *paraseptal*. Such paraseptal areas, which will become significant when attention is paid to accessory myocardial atrioventricular pathways, are to be found antero-superiorly and -inferiorly in the right atrioventricular junction (Figure 12.6 panel A). In the left atrioventricular orifice, insulation between the left atrial vestibule and the base of the left ventricular cone is found in relation to the mural leaflet of the mitral valve. The aortic leaflet of the mitral valve, in almost all individuals, is in fibrous continuity with the non-coronary and left coronary leaflets of the aortic valve. The area of fibrous continuity thus formed spans the roof of the left ventricle, removing any potential for atrioventricular myocardial continuity. In rare circumstances, nonetheless, it is possible to find otherwise normal individuals with completely muscular subaortic infundibulums.[18] It may then be significant that such discontinuity between the leaflets of the aortic and mitral valves has been observed in the setting of hypertrophic cardiomyopathy.[19]

With regard to the mural component of the left junction, it is frequent to find fibrous shelves supporting the mural leaflet of the mitral valve. When present, the fibrous tissues also serve to separate the left atrial vestibule from the crest of the left ventricular wall. In other areas, as in the right side, the insulation is provided by the fibroadipose tissues of the junction. Taken together, because of the insulation, the key feature of normal atrioventricular conduction is the presence of a solitary tract of specialized conducting cardiomyocytes that provides continuity between the atrial and ventricular myocardial masses. At the site of insulation of the axis itself, which when insulated is then no longer in contact with atrial cardiomyocytes, the atrioventricular node becomes the non-branching atrioventricular bundle (Figure 12.7 panel A). The ventricular component of the axis then subsequently branches astride the crest of the muscular ventricular septum (Figure 12.7 panel B). The ***right*** and ***left bundle***

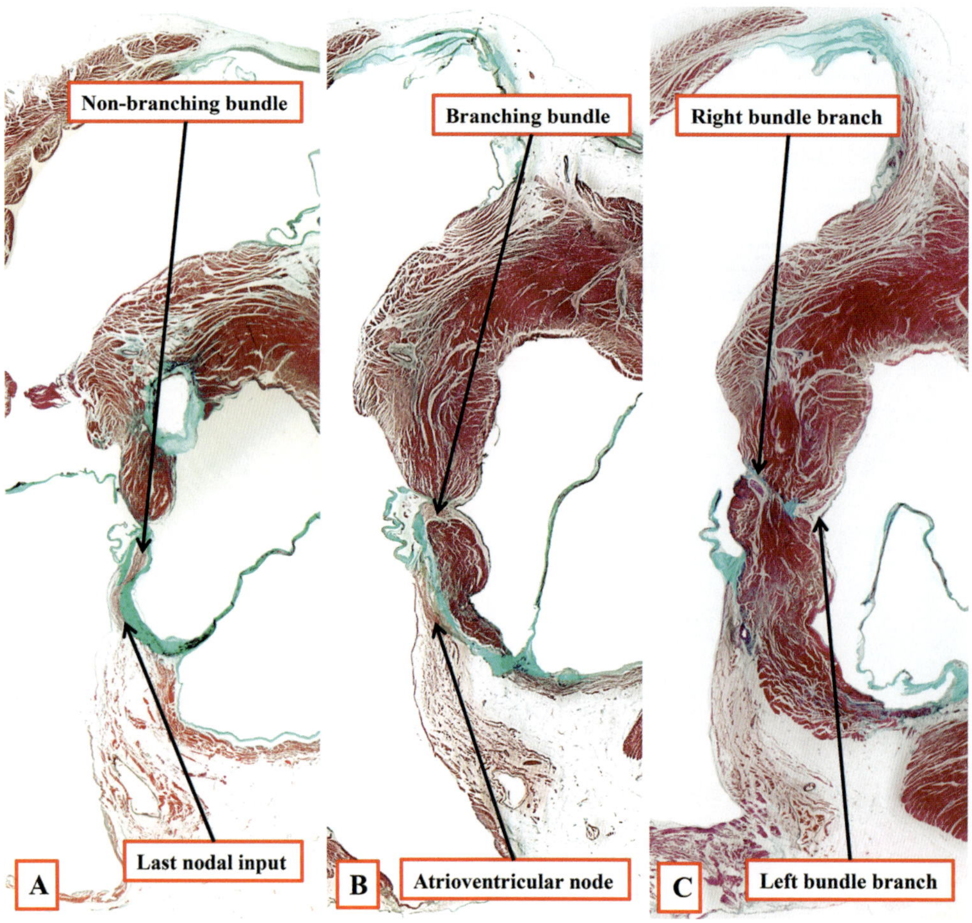

Figure 12.7. The images show serial sections from an adult heart cut in the short axis of the ventricular mass, with the images viewed from the cardiac apex looking towards the base of the heart. Panel A shows how the atrioventricular conduction axis penetrates the insulating plane to transition from the atrioventricular node to become the non-branching bundle. Panel B shows the axis branching on the crest of the muscular ventricular septum, with the branch point being centrally located within the ventricular mass. Panel C shows the insulated nature of the right and left bundle branches.

branches continue as insulated tracts (Figure 12.7 panel C) before ramifying with the working ventricular cardiomyocytes within the apexes of the ventricular chambers (Figure 12.1). In terms of gross anatomy, the transition between the atrial and ventricular myocardial components is found at the site where the superior apex of the inferior pyramidal space overlaps the inferior extent of the infero-septal recess of the left ventricle (Figure 12.6).[20]

The major ***atrial inputs*** to the atrioventricular node are found within the vestibules of the tricuspid and mitral valves. As described, the vestibules form the right-sided and left-sided parietal atrial boundaries of the pyramid of Koch (Figure 12.8 panel A). The cardiomyocytes forming these nodal inputs are histologically discrete (Figure 12.9 panel A), but it is the manner of their aggregation that permits them to be recognized as being "specialized", since they are

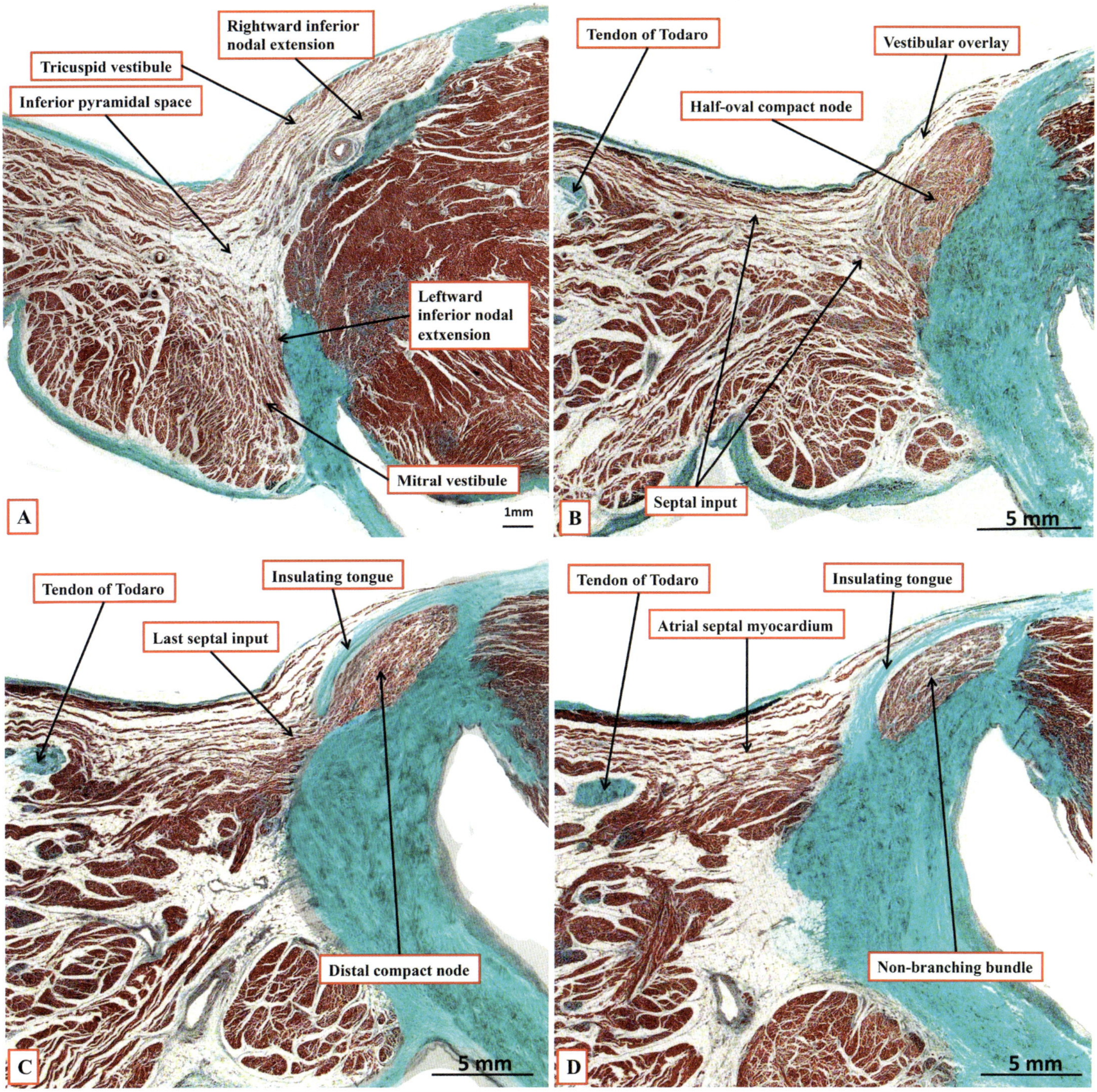

Figure 12.8. The serial sections are taken from an adult heart, moving from panel A, which is the most inferior section taken at the base of the triangle of Koch, to panel D, which shows how the axis has become insulated by the formation of a tongue of fibrous tissue that produces continuity between the leaflets of the mitral and tricuspid valves via the roof of the infero-septal recess. They are orientated in attitudinally appropriate fashion, with the right-sided chambers to the top. Panel A shows the inferior nodal extensions, with panel B showing extensive septal inputs to the compact atrioventricular node. Panel C then shows the final input to the node, before the axis becomes insulated as shown in panel D. The septal inputs form the fast pathway into the node, with the inferior extensions providing the slow pathways.

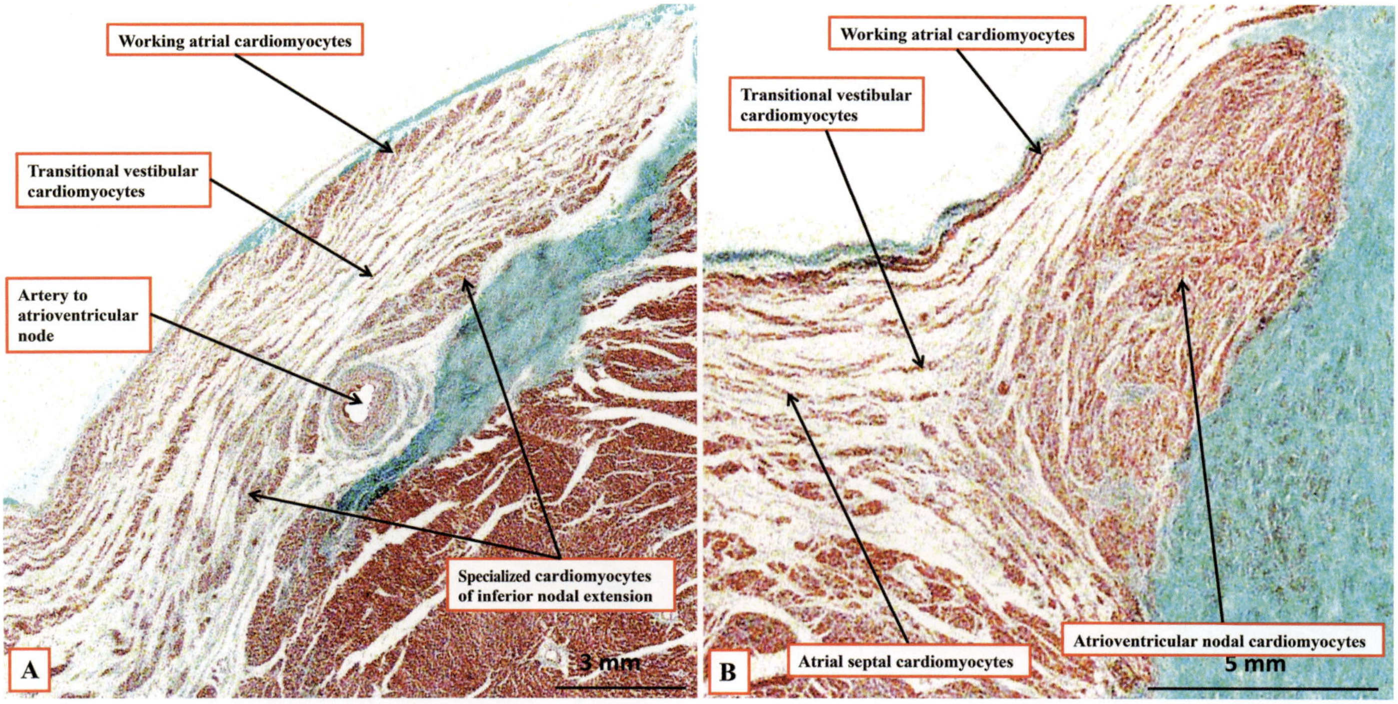

Figure 12.9. The higher-power images taken from panels A and B of Figure 12.8 show how the Aschoff–Monkeberg criterions permit distinction of the specialized cardiomyocytes making up the inferior nodal extensions (panel A) and the characteristic cells of the atrioventricular node (panel B). In this dataset, it is also possible to recognize cardiomyocytes intermediate in cellular histology between the nodal and the working cells. These are the transitional cardiomyocytes.

not insulated from the adjacent working vestibular cardiomyocytes. They can, nonetheless, be traced from section to section within the histological datasets. Hence, they are ***nodal extensions*** rather than specific tracts. When traced cranially through the serial sections, the inferior extensions merge to form the compact atrioventricular node (Figure 12.8 panel B).[21] The compact node is again recognized primarily because of the obvious arrangement of its contained specialized cardiomyocytes, which form a half-oval set against the supporting plane of fibrous atrioventricular insulation (Figure 12.8 panel B). The specialized cardiomyocytes are linked together in the form of a random three-dimensional meshwork, with no obvious alignment of their contained chains (Figure 12.9 panel B). In terms of their size, the nodal cardiomyocytes are smaller than the adjacent atrial working cardiomyocytes. Additional inputs then merge with the node from the buttress of the atrial septum, which forms the posterior atrial wall of the inferior pyramidal space (Figure 12.8 panel B). These septal inputs, and particularly the final one observed prior to the site of insulation (Figure 12.8 panel C), are composed of ordinary working atrial cardiomyocytes, although often the cells adopt a transitional appearance before merging to become part of the compact node (Figure 12.9 panel B).[13] It is difficult to provide a precise morphological criterion for a "***transitional cardiomyocyte***". The cells forming parts of the tricuspid vestibule have comparable appearances to those providing the inputs to the atrioventricular node. The transitional appearances of the inputs to the node themselves are also much more obvious in datasets obtained from infant and paediatric hearts than from adult datasets. Irrespective of such considerations, it is the inferior extensions of the node, and the atrial cardiomyocytes which feed them, that represent the anatomic substrates of the slow pathway into the node.[22,23]

When considering the nodal extensions, the ***left inferior extension*** is derived exclusively from myocardium that initially belonged to the atrioventricular canal (Figure 12.10). The ***right inferior extension***, in contrast, is a combination of atrioventricular canal myocardium and the atrial component of the developmental primary interventricular ring of specialized cardiomyocytes (Figure 12.10). As such, it has been speculated that the rightward extension is capable of both slow and fast conduction.

This notion is further supported by connexin genotyping studies, which have identified the right inferior extension as an area of high expression of connexin 43, and thus capable of providing faster conduction than the cardiomyocytes of the node itself. Expression of connexin 43 is low, in contrast, in the left extension.[23,24] During development, however, the entirety of the atrioventricular canal is known to be composed of primary myocardium, which also conducts slowly. Hence, the likelihood is that both nodal extensions can provide the so-called slow nodal pathway.[23] It is the inputs to the node from the buttress of the atrial septum, especially the final connection prior to insulation of the axis, that act as the fast pathway.[25,26] Variable gap junction connectivity due to differential expression of connexin isoforms in the area of the nodal extensions, and involvement in the circuit of remnants of the primary ring, described as "ring tissues",[27,28] are also likely to play a role in the production of atrioventricular nodal arrhythmias. A probabilistic model of the tachycardia circuit for all forms of atrioventricular nodal re-entrant tachycardia has been proposed based on the concept of variable atrio-nodal inputs, along with the varied expression of connexins (Figure 12.11).[16,29,30]

Little difference, if any, is to be found in the histological appearance of the specialized cardiomyocytes making up the conduction

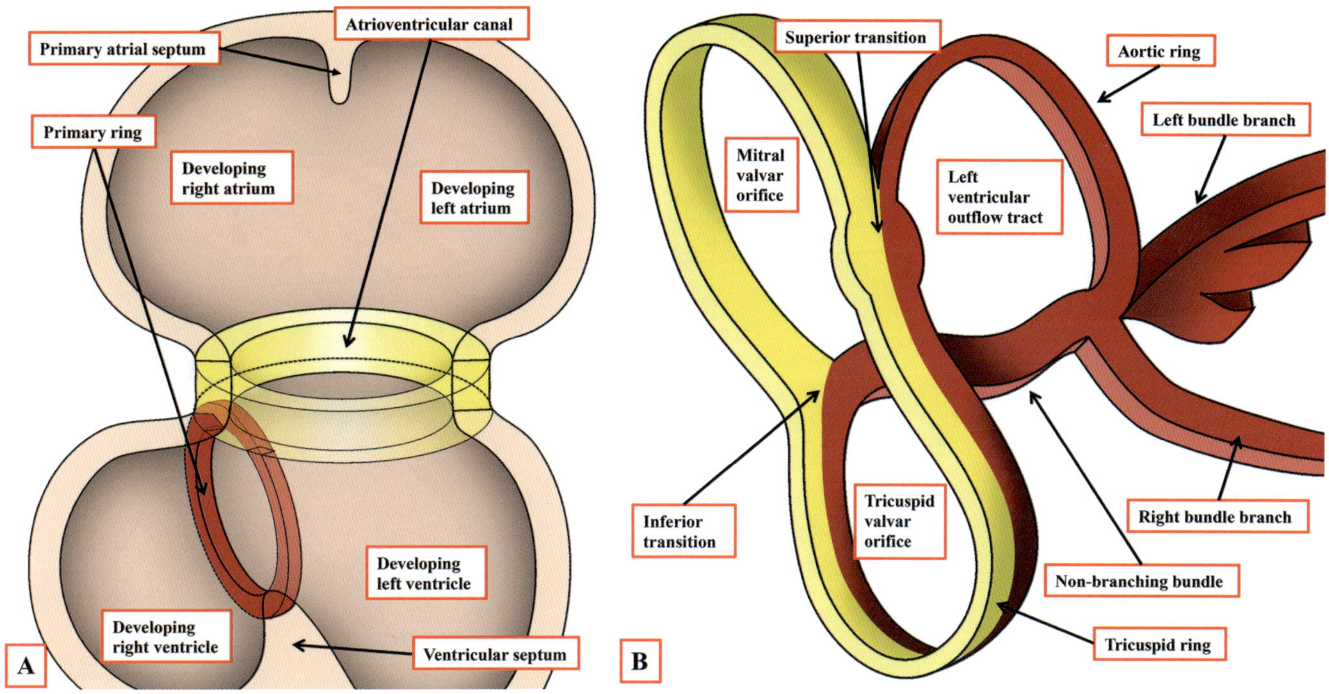

Figure 12.10. The components of the atrioventricular conduction axis and the atrial vestibules (see Chapter 2). The conduction axis is built on the basis of the primary ring of cardiomyocytes, shown in red, which encircles the embryonic interventricular communication. The atrioventricular canal myocardium itself, shown in yellow, is sequestrated during development on the atrial aspect of the atrioventricular junctions to become the vestibular myocardium. It is only the right atrial vestibule that has contributions from both the primary ring and the atrioventricular canal myocardium. The original drawings were made by Mrs Gemma Price and have been relabelled with her permission.

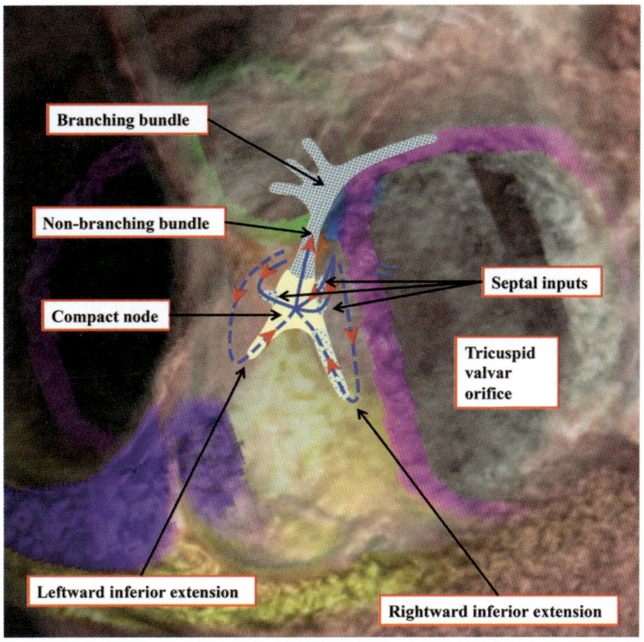

Figure 12.11. A proposed model is shown for conduction across the atrioventricular axis during sinus rhythm as mapped on the right septum. Normally, the impulse travels to the node via the septal inputs. With increasingly faster rates, the node expresses its decremental conduction properties. When the septal input becomes refractory, conduction shifts to the inferior extensions and the inputs they facilitate, and a jump may be seen. The right and left bundles and the bundle of His have been superimposed from the histological sections. The density of blue dots corresponds to relative conduction velocities, as indicated by experimental measurements, embryologic data, and connexin expression in relevant tissues.

axis when comparisons are made between the most distal extent of the atrioventricular node (Figure 12.12 panel A) and the non-branching ventricular bundle (Figure 12.12 panel B). As was emphasized by Tawara, when he first described the extent of the atrioventricular conduction axis, it is the insulation provided by the fibrous tissues of the atrioventricular junction that serves to distinguish between the node and the non-branching bundle.[2]

The arrangement is particularly evident when interrogating datasets prepared subsequent to scanning using the Synchrotron technique (Figure 12.13 panel A). This technique also now permits reconstructions to be made so as to put the conduction axis accurately back into the heart (Figure 12.13 panel B).

Conduction in the Ventricles

The solitary pathway permitting conduction to the ventricular mass in the normal heart is initially through a ***non-branching component*** of the insulated axis. It was this pathway that was first described by Wilhelm His the Younger, although it took quite some time before the accuracy of his observations was fully appreciated.[31] The pathway nowadays is usually described as the ***bundle of His***. Greater specificity is required if its anatomical arrangement is properly to be appreciated by those seeking selectively to pace the axis. Thus, oftentimes this part of the axis is also described as the "***penetrating bundle***". The area of penetration, however, is better considered as the transition from the distal part of the atrioventricular node to the non-branching part of the ventricular component of the axis (Figures 12.13, 12.14). Having become insulated from the myocardium of the antero-inferior buttress of the atrial septum (Figure 12.14 panel D),

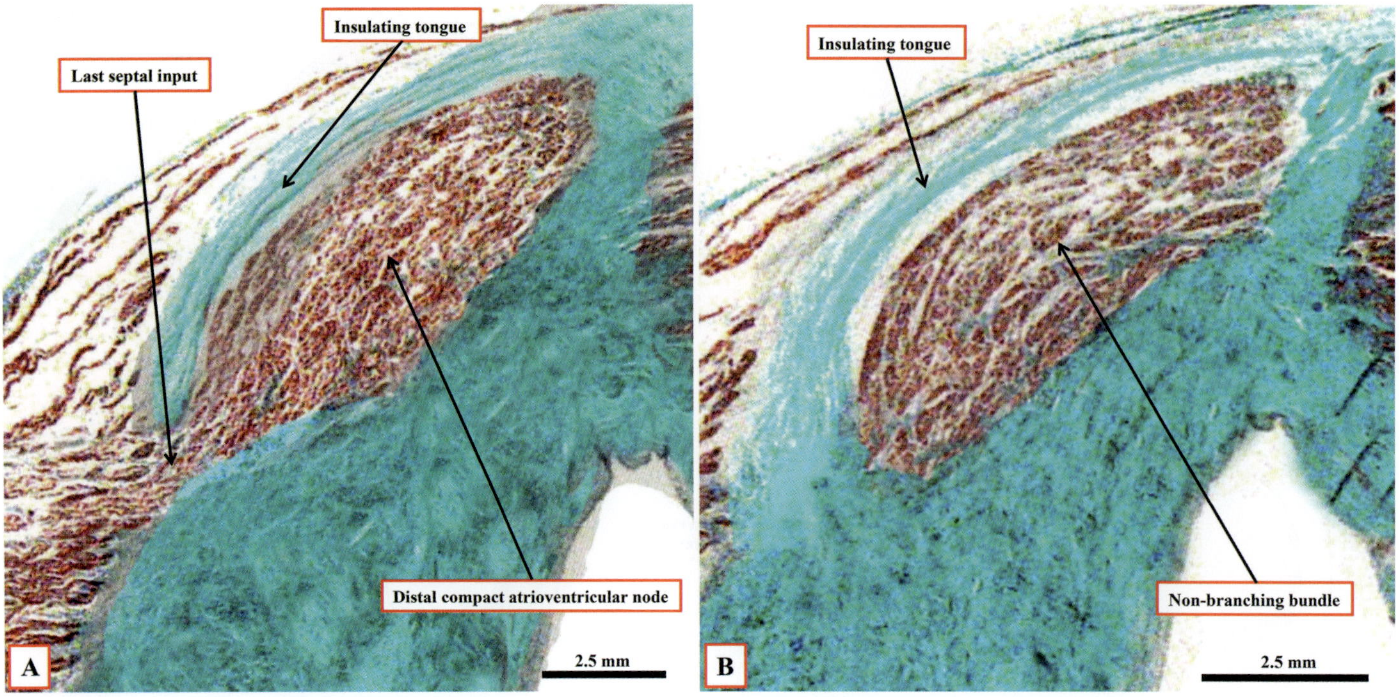

Figure 12.12. The images show the features of two adjacent sections from the dataset also shown in Figures 12.8 and 12.9. They show that, although the axis retains a septal input in panel A, but is insulated in the section shown in panel B, there is no difference in the histological make-up of the axis itself. It is the point of insulation that serves to distinguish between the distal extent of the node (panel A) and the origin of the ventricular component of the conduction axis (panel B).

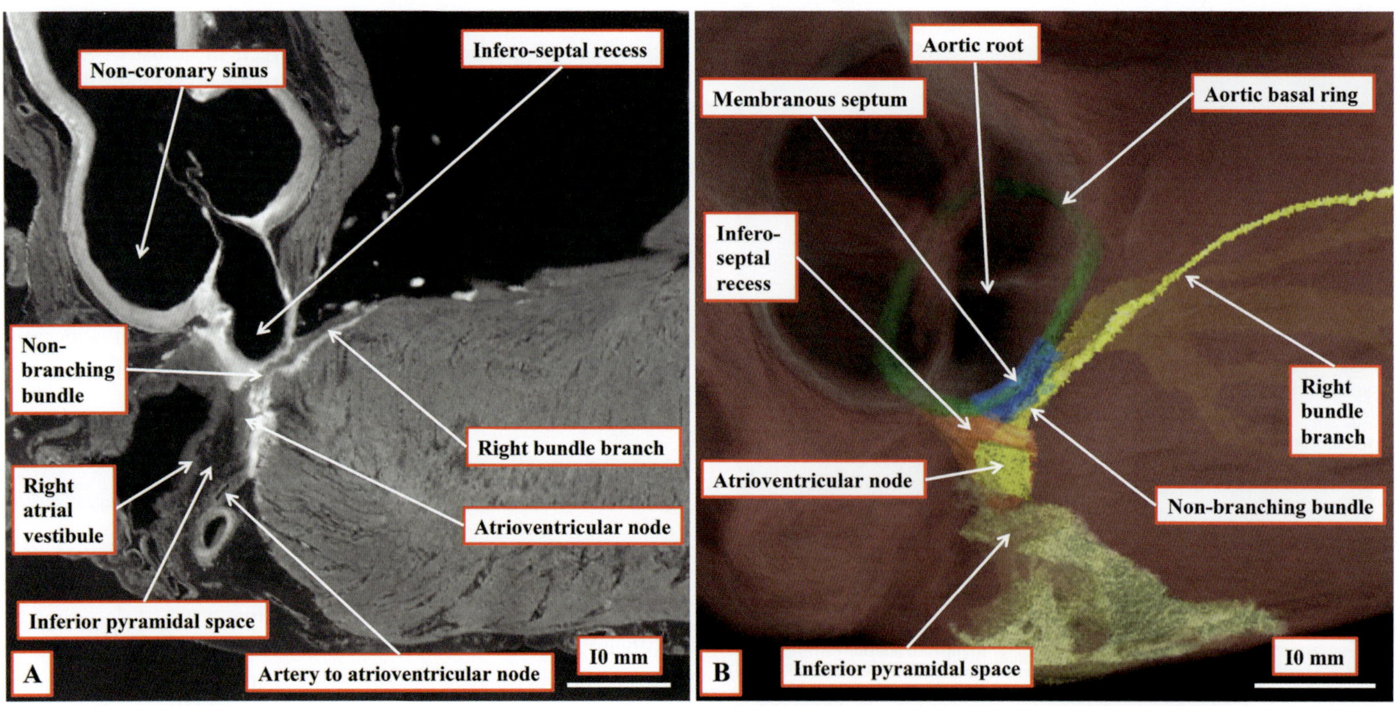

Figure 12.13. Panel A is a section taken from a publicly available dataset prepared subsequent to Synchrotron scanning to produce a HiP-CT image. It shows how the point of insulation of the atrioventricular conduction axis serves to distinguish the distal extent of the atrioventricular node from the non-branching atrioventricular bundle, with the transition occurring where the apex of the inferior pyramidal space overlaps the apex of the infero-septal recess of the left ventricular outflow tract. Panel B shows how the axis can be reconstructed and placed back into the heart. The fascicles of the left bundle branch are shown in "ghosted" fashion.

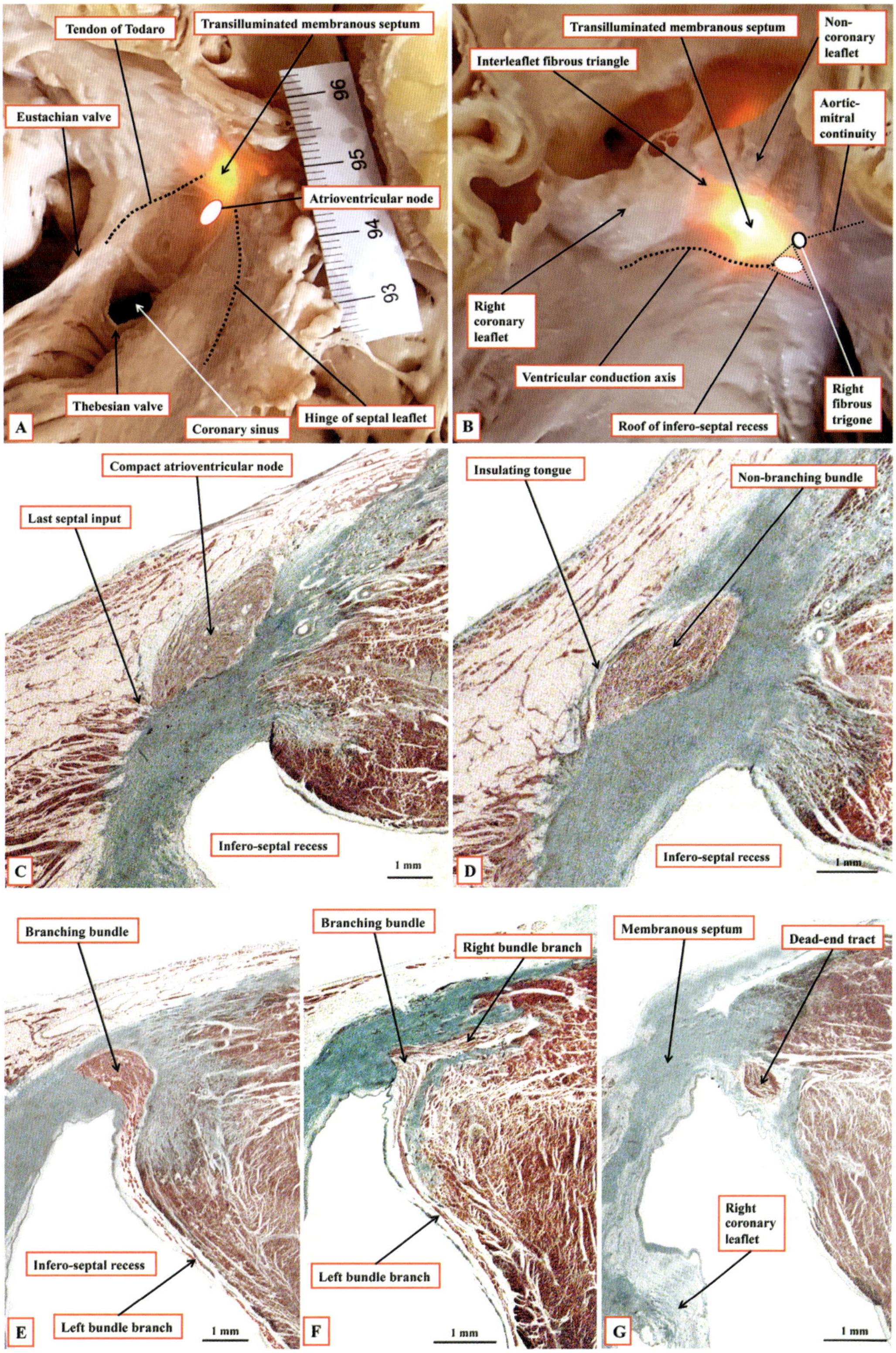

Figure 12.14. The images show the arrangement of the atrioventricular conduction axis in the pattern which, until very recently, was considered to be present in the majority of individuals. Panels A and B show gross images, revealing how the apex of the triangle of Koch (panel A) matches the apex of the infero-septal recess of the left ventricle (panel B), with the transilluminated membranous septum seen from both sides. Panels C through G then show histological sections cut from the same heart, orientated in attitudinal fashion, and stained using the trichrome technique, to reveal the features of the conduction axis as it extends from the distal atrioventricular node (panel C), through the non-branching bundle (panel D), to branch on the crest of the ventricular septum by giving off the left bundle branch (panel E). The axis then gives rise to the insulated right bundle branch (panel F), but in this heart then continues as the dead-end tract (panel G).

the non-branching bundle is usually positioned on the crest of the muscular ventricular septum, lying on the right wall of the inferoseptal recess of the left ventricular outflow tract (Figure 12.14 panel B). After a short non-branching course, shown in one study to be 3.6 ± 1.7 mm in length, with variation from 1.7 to 7.2 mm,[32] the axis then usually begins to branch by giving off the fascicles of the ***left bundle branch*** (Figure 12.14 panel E). The ***right bundle*** then takes its origin from the branching part of the axis (Figure 12.14 panel F). It used to be thought that the axis "bifurcated". The right bundle branch, however, can take its origin from the axis at various points along the crest of the muscular ventricular septum.[33] The axis itself, in some individuals, can also continue beyond the take-off of the bundle branches as a dead-end tract (Figure 12.14 panel G).[33]

It has now become appreciated that, in most individuals, the arrangement of the ventricular components of the axis is much more complex than the arrangement shown in Figure 12.14. This is because in the majority of human datasets recently examined using serial histological sections, additional pathways were identified between the ventricular components of the conduction axis and the crest of the muscular ventricular septum.[32] Such pathways were first identified by Mahaim in the mid-1930s and subsequently named by him as the ***paraspecific connections***.[34] This was because, based on his electrocardiographic experiments, he believed that the pathways offered an alternative route from the bundle branches themselves by which the working ventricular myocardium might become activated. In their review of the atrioventricular conduction axis published in the 1960s, Hecht and colleagues acknowledged the presence of the connections, naming them as the ***superior septal pathways***.[35]

Since that time, their significance as a substrate for normal conduction has received little attention. Along with persistent nodoventricular connections, they have been invoked as potential pathways for ventricular pre-excitation.[36] It is now suggested that the pathways may be activated during so-called selective pacing of the ventricular conduction system.[37] Further investigations will be required to validate this hypothesis. Attempts to achieve direct pacing of the components of the atrioventricular conduction axis, nonetheless, have now emerged as a more physiological alternative to right ventricular pacing for atrioventricular block. The technique is also being used in selected cases for cardiac resynchronization therapy.[38,39] Those using the "direct" approach seek either to stimulate the *non-branching bundle* or the *left bundle branch*, or simply to achieve *deep septal* stimulation.[40] In this regard, specific pacing of the non-branching bundle is well established as being superior to apical right ventricular pacing when treating atrioventricular block.[41] It also offers comparable, or even better, results when compared to biventricular pacing so as to achieve cardiac resynchronization.[42] Capture of the non-branching bundle, however, is hindered by the need for higher pacing thresholds. It also carries the potential for development of distal conduction block that may necessitate placement of a "backup" ventricular lead.[43] Its associated rate of complications is also higher than those encountered during apical or left bundle branch pacing.[44]

It was because of these constraints that attempted direct capture of the left bundle branch emerged as an alternative method for delivering physiological pacing, especially in patients with infranodal atrioventricular or left bundle branch block.[38,41] When successful, the technique has proved to be superior in providing improved left ventricular function in patients with heart failure.[45,46] It carries fewer late lead-related complications than attempted capture of the non-branching bundle in patients with atrial fibrillation and in those undergoing ablation of the atrioventricular node.[47] It follows that those seeking selectively to pace the different components of the conduction axis must take note of their known variability. This then obviously influences the site of the transition of the axis to become the non-branching bundle.[48] The non-branching bundle has long been known to vary in its own position relative to the crest of the muscular ventricular septum.[49] It has now been established that further variation is to be found in the relationship of the non-branching and branching components of the axis to the aortic root. These differences reflect the variation in the rotational position of the root within the base of the ventricular mass, along with the extent of the fibrous components that merge together to form the so-called central fibrous body (Figure 12.15).[50–52]

The anatomical investigations have now provided rules permitting the clinician to predict, with reasonable accuracy, the location of the axis relative to the gross cardiac landmarks. The gross landmarks themselves can now be established using clinical computed tomography. Thus, identification of the apex of the inferior pyramidal space, which is adjacent to the inferomedial commissure of the mitral valve, provides an accurate guide to the location of the atrioventricular node. Knowing that the node transitions to become the non-branching bundle by penetrating the atrioventricular component of the membranous septum permits points to be taken along the inferior margin of the membranous septum to show the course of the non-branching and branching bundles. A line connecting these points can be taken to represent the extent of the axis from the node to the origins of the bundle branches. The superior, septal, and inferior fascicles of the left bundle branch then course towards the base of the superolateral papillary muscle of the mitral valve, the left ventricular apex, and the inferomedial papillary muscle, respectively. The right bundle branch, in turn, courses towards the origin of the medial papillary muscle, and then extends down the septomarginal trabeculation, crossing the right ventricular cavity as part of the moderator band. When using this information, the clinician is now able to superimpose the anticipated location of components of the axis over the landmarks obtained using clinical cardiac computed tomography (Figure 12.16).

Irrespective of the variations described above relative to the location of the generally accepted components of the conduction axis, and even though their function has yet to be established, there can no longer be doubt regarding the presence, in the majority of individuals, of ***fasciculo-ventricular*** pathways as described by Mahaim.[53] In most instances, the pathways are relatively small and take their origin from the beginning of the branching bundle (Figure 12.17 panel A). In hearts showing this pattern, the axis itself then continues distally along the crest of the muscular septum before it gives rise in typical fashion to the cord-like right bundle branch (Figure 12.17 panel B).

In some instances, the arrangement is much more complex. In the most florid example observed in the series of cases studied using serial histological sectioning (Figure 12.18), the axis gave rise to multiple fasciculo-ventricular pathways before it became insulated as the cord-like right bundle branch (Figure 12.18 panel E). One of the pathways reconnected with the left bundle branch to form a ***fasciculo-fascicular connection***, producing an insulated loop of specialized cardiomyocytes which surrounded a block of working septal myocardium (Figure 12.18 panel C). The presence of such

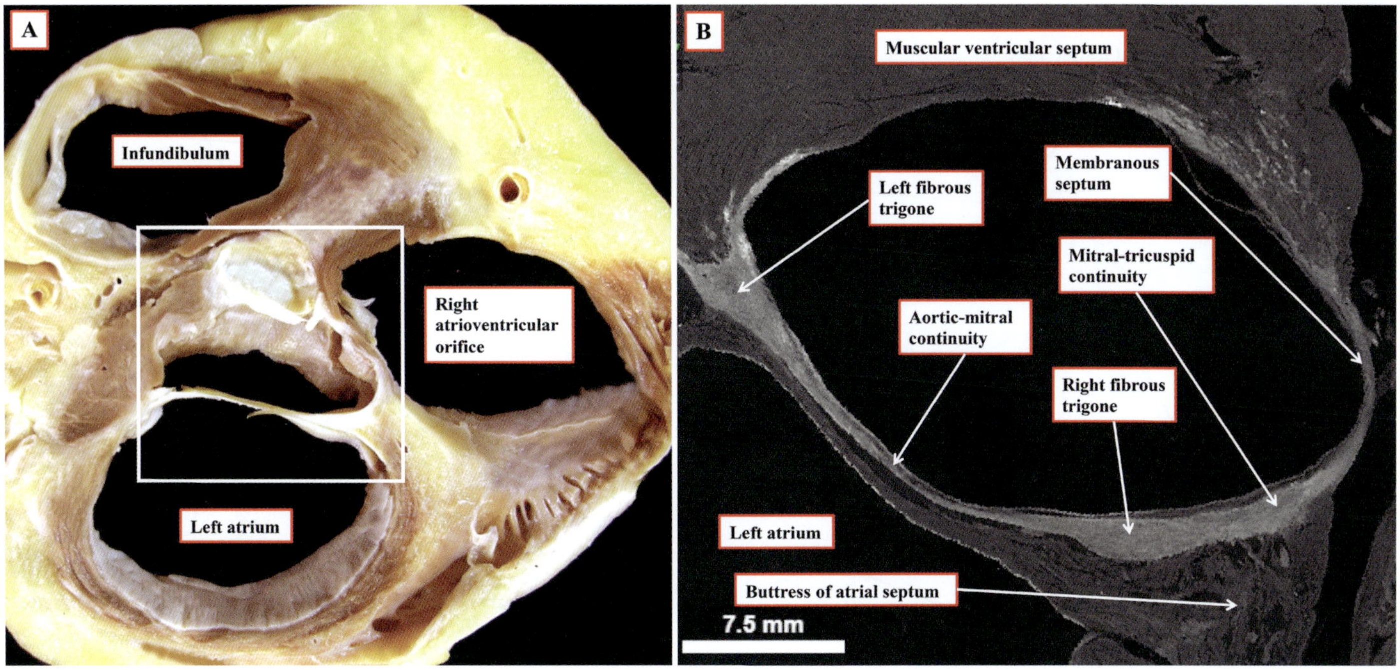

Figure 12.15. Panel A shows a view of the short axis of the ventricular mass, having removed the aortic root, leaving behind the base of the right coronary aortic sinus. The area shown by the white square has then been matched with the image shown in panel B. It is taken from an HiP-CT dataset, showing the area of mitral-to-aortic fibrous continuity and the so-called central fibrous body. The fibrous body has three parts, made up of the right fibrous trigone, the fibrous roof of the infero-septal recess, and the membranous septum. The dimensions of each part can vary within different individuals, with consequences for the relationship of the conduction axis to the aortic root.

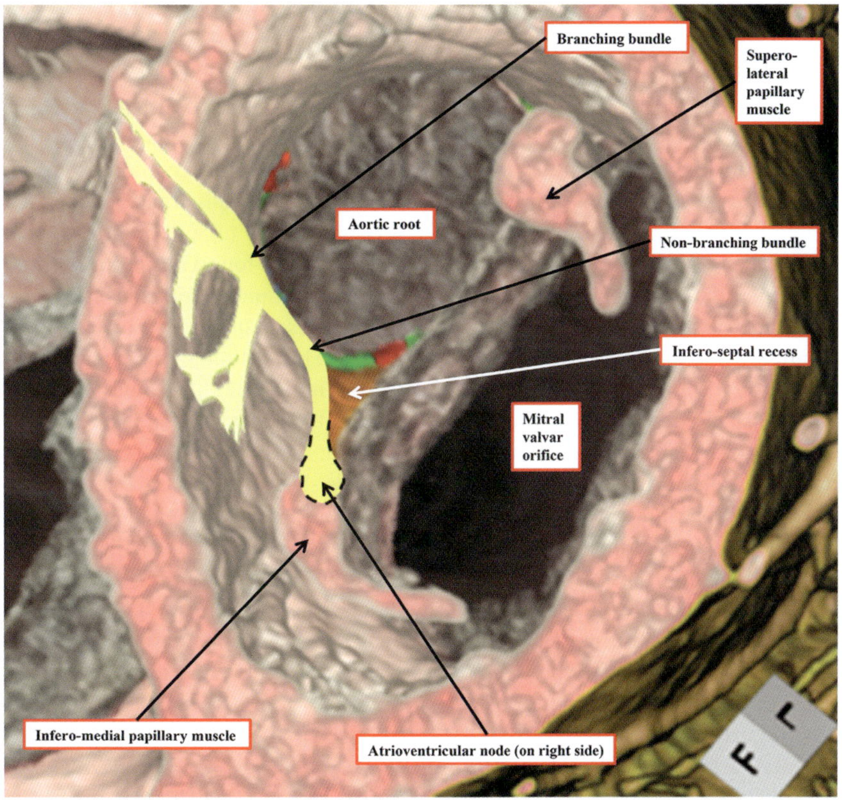

Figure 12.16. The image shows the short axis of the ventricular mass as seen from the apex of the left ventricle revealed by a clinical computed tomogram. Using the known landmarks, the estimated conduction axis has been placed within the heart, providing an indication of the likely disposition in the patient from whom the computed tomogram was obtained. Note that the components of the axis shown in the dashed lines are within the buttress of the atrial septum, at the apex of the inferior pyramidal space.

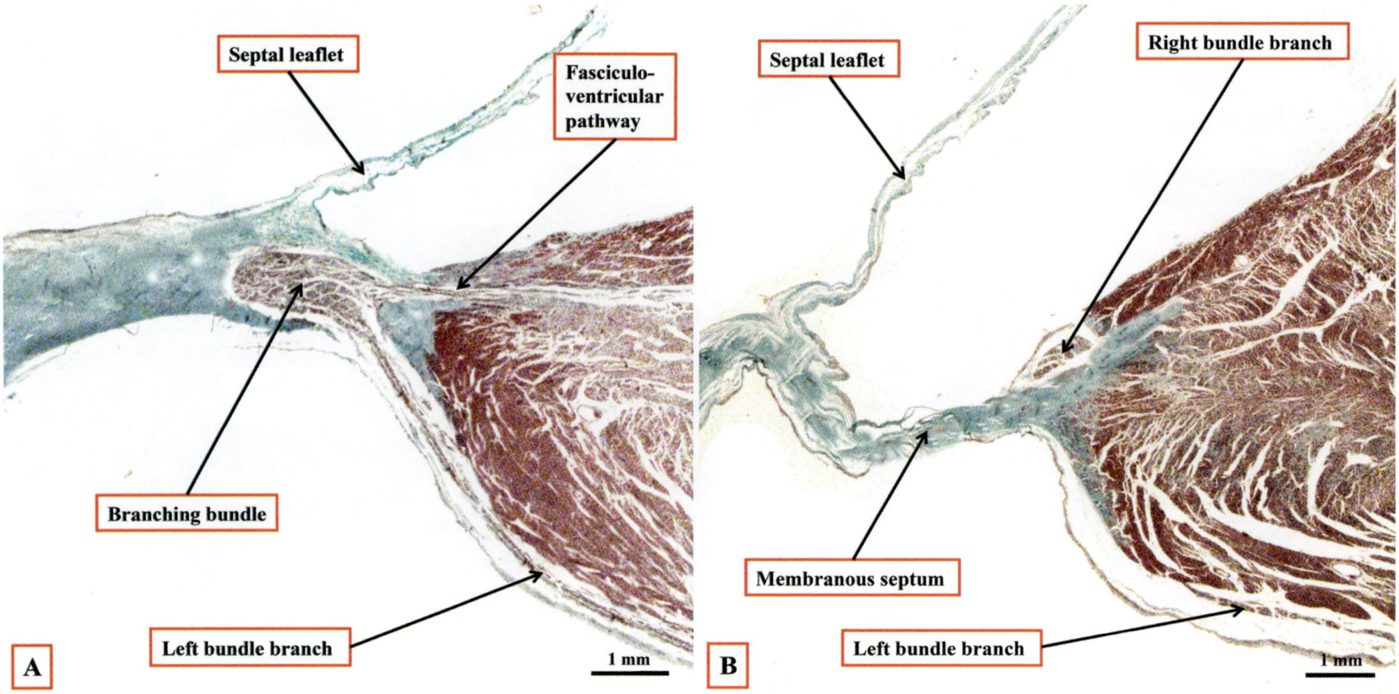

Figure 12.17. The images show the typical fasciculo-ventricular pathway as found in the majority of a series of adult human hearts examined using serial histological sections. As seen in panel A, the branching bundle gives rise to both the left bundle branch and a second pathway that extends into the crest of the muscular ventricular septum. At first sight, the second pathway is the right bundle branch. The pathway is no longer recognizable, however, in the subsequent distal serial sections, whereas the branching bundle itself subsequently gives rise to the cord-like right bundle branch, as shown in panel B.

loops, also found in several other of the cases studied using serial histological sections, produces the obvious potential for re-entry circuits. The function of these fasciculo-ventricular pathways remains to be clarified.

Having taken its origin from the branching bundle, the left bundle usually separates into three interconnected fascicles. When assessed in an attitudinal fashion, the fascicles extend in inferior, septal, and superior directions, with the inferior and superior fascicles running towards the infero-medial and supero-lateral papillary muscles of the mitral valve, respectively. Histological studies have revealed variation in the extent and dominance of the three fascicles.[54] Despite this variability, there is a relatively uniform overall pattern (Figure 12.19). The ***left superior fascicle***, usually described incorrectly as being anterior, courses towards the supero-lateral papillary muscle.

At its origin from the branching bundle, it can achieve a particularly close relationship to the nadir of the right coronary leaflet of the aortic valve (Figure 12.20). The closeness of this relationship is of major significance for those undertaking transcatheter replacement or surgical repair of the diseased aortic valve. The ***left inferior fascicle*** is directed to the infero-medial, or infero-septal, papillary muscle. The ***septal fascicle*** descends the septal surface between the superior and inferior fascicles, with its branches ramifying so as to connect with the other fascicles (Figure 12.19).

As the fascicles descend the septal surface, they are insulated from the underlying septal myocardium (Figure 12.21 panel A). Their contained cardiomyocytes, although histologically distinct, are no larger than the working cardiomyocytes of the septum (Figure 12.21 panel B). It is a mistake to describe the cardiomyocytes as "***Purkinje cells***". The cells described by Purkinje are to be found only within the ventricular components of the conduction systems of ungulates. Having reached the apex of the left ventricle, the fascicles lose their insulation, merging with the apical trabeculations (Figure 12.21 panel B). It is not possible, when using histological sections stained using the trichrome technique, to trace the specialized cells into the left ventricular walls. There is no evidence from the standard histological sections to support the current speculation that "Purkinje cells" are to be found ramifying within the septal myocardium.[55]

The right bundle branch usually takes its origin from the conduction axis as a cord-like insulated strand, emerging within the right ventricle in relation to the medial papillary complex of the tricuspid valve (Figure 12.22). In some hearts, the branch is much more extensive, and can be traced as a sheet descending intramyocardially within the right side of the muscular ventricular septum (Figure 12.23 panel A). The sheet-like variant is reminiscent of the pattern seen during embryonic development, albeit that the sheet is subendocardial during development. The variant is the exception rather than the rule in adult datasets examined histologically. Irrespective of whether descending as a cord or a sheet, the bundle eventually crosses the ventricular cavity as part of the moderator band. It then ramifies within the right ventricular apex (Figure 12.23 panel B). Some of its branches can be traced cranially into the infundibulum.[56]

Accessory Muscular Atrioventricular Pathways

In the normal heart, the atrioventricular conduction axis is the solitary myocardial pathway which provides electrical continuity between

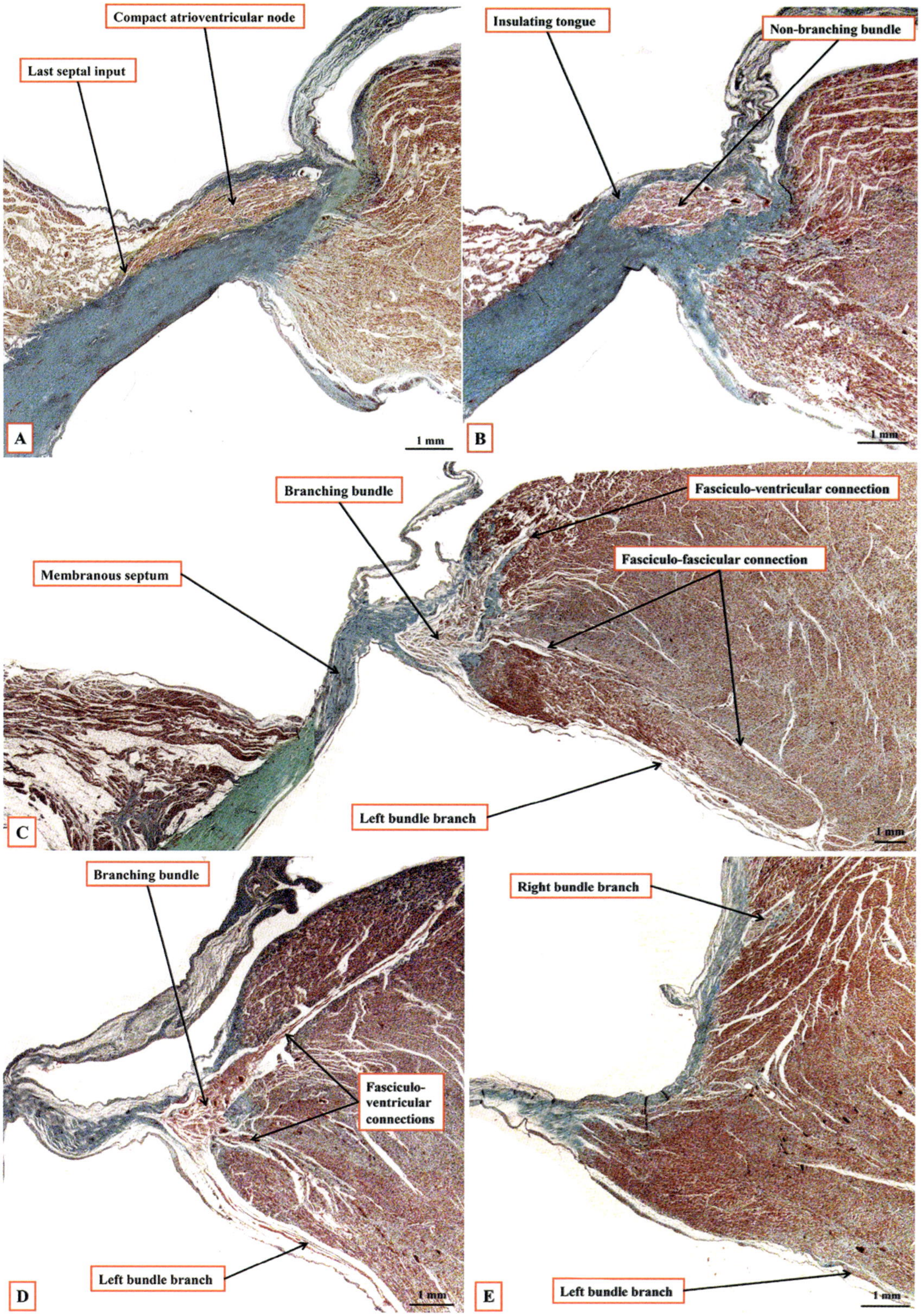

Figure 12.18. The images from this dataset, orientated in attitudinal fashion, reveal the features of the most florid example of fasciculo-ventricular pathways found in the series of adult hearts examined using serial histological sections. Panels A and B show the transition from the distal atrioventricular node to the non-branching bundle, which is comparable to the arrangement shown in Figure 12.14. In this example, however, as the axis branches on the crest of the muscular ventricular septum, not only does it give rise to the left bundle branch, but also, as shown in Figure 12.15, it provides direct connections with the crest of the muscular ventricular septum (panel C). One of the connections then forms a fasciculo-fascicular loop. When traced further distally (panel D), the axis continues to give rise to the pathway that formed the loop but also gives rise to additional connections to the crest of the septum (panel D). Only when traced still further distally does the axis eventually become insulated as the cord-like right bundle branch (panel E).

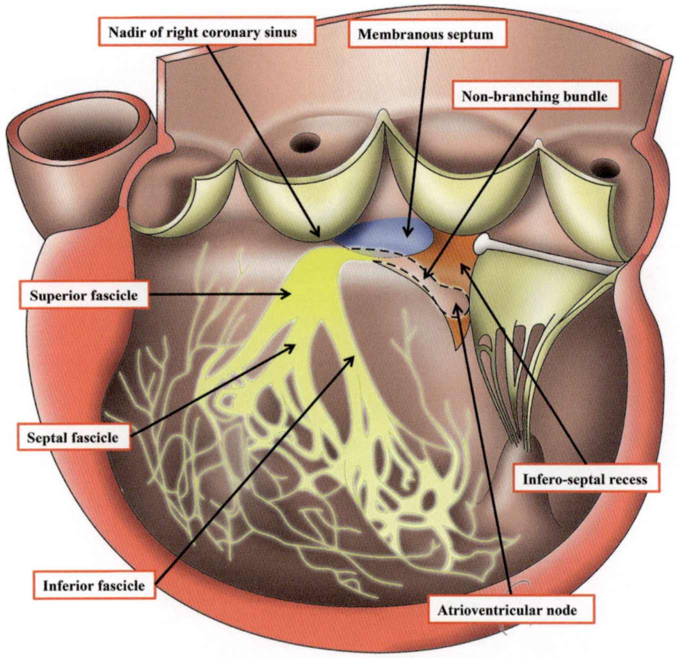

Figure 12.19. The drawing shows the arrangement of the fascicles of the left bundle branch. The superior fascicle, having descended with varying proximity to the nadir of the right coronary leaflet of the aortic root, extends towards the supero-lateral papillary muscle of the mitral valve, not shown in the drawing. The inferior fascicle is shown as extending towards the infero-medial papillary muscle. The original drawing was made by Mrs Gemma Price and has been relabelled with her permission.

the atrial and ventricular myocardial masses. On occasion, additional myocardial pathways can be present crossing the plane of atrioventricular insulation. Such pathways are themselves usually solitary, but they can be multiple. When present, the pathways produce the potential for ventricular pre-excitation and create the situation for atrioventricular re-entry tachycardia. The abnormal rhythms can be produced by several anatomical substrates.[36] The possibility for the presence of such pre-excitation was predicted by Mines long before the anatomical pathways themselves had been identified.[57] Having read the experience of A.G. Mayer in producing circus rhythms by stimulating the muscular umbrella of the jellyfish, Mines showed it was also possible experimentally to create circus movements in the hearts of various experimental animals. Noting the suggestion made by Kent that multiple pathways could be found crossing the atrioventricular junctions in normal hearts, Mines predicted the potential for atrioventricular re-entry. This was also long before Wolff, Parkinson, and White described the syndrome now known in their name.[58] Kent, however, had been wrong when suggesting that multiple atrioventricular pathways were to be found in the normal heart. To emphasize yet again, the atrioventricular conduction axis is the only pathway in the normal heart that provides for ventricular activation from the sinus node. But the findings of Kent were not entirely without substance. The entities he illustrated do exist. They are found within the vestibule of the normal tricuspid valve and are remnants of the primary interventricular ring (Figure 12.10). In the normal heart they are sequestrated on the atrial side of the plane of atrioventricular insulation (Figure 12.24). They are of significance in understanding the potential anatomical substrates for pre-excitation.

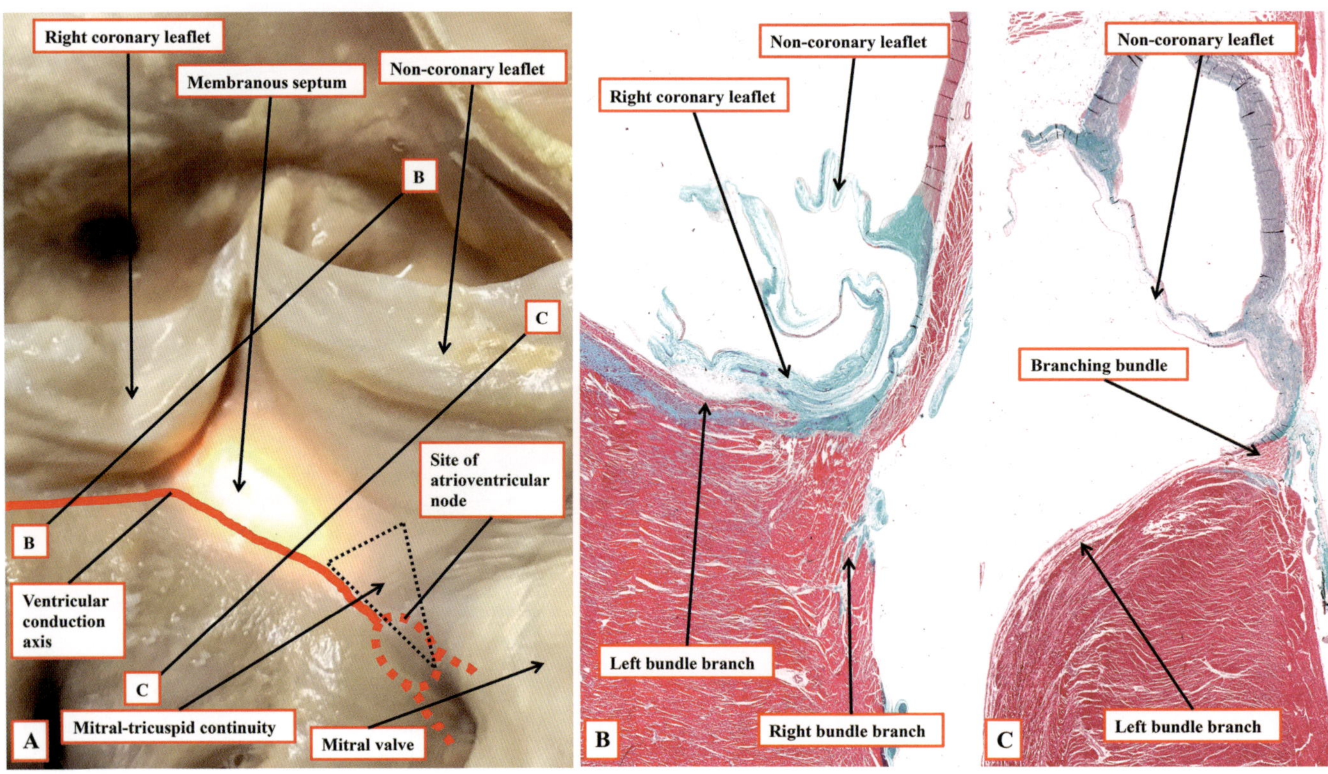

Figure 12.20. The images show the relationship of the superior fascicle of the left bundle branch to the nadir of the right coronary leaflet in one of the adult hearts studied using histological serial sections, having photographed the left ventricular outflow tract (panel A). The lines B–B and C–C demonstrate the approximate locations of the histological sections shown in panels B and C. The sections are stained using the trichrome technique. As can be seen, in this heart the superior fascicle is directly related to the hinge of the valvar leaflet. The dashed red lines show the location of the atrioventricular node within the pyramid of Koch.

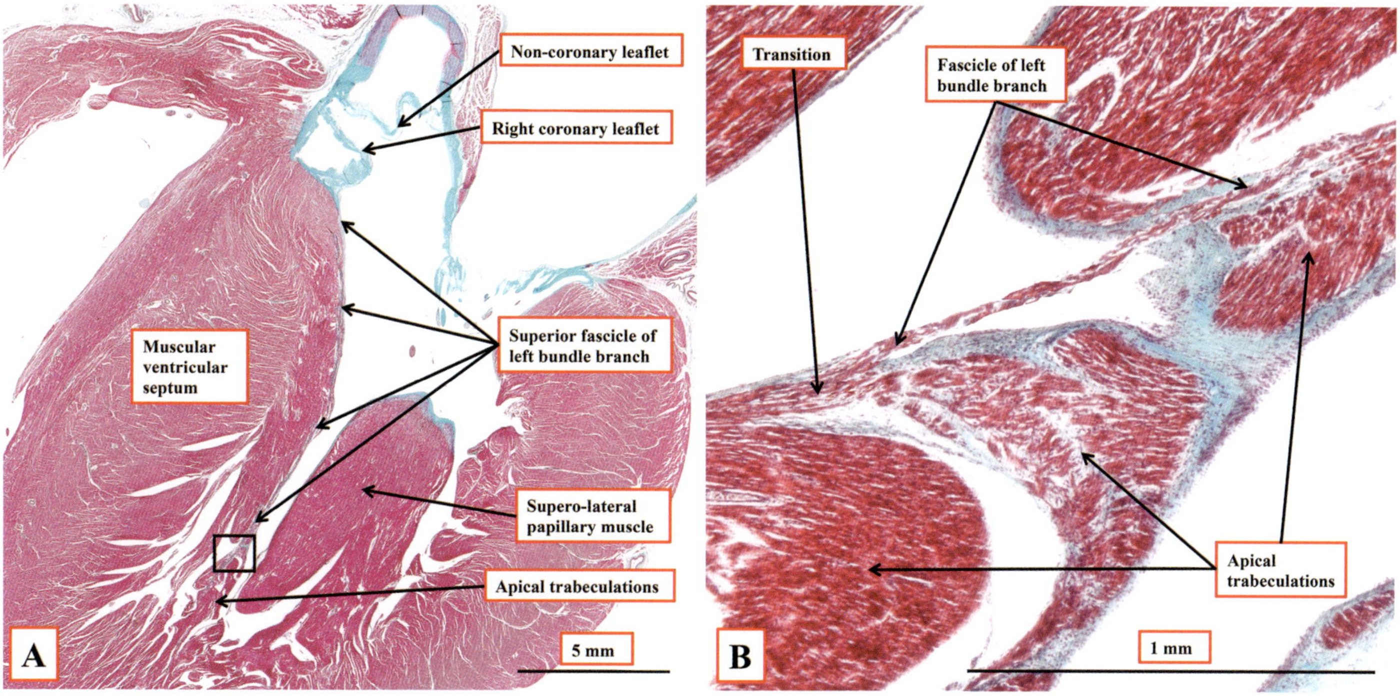

Figure 12.21. The histological section across the left ventricle shown in panel A, stained with the trichrome technique, and orientated in "four-chamber" fashion, demonstrates the course of the superior fascicle of the left bundle branch. In this heart, it runs within 2 mm of the nadir of the right coronary leaflet of the aortic valve and extends towards the supero-lateral papillary muscle of the mitral valve, where it ramified into the apical trabeculations. The black open square is magnified to produce panel B, which shows that the cardiomyocytes of the left bundle branch are no larger than the adjacent working ventricular cardiomyocytes. It is a mistake to describe the specialized cardiomyocytes as being "Purkinje cells".

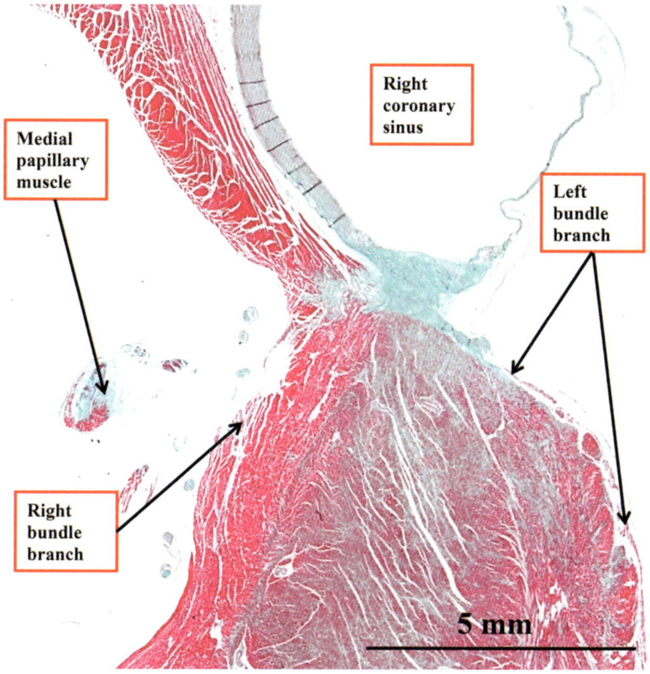

Figure 12.22. The image shows the typical arrangement of the right bundle branch, with the section orientated in four-chamber fashion to compare with Figure 12.23. The right bundle is cord-like, as also shown in Figure 12.17. In this image, it is possible to recognize its relationship to the medial papillary muscle of the tricuspid valve.

Some of the connections that can potentially provide an anatomical circuit for re-entry tachycardia arise from the atrioventricular conduction axis itself. Such connections between the branching atrioventricular bundle and the crest of the muscular septum, if searched for diligently, are found in the majority of normal hearts (Figures 12.17, 12.18). These ***fasciculo-ventricular*** connections are the pathways initially identified by Mahaim[34] and described as being superior septal by Hecht and colleagues.[35] It remains to be established whether they are of greater significance in providing an explanation for the success of so-called selective pacing of the conduction system as opposed to functioning as substrates for pre-excitation.[37] Persistent ***fasciculo-ventricular*** pathways, on the other hand, have been identified histologically as providing the anatomical substrate for pre-excitation.[53] Unlike the fasciculo-ventricular connections, it is exceedingly rare to find nodoventricular pathways in otherwise normal adult hearts. They have been identified, nonetheless, with some frequency in the setting of Ebstein's malformation (Figure 12.25).[53,59]

If the significance of the superior septal pathways has yet fully to be established in the setting of ventricular pre-excitation, there can be no doubt that it is accessory myocardial atrioventricular pathways that underscore the presence of the Wolff–Parkinson–White syndrome and its related arrhythmias. As emphasized, the potential for such pathways providing the circuits for atrioventricular re-entry had been predicted by Mines prior to the description of the syndrome.[57] The presence of such a pathway was eventually demonstrated histologically by Öhnell.[60] The account and iconography

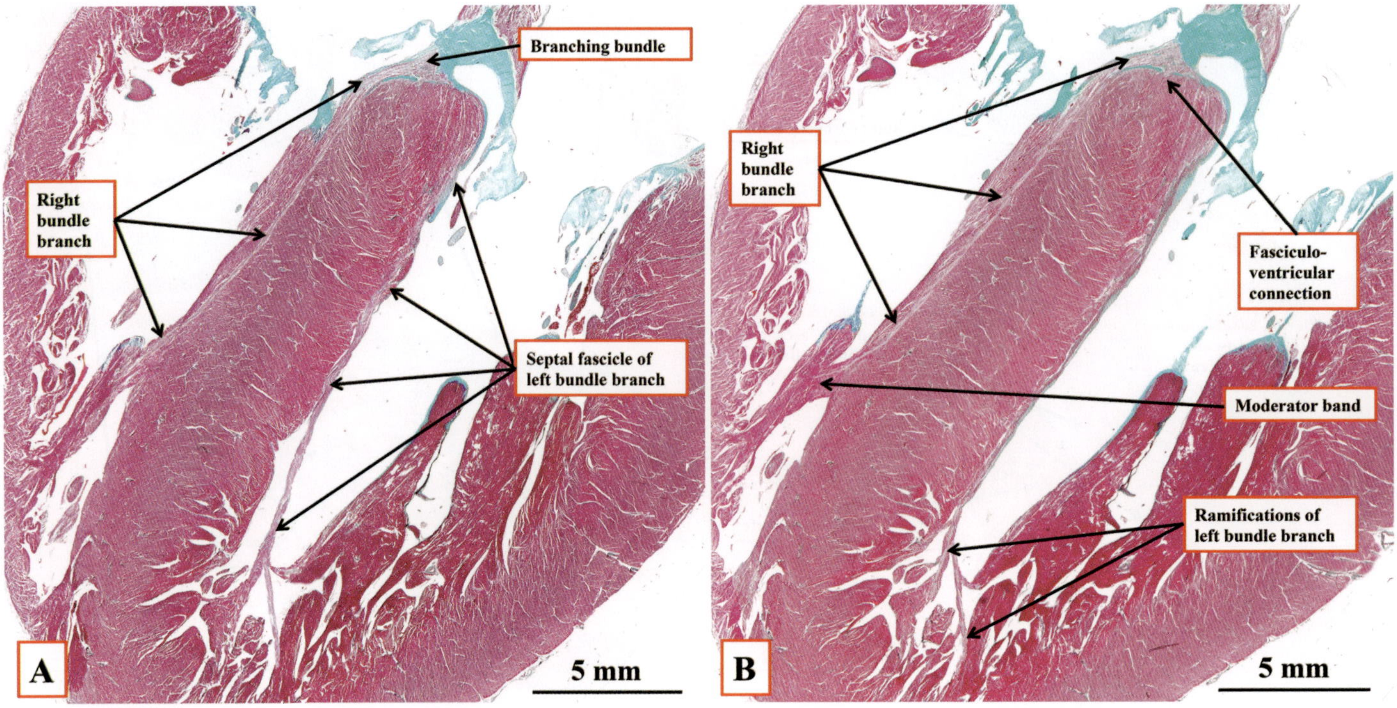

Figure 12.23. These images are serial sections from the same dataset as used to provide Figure 12.21, again orientated in four-chamber fashion. They are 1 mm apart, showing that, in this heart, the right bundle branch is formed as a sheet of insulated cardiomyocytes located intramyocardially within the ventricular septum. As can be seen in panel B, the right bundle crosses the cavity of the right ventricle as part of the moderator band. The sections also show well the ramifications of the fascicles of the left bundle at the apex of the left ventricle. Note the presence of the fasciculo-ventricular connection from the base of the branching bundle in panel B.

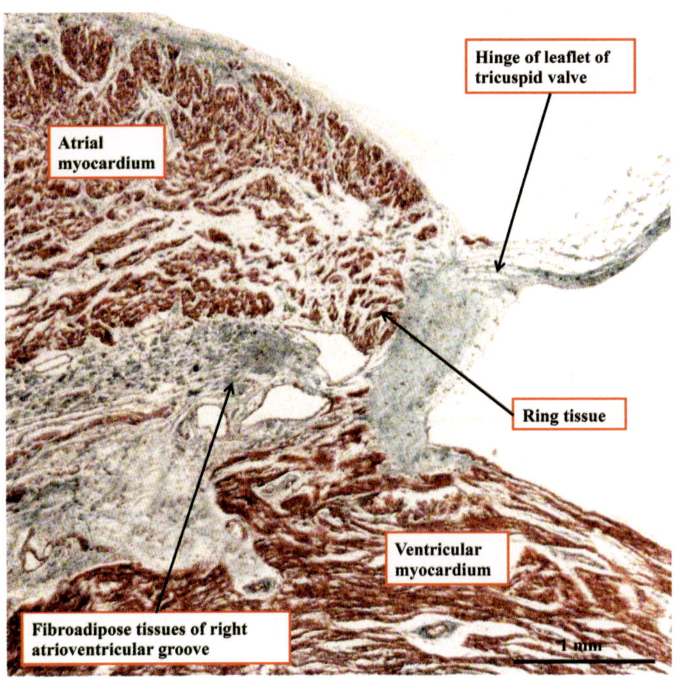

Figure 12.24. The image shows the inferior right atrioventricular junction of a normal heart. There is a node-like structure sequestrated on the atrial side of the plane of atrioventricular insulation. Such structures are remnants of the ring of specialized myocardium that, early in development, surround the embryonic interventricular foramen (see Figure 12.10). It was structure of this kind that Kent incorrectly identified as multiple atrioventricular pathways in the normal heart. As can be seen, the structure does not cross the plane of atrioventricular insulation.

provided by Öhnell were remarkably accurate. As he showed, when found in the left atrioventricular junction, the accessory pathways, composed of working cardiomyocytes, can skirt a well-formed fibrous shelf within the junction (Figure 12.26).

The pathways tend to become smaller when traced from their atrial origin to the ventricular insertion, but they can branch prior to inserting into the ventricular myocardium. Although the accessory pathways can be found anywhere within the mural ***left atrioventricular groove***, on occasion pathways have been described in relation to the aortic leaflet of the mitral valve. Again, as already discussed, in almost all individuals this leaflet is in fibrous continuity with two of the leaflets of the aortic valve. It is difficult, therefore, to envisage how an accessory myocardial pathway could extend from the atrial to the ventricular myocardial masses in this area. The obvious explanation is that the pathways are found in the rare circumstances where the aortic root remains supported by the myocardium of the inner heart circumference. Such myocardium is present during the early stages of embryonic life, but attenuates during the initial stages of foetal development.[61] Should such myocardium persist postnatally, as has now been recognized in the setting of hypertrophic cardiomyopathy, then it would provide a potential substrate for an accessory atrioventricular pathway.[19] Unlike the arrangement in the left atrioventricular junction, it is rare in the right atrioventricular junction to find fibrous shelves separating the atrial and ventricular myocardial masses. Hence, when found within the right atrioventricular junction, accessory pathways, which again can be multiple, simply cross through the layer of fibro-adipose tissue that usually insulates the atrial and ventricular myocardial components (Figure 12.27).

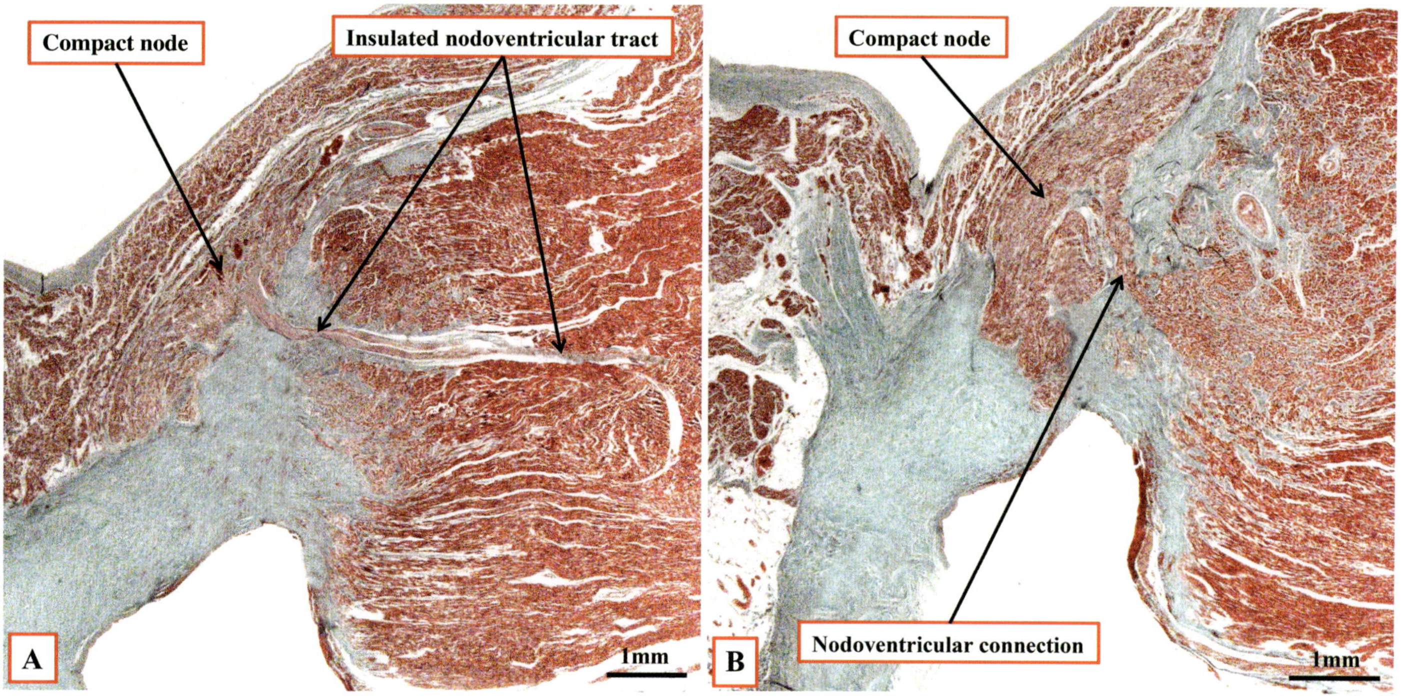

Figure 12.25. The sections are taken from serially sectioned hearts from neonates dying with Ebstein's malformation. They show examples of nodoventricular pathways, with the variant shown in panel A producing an insulated tract extending into the crest of the ventricular septum. The example shown in panel B is more reminiscent of so-called foetal dispersion of the developing conduction axis.

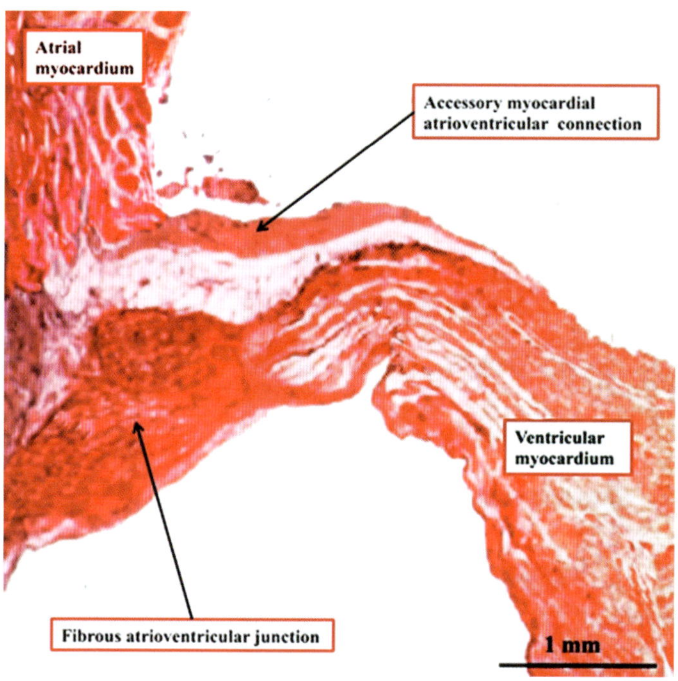

Figure 12.26. The image shows a left-sided accessory myocardial atrioventricular pathway from a patient known to have suffered with Wolff–Parkinson–White syndrome. The pathway, made of working myocardium, skirts a well-formed fibrous shelf separating the atrial and ventricular myocardial components of the junction.

The accessory pathways responsible for pre-excitation can be found anywhere within the atrioventricular junctions where the distal components of the ***atrial walls are adjacent to the crest of the ventricular walls***. In the past, description of the location of the pathways was bedevilled by use of cardiocentric as opposed to attitudinally appropriate terms. Further problems were produced by the failure to recognize that the areas directly superior and inferior to the membranous part of the septum were themselves paraseptal, rather than being septal.[62] The pathways that had conventionally been described as being located "posteriorly" are located inferiorly when assessed in attitudinally appropriate fashion (Figure 12.28). In the same way, pathways currently supposed to be "antero-septal" are located superiorly and in paraseptal location. These pathways are directly adjacent to the right coronary sinus of the aortic root. The only septal component of the atrioventricular junctions is the atrioventricular component of the membranous septum, although this is often overlaid by atrial vestibular myocardium to produce a fibromuscular septum. This area frequently includes the atrioventricular conduction axis itself. It is unlikely that true septal accessory muscular connections could exist in this area to produce the Wolff–Parkinson–White syndrome. Hence, those pathways previously labelled as being "mid-septal" are better considered to be mid-paraseptal (Figure 12.28).[62]

There are then additional entities found in the ***right atrioventricular junction*** that are of significance to the understanding of the variants of the Wolff–Parkinson–White syndrome. These structures are remnants of the primary ring of conduction tissue found during embryonic development (Figure 12.10). As has been explained, it was the remnants of this ring that were incorrectly identified by Kent as producing accessory atrioventricular connections in the normal heart.[63] On occasion, the remnants can, indeed, persist as parts of right-sided accessory atrioventricular pathways. These are the so-called ***atriofascicular*** tracts (Figure 12.29).[64]

The ventricular parts of the tracts can insert into the right bundle branch. They are insulated as they join the ventricular walls, usually

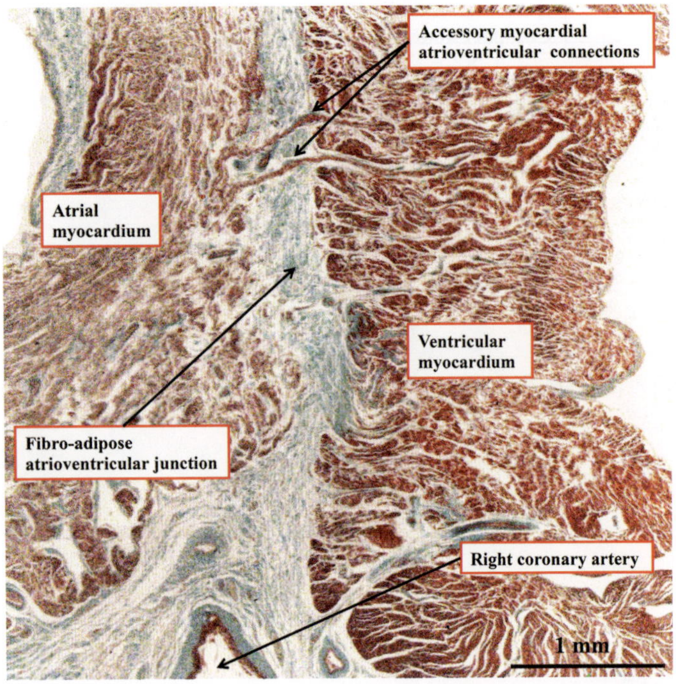

Figure 12.27. The image shows dual accessory myocardial pathways crossing the right-sided atrioventricular junction. The pathways are composed of working myocardium.

adjacent to the hinge of the antero-superior leaflet of the tricuspid valve at the acute margin of the right atrioventricular junction. The pathways, made up of working myocardium, can traverse the epicardial tissues of the junction at any site from the hinge of the leaflet to the epicardial covering, and can be found anywhere within the parietal parts of the right junction. The feature of the atriofascicular tracts is that they conduct in decremental fashion. Because of this, they have frequently been described as producing the "Mahaim" variant of pre-excitation.[53] As has also been explained, Mahaim described the superior septal pathways as producing a second system for atrioventricular conduction which involved the atrioventricular conduction axis itself. And as has again already been explained, on occasion the pathways that he described can, indeed, produce pre-excitation. Mahaim, however, did not describe atriofascicular tracts. It is preferable, therefore, to avoid using the eponym in the context of the atriofascicular tracts, whilst accepting that the electrophysiological features of the pre-excitation can be similar. Decrementally conducting tracts can also be found producing pre-excitation in the left atrioventricular junction.[65] Whatever is responsible for the decremental features of these pathways, it cannot be because they originate in remnants of the primary ring. The vestibular myocardium of the left atrioventricular junction, nonetheless, is derived from the embryonic atrioventricular canal, and it does have the capacity to delay atrioventricular conduction. Although the primary

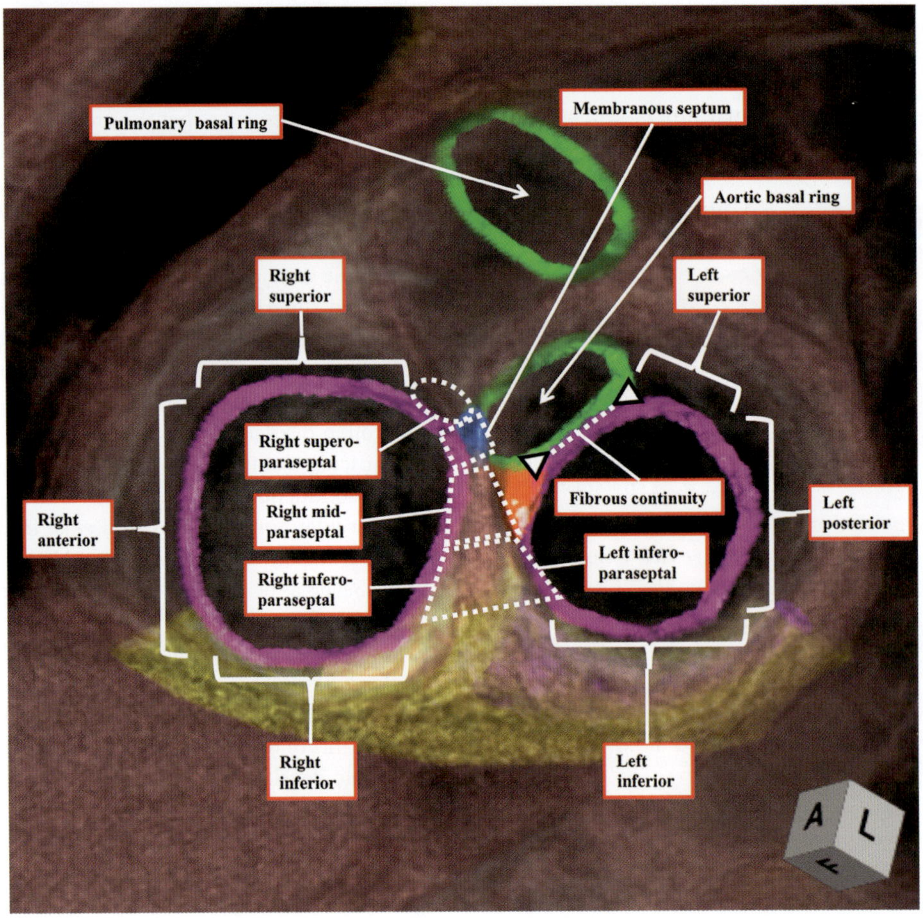

Figure 12.28. The segmented computed tomographic image previously shown in Figure 12.6 panel A has been re-labelled to show the correct way of describing the atrioventricular junctions in attitudinally appropriate fashion, and in distinguishing the components of the junctions that are paraseptal rather than representing true septal areas. The only true septal component is the part related to the membranous septum, which has been segmented in blue.

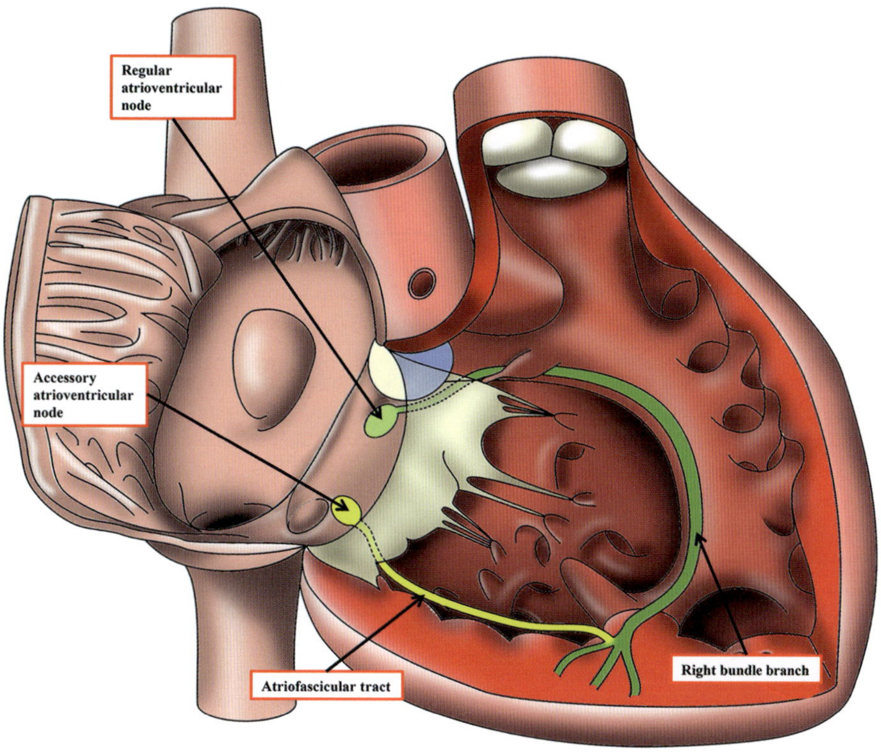

Figure 12.29. Features of the so-called atriofascicular tract. The pathway takes its origin from one of the remnants of the primary interventricular ring, as shown in Figure 12.24. When fully formed, it is presumed to insert into the right bundle branch. Lesser variants can produce decrementally conducting pathways. The original drawing was made by Mrs Gemma Price and has been relabelled with her permission.

ring encircles only the right atrioventricular junction, it is of note that, during its development, it included a second nodal remnant formed within the base of the atrial septum. This is the ***retro-aortic node***.[27] As yet, the function of the node during normal atrioventricular conduction has yet to be established. It is likely involved in some of the arrhythmias that are cured by ablation from the non-coronary sinus of the aortic root.[66]

When considered as an overall group, approximately half of the accessory myocardial pathways are able to conduct both antegradely and retrogradely. The majority of the other half conducted only in the retrograde direction. They are labelled as being ***concealed***, since they produce no evidence of pre-excitation on the surface electrocardiogram. A small percentage of pathways conduct only in the anterograde direction. Concealed pathways give rise only to orthodromic re-entry and occasionally have decremental properties.[67] They are not associated with an increased risk of sudden cardiac death. No gender predilection is found and these pathways tend to become clinically apparent at an earlier age than those responsible for atrioventricular nodal re-entry. There is, nonetheless, significant overlap between the different forms.[68] Those pathways that are concealed are predominantly localized along the left free wall, being found less frequently in paraseptal and right-sided locations.[67,69]

REFERENCES

1. Anderson RH, Christoffels VM, Moorman AF. Controversies concerning the anatomical definition of the conduction tissues. *Anat Rec B New Anat*. 2004;**280**:8–14. doi: 10.1002/ar.b.20028
2. Tawara S. *Das Reizleitungssystem des Säugetierherzens*. Jena: G. Fischer; 1906.
3. Keith A, Flack M. The form and nature of the muscular connections between the primary divisions of the vertebrate heart. *J Anat Physiol*. 1907;**41**:172–189. PMID: 17232727
4. Anderson KR, Ho SY, Anderson RH. Location and vascular supply of sinus node in human heart. *Br Heart J*. 1979;**41**:28–32. doi: 10.1136/hrt.41.1.28
5. Sanchez-Quintana D, Cabrera JA, Farre J, Climent V, Anderson RH, Ho SY. Sinus node revisited in the era of electroanatomical mapping and catheter ablation. *Heart*. 2005;**91**:189–194. doi: 91/2/189 [pii]10.1136/hrt.2003.031542
6. Park DS, Fishman GI. The cardiac conduction system. *Circulation*. 2011;**123**:904–915. doi: 10.1161/CIRCULATIONAHA.110.942284123/8/904 [pii]
7. Pauza DH, Skripka V, Pauziene N, Stropus R. Morphology, distribution, and variability of the epicardiac neural ganglionated subplexuses in the human heart. *Anat Rec*. 2000;**259**:353–382. doi: 10.1002/1097-0185(20000801)259:4<353::AID-AR10>3.0.CO;2-R
8. Fedorov VV, Glukhov AV, Chang R, Kostecki G, Aferol H, Hucker WJ, Wuskell JP, Loew LM, Schuessler RB, Moazami N, et al. Optical mapping of the isolated coronary-perfused human sinus node. *J Am Coll Cardiol*. 2010;**56**:1386–1394. doi: 10.1016/j.jacc.2010.03.098S0735-1097(10)03457-1 [pii]
9. Ho SY, Anderson RH, Sánchez-Quintana D. Atrial structure and fibres: morphologic bases of atrial conduction. *Cardiovasc Res*. 2002;**54**:325–336. doi: 10.1016/S0008-6363(02)00226-2
10. James TN. The connecting pathways between the sinus node and A-V node and between the right and the left atrium in

the human heart. *Am Heart J*. 1963;**66**:498–508. doi: 10.1016/0002-8703(63)90382-x

11. Anderson RH, Sanchez-Quintana D, Spicer DE, Farre J, Back Sternick E. How does the cardiac impulse pass from the sinus to the atrioventricular node? *Heart Rhythm*. 2022;**19**:1738–1746. doi: 10.1016/j.hrthm.2022.05.032
12. Power DA, Lampert J, Camaj A, Bienstock SW, Kocovic N, Bayes-Genis A, Miller MA, Bayes-de-Luna A, Fuster V. Cardiovascular complications of interatrial conduction block: JACC state-of-the-art review. *J Am Coll Cardiol*. 2022;**79**:1199–1211. doi: 10.1016/j.jacc.2022.01.030
13. Chandler N, Aslanidi O, Buckley D, Inada S, Birchall S, Atkinson A, Kirk D, Monfredi O, Molenaar P, Anderson R, et al. Computer three-dimensional anatomical reconstruction of the human sinus node and a novel paranodal area. *Anat Rec*. 2011;**294**:970–979. doi: 10.1002/ar.21379
14. Anderson RH, Mori S, Spicer DE, Sanchez-Quintana D, Jensen B. The anatomy, development, and evolution of the atrioventricular conduction axis. *J Cardiovasc Dev Dis*. 2018;**5**:44. doi: 10.3390/jcdd5030044
15. Tretter JT, Koneru JN, Spicer DE, Ellenbogen KA, Anderson RH, Ben-Haim S. A new dimension in cardiac imaging: three-dimensional exploration of the atrioventricular conduction axis with hierarchical phase-contrast tomography. *Heart Rhythm*. 2024;**21**:2388–2396. doi: 10.1016/j.hrthm.2024.10.002
16. Kuniewicz M, Ostrowski P, Bonczar M, Kwiecinska M, Mozdzen K, Murawska A, Dziedzic M, Zytkowski A, Goncerz G, Walocha J, et al. The anatomy of the atrioventricular nodal artery: a meta-analysis with implications for cardiothoracic surgery and ablation procedures. *Clin Anat*. 2023;**36**:951–957. doi: 10.1002/ca.24072
17. Tretter JT, Spicer DE, Sanchez-Quintana D, Back Sternick E, Farre J, Anderson RH. Miniseries 1—Part III: 'Behind the scenes' in the triangle of Koch. *Europace*. 2022;**24**:455–463. doi: 10.1093/europace/euab285
18. Rosenquist GC, Clark EB, Sweeney LJ, McAllister HA. The normal spectrum of mitral and aortic valve discontinuity. *Circulation*. 1976;**54**:298–301. doi: 10.1161/01.cir.54.2.298
19. Ferrazzi P, Spirito P, Binaco I, Zyrianov A, Poggio D, Vaccari G, Grillo M, Pezzoli L, Scatigno A, Dorobantu L, et al. Congenital muscular mitral-aortic discontinuity identified in patients with obstructive hypertrophic cardiomyopathy. *J Am Coll Cardiol*. 2020;**76**:2238–2247. doi: 10.1016/j.jacc.2020.09.534
20. Macias Y, de Almeida MC, Tretter JT, Anderson RH, Spicer DE, Mohun TJ, Sanchez-Quintana D, Farre J, Back Sternick E. Miniseries 1—Part II: The comparative anatomy of the atrioventricular conduction axis. *Europace*. 2022;**24**:443–454. doi: 10.1093/europace/euab291
21. Inoue S, Becker AE. Posterior extensions of the human compact atrioventricular node: a neglected anatomic feature of potential clinical significance. *Circulation*. 1998;**97**:188–193. doi: 10.1161/01.cir.97.2.188
22. Katritsis DG, Josephson ME. Classification of electrophysiological types of atrioventricular nodal re-entrant tachycardia: a reappraisal. *Europace*. 2013;**15**:1231–1240. doi: 10.1093/europace/eut100
23. Katritsis DG, Anderson RH. New insights into the mechanisms of fast and slow conduction in the atrioventricular node. *Heart Rhythm*. 2023;**20**:627–630. doi: 10.1016/j.hrthm.2022.08.025
24. Katritsis DG, Efimov IR. Cardiac connexin genotyping for identification of the circuit of atrioventricular nodal re-entrant tachycardia. *Europace*. 2019;**21**:190–191. doi: 10.1093/europace/euy099
25. Katritsis DG, Becker A. The atrioventricular nodal reentrant tachycardia circuit: a proposal. *Heart Rhythm*. 2007;**4**:1354–1360. doi: S1547-5271(07)00603-0 [pii]10.1016/j.hrthm.2007.05.026
26. Anderson RH, Sanchez-Quintana D, Mori S, Cabrera JA, Back Sternick E. Re-evaluation of the structure of the atrioventricular node and its connections with the atrium. *Europace*. 2020;**22**:821–830. doi: 10.1093/europace/euaa031
27. Yanni J, Boyett MR, Anderson RH, Dobrzynski H. The extent of the specialized atrioventricular ring tissues. *Heart Rhythm*. 2009;**6**:672–680. doi: 10.1016/j.hrthm.2009.01.021
28. Katritsis DG, al. e. Spatial characterization of the tachycardia circuit of atrioventricular nodal reentrant tachycardia. *Europace*. 2021;**23**:1596–1602. doi: 10.1093/europace/euab130
29. Katritsis DG. A unified theory for the circuit of atrioventricular nodal re-entrant tachycardia. *Europace*. 2020;**22**:1763–1767. doi: 10.1093/europace/euaa196
30. Katritsis DG, Calkins H, Anderson RH. The specialized atrioventricular ring tissues participate in the circuit of atrioventricular nodal reentrant tachycardia. *J Am Heart Assoc*. 2021;**10**:e022811. doi: 10.1161/JAHA.121.022811
31. Anderson RH, Mori S. Wilhelm His Junior and his bundle. *J Electrocardiol*. 2016;**49**:637–643. doi: 10.1016/j.jelectrocard.2016.06.003
32. Macias Y, Tretter JT, Anderson RH, Sanchez-Quintana D, Soares Correa F, Farre J, Back Sternick E. Miniseries 1—Part IV: How frequent are fasciculo-ventricular connections in the normal heart? *Europace*. 2022;**24**:464–472. doi: 10.1093/europace/euab286
33. Massing GK, James TN. Anatomical configuration of the His bundle and bundle branches in the human heart. *Circulation*. 1976;**53**:609–621. doi: 10.1161/01.cir.53.4.609
34. Mahaim I. Kent's fibers and the A-V paraspecific conduction through the upper connections of the bundle of His-Tawara. *Am Heart J*. 1947;**33**:651–653. doi: 10.1016/0002-8703(47)90080-x
35. Hecht HH, Kossmann CE, Childers RW, Langendorf R, Lev M, Rosen KM, Pruitt RD, Truex RC, Uhley HN, Watt TB, Jr. Atrioventricular and intraventricular conduction. Revised nomenclature and concepts. *Am J Cardiol*. 1973;**31**:232–244. doi: 10.1016/0002-9149(73)91036-9
36. Anderson RH, Becker AE, Brechenmacher C, Davies MJ, Rossi L. Ventricular preexcitation. A proposed nomenclature for its substrates. *Eur J Cardiol*. 1975;3:27–36. PMID: 1132407
37. Mahmud R, Sanchez-Quintana D, Macias Y, de Almeida MC, Anderson RH, Back Sternick E. Correction of bundle branch block by so-called nonselective His bundle pacing: the potential role of accessory connections in the ventricular septal crest. *Heart Rhythm*. 2024;**21**:647–654. doi: 10.1016/j.hrthm.2024.01.003
38. Burri H, Jastrzebski M, Cano O, Curila K, de Pooter J, Huang W, Israel C, Joza J, Romero J, Vernooy K, et al. EHRA clinical consensus statement on conduction system pacing implantation: executive summary. Endorsed by the Asia-Pacific Heart Rhythm Society (APHRS), Canadian Heart Rhythm Society (CHRS) and Latin-American Heart Rhythm Society (LAHRS). *Europace*. 2023;**25**:1237–1248. doi: 10.1093/europace/euad044
39. Vijayaraman P, Chelu MG, Curila K, Dandamudi G, Herweg B, Mori S, Jastrzebski M, Sharma PS, Shivkumar K, Tung R, et al. Cardiac conduction system pacing: a comprehensive update.

JACC Clin Electrophysiol. 2023;**9**:2358–2387. doi: 10.1016/j.jacep.2023.06.005
40. Gonzalez-Matos CE, Rodriguez-Queralto O, Zaraket F, Jimenez J, Casteigt B, Valles E. Conduction system stimulation to avoid left ventricle dysfunction. *Circ Arrhythm Electrophysiol.* 2024;**17**:e012473. doi: 10.1161/CIRCEP.123.012473
41. Tan ESJ, Soh R, Lee JY, Boey E, Ho KH, Aguirre S, de Leon J, Chan SP, Seow SC, Kojodjojo P. Clinical outcomes in conduction system pacing compared to right ventricular pacing in bradycardia. *JACC Clin Electrophysiol.* 2023;**9**:992–1001. doi: 10.1016/j.jacep.2022.10.016
42. Slotwiner DJ, Raitt MH, Del-Carpio Munoz F, Mulpuru SK, Nasser N, Peterson PN. Impact of physiologic pacing versus right ventricular pacing among patients with left ventricular ejection fraction greater than 35%. A systematic review for the 2018 ACC/AHA/HRS Guideline on the evaluation and management of patients with bradycardia and cardiac conduction delay. A report of the American College of Cardiology/American Heart Association Task Force on Clinical Practice Guidelines and the Heart Rhythm Society. *J Am Coll Cardiol.* 2019;**74**:988–1008. doi: 10.1016/j.jacc.2018.10.045
43. Glikson M, Nielsen JC, Kronborg MB, Michowitz Y, Auricchio A, Barbash IM, Barrabes JA, Boriani G, Braunschweig F, Brignole M, et al. 2021 ESC Guidelines on cardiac pacing and cardiac resynchronization therapy. *Eur Heart J.* 2021;**42**:3427–3520. doi: 10.1093/eurheartj/ehab364
44. Ponnusamy SS, Basil W, Vijayaraman P. Electrophysiological characteristics of septal perforation during left bundle branch pacing. *Heart Rhythm.* 2022;**19**:728–734. doi: 10.1016/j.hrthm.2022.01.018
45. Vijayaraman P, Sharma PS, Cano Ó, Ponnusamy SS, Herweg B, Zanon F, Jastrzebski M, Zou J, Chelu MG, Vernooy K, et al. Comparison of left bundle-branch area pacing to biventricular pacing in candidates for resynchronization therapy. *J Am Coll Cardiol.* 2023;**82**:228–241. doi: 10.1016/j.jacc.2023.05.006
46. Gin J, Chow CL, Voskoboinik A, Nalliah C, Wong C, Van Gaal W, Farouque O, Mohamed U, Lim HS, Kalman JM, et al. Improved outcomes of conduction system pacing in heart failure with reduced ejection fraction: a systematic review and meta-analysis. *Heart Rhythm.* 2023;**20**:1178–1187. doi: 10.1016/j.hrthm.2023.05.010
47. Cai M, Wu S, Wang S, Zheng R, Jiang L, Lian L, He Y, Zhu L, Xu L, Ellenbogen KA, et al. Left bundle branch pacing postatrioventricular junction ablation for atrial fibrillation: propensity score matching with His bundle pacing. *Circ Arrhythm Electrophysiol.* 2022;**15**:e010926. doi: 10.1161/CIRCEP.122.010926
48. Cabrera JA, Anderson RH, Macias Y, Nevado-Medina J, Porta-Sanchez A, Rubio JM, Sanchez-Quintana D. Variable arrangement of the atrioventricular conduction axis within the triangle of Koch: implications for permanent His bundle pacing. *JACC Clin Electrophysiol.* 2020;**6**:362–377. doi: 10.1016/j.jacep.2019.12.004
49. Kawashima T, Sato F. Visualizing anatomical evidences on atrioventricular conduction system for TAVI. *Int J Cardiol.* 2014;**174**:1–6. doi: 10.1016/j.ijcard.2014.04.003
50. Tretter JT, Mori S, Saremi F, Chikkabyrappa S, Thomas K, Bu F, Loomba RS, Alsaied T, Spicer DE, Anderson RH. Variations in rotation of the aortic root and membranous septum with implications for transcatheter valve implantation. *Heart.* 2018;**104**:999–1005. doi: 10.1136/heartjnl-2017-312390
51. Tretter JT, Mori S, Anderson RH, Taylor MD, Ollberding N, Truong V, Choo J, Kereiakes D, Mazur W. Anatomical predictors of conduction damage after transcatheter implantation of the aortic valve. *Open Heart.* 2019;**6**:e000972. doi: 10.1136/openhrt-2018-000972
52. Tretter JT, Spicer DE, Macias Y, Talbott C, Kasten JL, Sanchez-Quintana D, Kapadia SR, Anderson RH. Vulnerability of the ventricular conduction axis during transcatheter aortic valvar implantation: a translational pathologic study. *Clin Anat.* 2023;**36**:836–846. doi: 10.1002/ca.24032
53. Katritsis DG, Wellens HJ, Josephson ME. Mahaim accessory pathways. *Arrh Electrophysiol Rev.* 2017;**6**:29–32. doi: 10.15420/aer.2016:35:1
54. Demoulin JC, Kulbertus HE. Histopathological examination of concept of left hemiblock. *Br Heart J.* 1972;**34**:807–814. doi: 10.1136/hrt.34.8.807
55. Hillestad ML, Amontree M, Mahlberg RC, Bagwell MS, Rizzo SA, Arrell DK, Kargaran PK, Crespo-Diaz RJ, Syed FF, Lockhart EN, et al. MYL4 identifies intramural anatomy of Purkinje fibers in human hearts. *JACC Clin Electrophysiol.* 2025;**11**:1718–1735. doi: 10.1016/j.jacep.2025.03.039
56. De Almeida MC, Stephenson RS, Anderson RH, Benvenuti LA, Loukas M, Aiello VD. Human subpulmonary infundibulum has an endocardial network of specialized conducting cardiomyocytes. *Heart Rhythm.* 2020;**17**:123–130. doi: 10.1016/j.hrthm.2019.07.033
57. Janse MJ. A tale of 2 arrhythmias: the early history of the arrhythmias involving the AV node. *JACC Clin Electrophysiol.* 2023;**9**:2412–2415. doi: 10.1016/j.jacep.2023.07.020
58. Wolff L, Parkinson J, White PD. Bundle-branch block with short P-R interval in healthy young people prone to paroxysmal tachycardia. 1930. *Ann Noninvasive Electrocardiol.* 2006;**11**:340–353. doi: 10.1111/j.1542-474X.2006.00127.x
59. Sanchez-Quintana D, Cabrera JA, Picazo-Angelin B, Cabrera A, Anderson RH. Histological examination of the potential arrhythmic substrates in the setting of Ebstein's malformation. *J Anat.* 2020;**237**:155–165. doi: 10.1111/joa.13179
60. Öhnell RF. The WPW-syndrome and related problems: preliminary communication. *Cardiology.* 1942;**6**: 332–334. doi: 10.1159/000164745
61. Anderson RH, Lamers WH, Hikspoors J, Mohun TJ, Bamforth SD, Chaudhry B, Eley L, Kerwin J, Crosier M, Henderson DJ. Development of the arterial roots and ventricular outflow tracts. *J Anat.* 2024;**244**:497–513. doi: 10.1111/joa.13973
62. Farre J, Anderson RH, Rubio JM, Garcia-Talavera C, Sanchez-Quintana D, Bansal R, Lokhandwala Y, Cabrera JA, Wellens HJJ, Back Sternick E. Miniseries 2—Septal and paraseptal accessory pathways—Part III: Mid-paraseptal accessory pathways—revisiting bypass tracts crossing the pyramidal space. *Europace.* 2022;**24**:662–675. doi: 10.1093/europace/euab294
63. Anderson RH, Ho SY, Gillette PC, Becker AE. Mahaim, Kent and abnormal atrioventricular conduction. *Cardiovasc Res.* 1996;**31**:480–491. PMID: 8689639
64. Anderson RH, Sanchez-Quintana D, Mori S, Lokhandwala Y, Correa FS, Wellens HJ, Sternick EB. Unusual variants of pre-excitation: from anatomy to ablation: Part I—Understanding the anatomy of the variants of ventricular pre-excitation. *J Cardiovasc Electrophysiol.* 2019;**30**:2170–2180. doi: 10.1111/jce.14106
65. Katritsis DG, Wellens HJ, Josephson ME. Mahaim accessory pathways. *Arrhythm Electrophysiol Rev.* 2017;**6**:29–32. doi: 10.15420/aer.2016:35:1

66. Bohora S, Lokhandwala Y, Sternick EB, Anderson RH, Wellens HJJ. Reappraisal and new observations on atrial tachycardia ablated from the non-coronary aortic sinus of Valsalva. *Europace.* 2018;**20**:124–133. doi: 10.1093/europace/euw324
67. Kuck KH, Friday KJ, Kunze KP, Schluter M, Lazzara R, Jackman WM. Sites of conduction block in accessory atrioventricular pathways. Basis for concealed accessory pathways. *Circulation.* 1990;**82**:407–417.
68. Katritsis DG, Boriani G, Cosio FG, Hindricks G, Jais P, Josephson ME, Keegan R, Kim Y-H, Knight BP, Kuck K-H, et al. European Heart Rhythm Association (EHRA) consensus document on the management of supraventricular arrhythmias, endorsed by Heart Rhythm Society (HRS), Asia-Pacific Heart Rhythm Society (APHRS), and Sociedad Latinoamericana de Estimulación Cardiaca y Electrofisiologia (SOLAECE). *Eur Heart J.* 2018;**39**:1442–1445. doi: 10.1093/eurheartj/ehw455
69. Ho SY. Accessory atrioventricular pathways: getting to the origins. *Circulation.* 2008;**117**:1502–1504. doi: 10.1161/circulationaha.107.764035

13 The Cardiac Nerves

The heart receives a rich autonomic innervation, with the cardiac nerves taking their origins from the sympathetic trunks and the vagus nerves. It was initially presumed that these nerves were cholinergic and adrenergic in terms of their neurotransmitters, with the two sets of nerves providing antagonism in terms of the various cardiac tropies, but primarily influencing control of the heart rate, or chronotropy. Later, it became obvious that the situation in terms of neurotransmission was much more complicated, with the identification of non-cholinergic and non-adrenergic neurons, particularly in relation to the pulmonary veins.[1] Irrespective of the neurotransmitters involved, the neural pathways remain the same.

The ***sympathetic nerves*** carry both efferent and afferent fibres, with the afferent fibres responding to pain. The preganglionic efferent fibres originate within the spine, with the postganglionic fibres then taking origin from the ganglions of the sympathetic chains. There are three such ganglions in the neck region, located in ***superior***, ***middle***, and ***inferior*** positions on both sides, along with an additional ganglion on each side related to the vertebral artery. The inferior cervical ganglion on each side is usually combined with the superior thoracic ganglion on the same side to produce the composite ***stellate ganglion***. Nerves arise from all of these ganglions on both sides and extend towards the heart, where they form the cardiac plexus in relation to the aortic arch and the extrapericardial arterial trunks.[2] Also contributing to the cardiac plexus are nerves arising bilaterally from the ***first five thoracic ganglions***. It had been suggested that the postganglionic sympathetic nerves originated only from the stellate ganglion, and the thoracic chain, but detailed dissections prepared using an operative stereomicroscope confirmed that significant contributions were made to the plexuses from each of the cervical ganglions.[3] The detailed stereomicroscopic study, whilst confirming the major route of the nerves into the cardiac plexuses along the brachiocephalic arteries, also showed that thoracic nerves entered the plexuses by ascending from both sides within the adventitia of the descending aorta. The ***cardiac plexus*** itself is usually described as having a superficial component, related to the aortic arch, and a deeper part related to the bifurcation of the trachea, but in reality the two parts intermingle to form a conjoined network. Note should also be taken of the ***subclavian loops***, or ansa subclavia, which are formed on both sides. These branches, which recur around the subclavian arteries, although not contributing directly to the cardiac plexuses, innervate the irises. They can be damaged during operations involving the brachiocephalic arteries, particularly the Blalock–Taussig–Thomas shunt should the surgeon choose to use the right subclavian artery,

The ***parasympathetic nerves*** originate from the vagal nerves or their recurrent laryngeal branches. The preganglionic fibres of these nerves have their cell bodies in the dorsal vagal nucleuses, while parasympathetic sensory nerves terminate in the nodose ganglions. The vagus nerves, of course, carry fibres to supply many other organs, but those supplying the heart originate predominantly from the cervical course of the nerves. The ***upper cervical branches*** descend along with the branches of the superior and middle sympathetic ganglions and run into the deeper part of the cardiac plexus. The ***lower cervical branches*** originate at the root of the neck and follow the brachiocephalic vessels to enter the superficial part of the plexus. ***Thoracic branches*** of the vagus nerves themselves then join branches from the recurrent laryngeal nerves to enter the deeper part of the plexus.

From the cardiac plexus itself, which is positioned extrapericardially, the ***intrinsic cardiac nerves*** enter the heart through the superior and posterior hilums (Figure 13.1).[4] The sympathetic

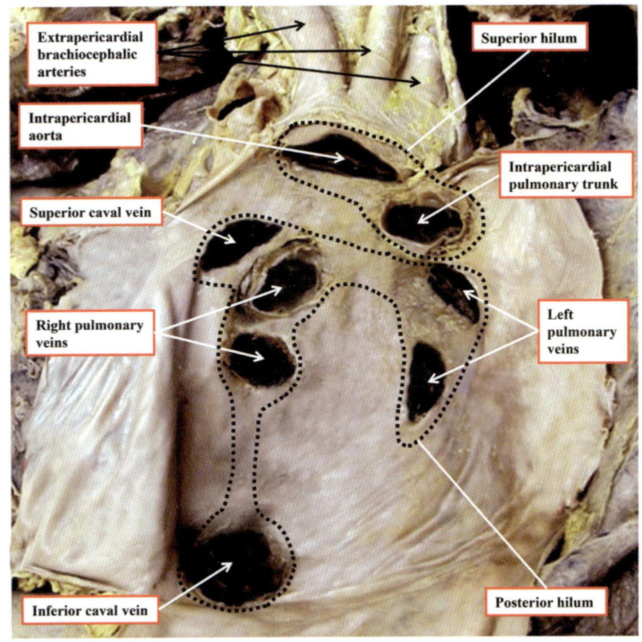

Figure 13.1. The heart has been removed from its pericardial cradle to provide this image, which shows the superior and posterior hilums. The cardiac nerves enter the heart through these two portals from the cardiac plexus, which is related to the arch of the aorta and the middle mediastinum directly behind the pericardial cavity at the site of bifurcation of the trachea. The sympathetic nerves enter primarily through the superior hilum, with the parasympathetic nerves entering mostly through the posterior hilum.

components of the plexus enter and leave the heart mostly through the superior hilum. As they extend into the heart, the nerves are contained within the adventitial coats of both the intrapericardial aorta and the pulmonary trunk. Some vagal nerves also enter through the superior hilum, having their cell bodies in the aortic root ganglions. The cardiac nerves then ramify into the ventricles along the coronary arteries. The larger part of the vagal component of the cardiac plexus, however, enters the heart through the much more extensive posterior hilum (Figure 13.1). These parasympathetic nerves then synapse in the extensive ganglionated plexuses, with the postganglionic vagal nerves largely supplying the atrial structures, with prominent plexuses formed in relation to the pulmonary veins and the sinus node. There are very few ganglions found within the ventricular component of the heart.

The Cardiac Ganglionated Plexuses

Having entered the heart through the hilums, mostly through the posterior hilum, the autonomic cardiac nerves ramify within the epicardial layer of the pericardium to form the ganglionated plexuses. In an initial study, it was suggested that there were ten specific ganglionated plexuses, five related to the atrial chambers and five supplying the ventricles. Those related to the ***atrial*** chambers were described as being related ***superiorly and posteriorly to the right atrium***, and superiorly, postero-medially, and postero-laterally to the left atrium (Figure 13.2 panel A). The ***ventricular*** plexuses were identified within the atrioventricular grooves and designated as being ***aortic***, ***anterior and inferior interventricular***, and ***right and obtuse marginally*** (Figure 13.2 panel B).[5] A subsequent more detailed study suggested that the number of plexuses could be reduced to seven, retaining the five atrial plexuses but naming those related to the ***left atrium as being anterior, posterior, and lateral***. The plexuses within the atrioventricular grooves were reduced to those feeding the right and left coronary arteries (Figure 13.3).[6]

The ganglionated plexuses are now recognized as having a major influence on the triggering and perpetuation of atrial fibrillation.[7,8] Knowledge of their location, therefore, is key for the interventionists who now seek to produce autonomic denervation by ablating their parasympathetic and sympathetic components. Such denervation can be accomplished either endocardially or epicardially, either during the surgical maze procedures or by using thoracoscopic approaches.[9] Recent evidence indicates that ablation of the plexuses at the relevant atrial sites is safe, and if successful improves the results of pulmonary venous isolation in patients with paroxysmal and persistent atrial fibrillation.[9,10] The plexuses are ablated endocardially at distances of 1 to 2 cm from the junctions of the individual pulmonary veins with the body of the left atrium, along with further ablations at the superior and inferior paraseptal areas.[11–14] Conventional isolation of the pulmonary veins also leads to modulation of the intrinsic cardiac autonomic nervous system. When using radiofrequency or cryoablation, the autonomic reaction has been reported as a surrogate marker for denervation, although this effect might be less prominent when using pulsed-field ablation.[15,16] The results of epicardial ablation achieved using cardiac surgery have

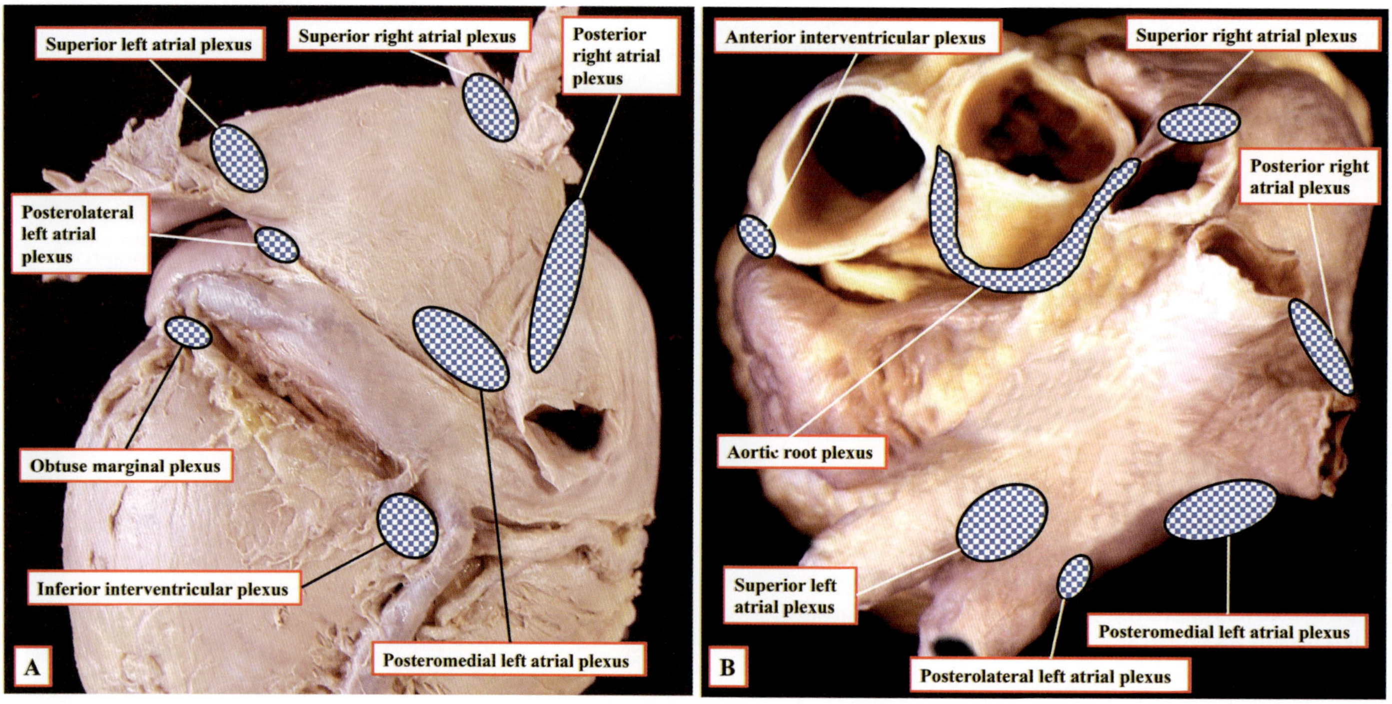

Figure 13.2. The locations of the ganglionated plexuses as initially identified by Armour and colleagues[5] have been superimposed on the inferior and posterior surfaces of the heart in panel A and on the atrial chambers and the origins of the arterial roots in panel B. These workers identified five atrial plexuses, as shown in panel A, along with five ventricular plexuses, which were located in the atrioventricular grooves. Of these ventricular plexuses, the sites of obtuse marginal and inferior plexuses are shown in panel A and the aortic root and anterior interventricular plexuses in panel B. The fifth plexus was described as occupying the right acute margin of the atrioventricular junctions.

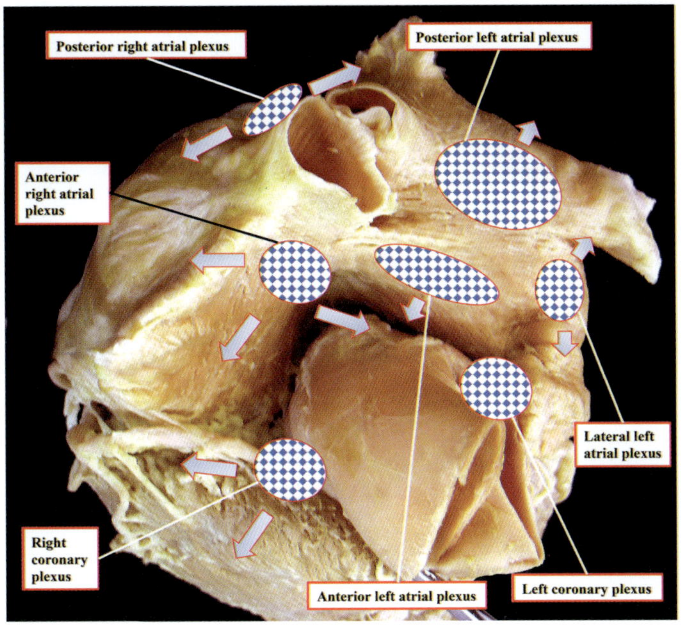

Figure 13.3. The image shows the location of the seven ganglionated plexuses as identified by Pauza and colleagues.[6] The atrial plexuses are more-or-less the same as initially identified by Armour and associates,[5] although given different names. The ventricular plexuses have been simplified into those related to the right and left coronary arteries.

been controversial,[17,18] but use of pulsed-field energy during coronary artery bypass grafting shows promising results.[19] It has now been shown, furthermore, that targeted modulation using magnetic nanoparticles or nanoformulated calcium is able to suppress atrial fibrillation by inducing apoptosis of the neurons contained within the plexuses, in this way inhibiting the vagosympathetic neural activity.[20,21]

REFERENCES

1. Vaitkevicius R, Saburkina I, Rysevaite K, Vaitkeviciene I, Pauziene N, Zaliunas R, Schauerte P, Jalife J, Pauza DH. Nerve supply of the human pulmonary veins: an anatomical study. *Heart Rhythm*. 2009;**6**:221–228. doi: 10.1016/j.hrthm.2008.10.027
2. Ellison JP, Williams TH. Sympathetic nerve pathways to the human heart, and their variations. *Am J Anat*. 1969;**124**:149–162. doi: 10.1002/aja.1001240203
3. Kawashima T. The autonomic nervous system of the human heart with special reference to its origin, course, and peripheral distribution. *Anat Embryol (Berl)*. 2005;**209**:425–438. doi: 10.1007/s00429-005-0462-1
4. Pauza DH, Pauziene N, Tamasauskas KA, Stropus R. Hilum of the heart. *Anat Rec*. 1997;**248**:322–324. doi: 10.1002/(SICI)1097-0185(199707)248:3<322::AID-AR3>3.0.CO;2-R
5. Armour JA, Murphy DA, Yuan BX, Macdonald S, Hopkins DA. Gross and microscopic anatomy of the human intrinsic cardiac nervous system. *Anat Rec*. 1997;**247**:289–298. doi: 10.1002/(SICI)1097-0185(199702)247:2<289::AID-AR15>3.0.CO;2-L
6. Pauza DH, Skripka V, Pauziene N, Stropus R. Morphology, distribution, and variability of the epicardiac neural ganglionated subplexuses in the human heart. *Anat Rec*. 2000;**259**:353–382. doi: 10.1002/1097-0185(20000801)259:4<353::AID-AR10>3.0.CO;2-R
7. Yang N, Zou Y, Wen B, Wang Y, Mei J, Jiang Z. Development of neuromodulation for atrial fibrillation: a narrative review. *J Thorac Dis*. 2024;**16**:3472–3483. doi: 10.21037/jtd-23-1981
8. Baykaner T, Zografos TA, Zaman JAB, Pantos I, Alhusseini M, Navara R, Krummen DE, Narayan SM, Katritsis DG. Spatial relationship of organized rotational and focal sources in human atrial fibrillation to autonomic ganglionated plexi. *Int J Cardiol*. 2017;**240**:234–239. doi: 10.1016/j.ijcard.2017.02.152
9. Katritsis GD, Katritsis DG. Cardiac autonomic denervation for ablation of atrial fibrillation. *Arrhythm Electrophysiol Rev*. 2014;**3**:113–115. doi: 10.15420/aer.2014.3.2.113
10. Gottlieb LA, Mahfoud F, Stavrakis S, Jespersen T, Linz D. Autonomic nervous system: a therapeutic target for cardiac end-organ damage in hypertension. *Hypertension*. 2024;**81**:2027–2037. doi: 10.1161/HYPERTENSIONAHA.123.19460
11. Katritsis DG, Giazitzoglou E, Zografos T, Pokushalov E, Po SS, Camm AJ. Rapid pulmonary vein isolation combined with autonomic ganglia modification: a randomized study. *Heart Rhythm*. 2011;**8**:672–678. doi: 10.1016/j.hrthm.2010.12.047
12. Pokushalov E, Romanov A, Katritsis DG, Artyomenko S, Shirokova N, Karaskov A, Mittal S, Steinberg JS. Ganglionated plexus ablation vs linear ablation in patients undergoing pulmonary vein isolation for persistent/long-standing persistent atrial fibrillation: a randomized comparison. *Heart Rhythm*. 2013;**10**:1280–1286. doi: 10.1016/j.hrthm.2013.04.016
13. Katritsis DG, Pokushalov E, Romanov A, Giazitzoglou E, Siontis GC, Po SS, Camm AJ, Ioannidis JP. Autonomic denervation added to pulmonary vein isolation for paroxysmal atrial fibrillation: a randomized clinical trial. *J Am Coll Cardiol*. 2013;**62**:2318–2325. doi: 10.1016/j.jacc.2013.06.053
14. Benabou L, Ascione C, Sore B, Cherbi M, Labrousse R, Tixier R, Bouyer B, Arnaud M, Buliard S, Pambrun T, et al. A computed tomography-based evaluation and comparison of ganglionated plexus targeting techniques for cardioneuroablation. *Heart Rhythm*. 2025. doi: 10.1016/j.hrthm.2025.01.013
15. Pappone C, Santinelli V, Manguso F, Vicedomini G, Gugliotta F, Augello G, Mazzone P, Tortoriello V, Landoni G, Zangrillo A, et al. Pulmonary vein denervation enhances long-term benefit after circumferential ablation for paroxysmal atrial fibrillation. *Circulation*. 2004;**109**:327–334. doi: 10.1161/01.CIR.0000112641.16340.C7
16. Yorgun H, Aytemir K, Canpolat U, Sahiner L, Kaya EB, Oto A. Additional benefit of cryoballoon-based atrial fibrillation ablation beyond pulmonary vein isolation: modification of ganglionated plexi. *Europace*. 2014;**16**:645–651. doi: 10.1093/europace/eut240
17. Barta J, Brat R. Assessment of the effect of left atrial cryoablation enhanced by ganglionated plexi ablation in the treatment of atrial fibrillation in patients undergoing open heart surgery. *J Cardiothorac Surg*. 2017;**12**:69. doi: 10.1186/s13019-017-0625-1
18. Avazzadeh S, McBride S, O'Brien B, Coffey K, Elahi A, O'Halloran M, Soo A, Quinlan LR. Ganglionated plexi ablation for the treatment of atrial fibrillation. *J Clin Med*. 2020;**9**:3081. doi: 10.3390/jcm9103081
19. Musikantow DR, Reddy VY, Shaburishvili T, van Zyl M, O'Brien B, Coffey K, Reilly J, Asirvatham S, de Groot JR. Epicardial pulsed field ablation for the treatment of paroxysmal atrial fibrillation

during cardiac surgery. *JACC Clin Electrophysiol*. 2024;**10**:2097–2099. doi: 10.1016/j.jacep.2024.06.012
20. Yu L, Scherlag BJ, Dormer K, Nguyen KT, Pope C, Fung KM, Po SS. Autonomic denervation with magnetic nanoparticles. *Circulation*. 2010;**122**:2653–2659. doi: 10.1161/CIRCULATIONAHA.110.940288
21. Jafree E, O'Quinn M, Shoureshi P, Rose B, Wang L, Nguyen N, Nguyen T, Dormer KJ, Nguyen KT, Das A, et al. Targeted ganglionated plexi ablation with nanoformulated calcium suppresses postoperative AF via vagosympatholytic and anti-inflammatory effects. *JACC Clin Electrophysiol*. 2025;**11**:56–70. doi: 10.1016/j.jacep.2024.09.035

14

Comparative Cardiac Anatomy

Although experimental animals remain widely used for the investigation of cardiac structure function, little attention has been given to the differences that exist between the cardiac anatomy of the major species used for these purposes when compared to the arrangements in the human heart described in the previous chapters of this book. When considering the precise make-up of the atrioventricular node, for example, or the relationship of the ventricular components of the atrioventricular conduction axis to the aortic root, or the relationship of the aortic root itself to the left ventricle, the differences in the anatomy and arrangement of the cardiac components become of major significance.

The Overall Arrangement of the Non-Primate Heart

In Chapter 1, emphasis was placed on the problems that had previously been created by anatomists using the "Valentine" approach, in which the heart was removed from the chest, with its components described as if the heart stood on its apex, rather than accounting for the location of the components in attitudinally appropriate fashion. When assessing the ***non-primate heart*** in the appropriate attitude of given species, however, the arrangement is indeed reminiscent of the heart as illustrated for the purposes of St Valentine's Day.[1] The apex does point downwards. And the atrial chambers are positioned directly above their appropriate ventricles, with far less spiralling of the arterial trunks as they extend from the heart into the mediastinum (Figure 14.1).

The aortic root, furthermore, although centrally positioned relative to the short axis of the ventricular base, is not wedged between the right and left atrioventricular junctions to the extent seen in the human heart (Figure 14.2). These differences reflect the location of the heart within the body according to the stance and gait of the animal. Despite the subtle differences when compared to the human heart, the overall arrangement of the cardiac components is more-or-less standardized across the mammalian species.[2] The atrial chambers continue to possess part of the body, derived from the primary heart tube, along with a venous component, appendage, and vestibule. The atrial chambers continue to be separated by the atrial septum. And the ventricles continue to be made up of inlet, apical, and outlet parts. But in all the species, there are subtle features that are not directly comparable with those observed in the human heart.

When considering the atrial chambers, a good example is the relationships of the venous tributaries at their junctions with the atrial chambers. These differences again reflect the stance of the specific animals. In the non-primate hearts, it is usual to find the superior and inferior caval veins entering the right atrium at right angles to each other (Figure 14.3 panel A). This is in contrast to the cranial and caudal arrangements as found in the human heart (see Chapter 4). In consequence, the orifice of the inferior caval vein in the non-primate hearts is more directly related to the oval fossa (Figure 14.3 panel B). The pulmonary veins also enter the morphologically left atrium close to the left atrioventricular junction, often through a common orifice. It is not possible to find the multiple openings to the atrial roof as observed in the human heart. This, in turn, reflects the relationship between the margins of the oval fossa and Bachmann's bundle.

As was shown in Chapter 4, in the human heart the right atrial rim of the oval fossa merges with the precaval band to produce Bachmann's bundle. In the ***porcine*** heart, in contrast, the right pulmonary venoatrial junction interposes between the cavoatrial junction and Bachmann's bundle (Figure 14.4). The differences in venoatrial connections, nonetheless, do not distort the arrangement of the atrial septum itself. As in the human heart, the larger part of the septum is made up by the flap valve, derived from the primary developmental septum (Figure 14.5).

The flap valve is bound to the atrioventricular junctions through its muscular buttress, with the remaining margins of the oval fossa being infoldings between the right and left atrial walls. And although in the non-primate animal species the shapes of the atrial appendages are not as strikingly different as seen in the human heart, when assessing the extent of the pectinate muscles relative to the atrial vestibules, as in the human heart it is an easy matter to distinguish between the morphologically right and morphologically left atrial appendages (Figure 14.6). In similar fashion, when direct comparisons are made in the same heart, the coarseness of the apical trabeculations, along with attachments of the tension apparatus of the atrioventricular valves and the characteristics of the septal surface, permit the distinction to be made between the morphologically right and left ventricles (Figure 14.6).

The overall arrangements of the leaflets of the atrioventricular and arterial valves are also comparable to the features anticipated in the human heart, albeit that the non-coronary leaflet of the aortic valve has a direct attachment to the ventricular septum in species such as the dog, pig, sheep, and ox.[3] This difference is particularly

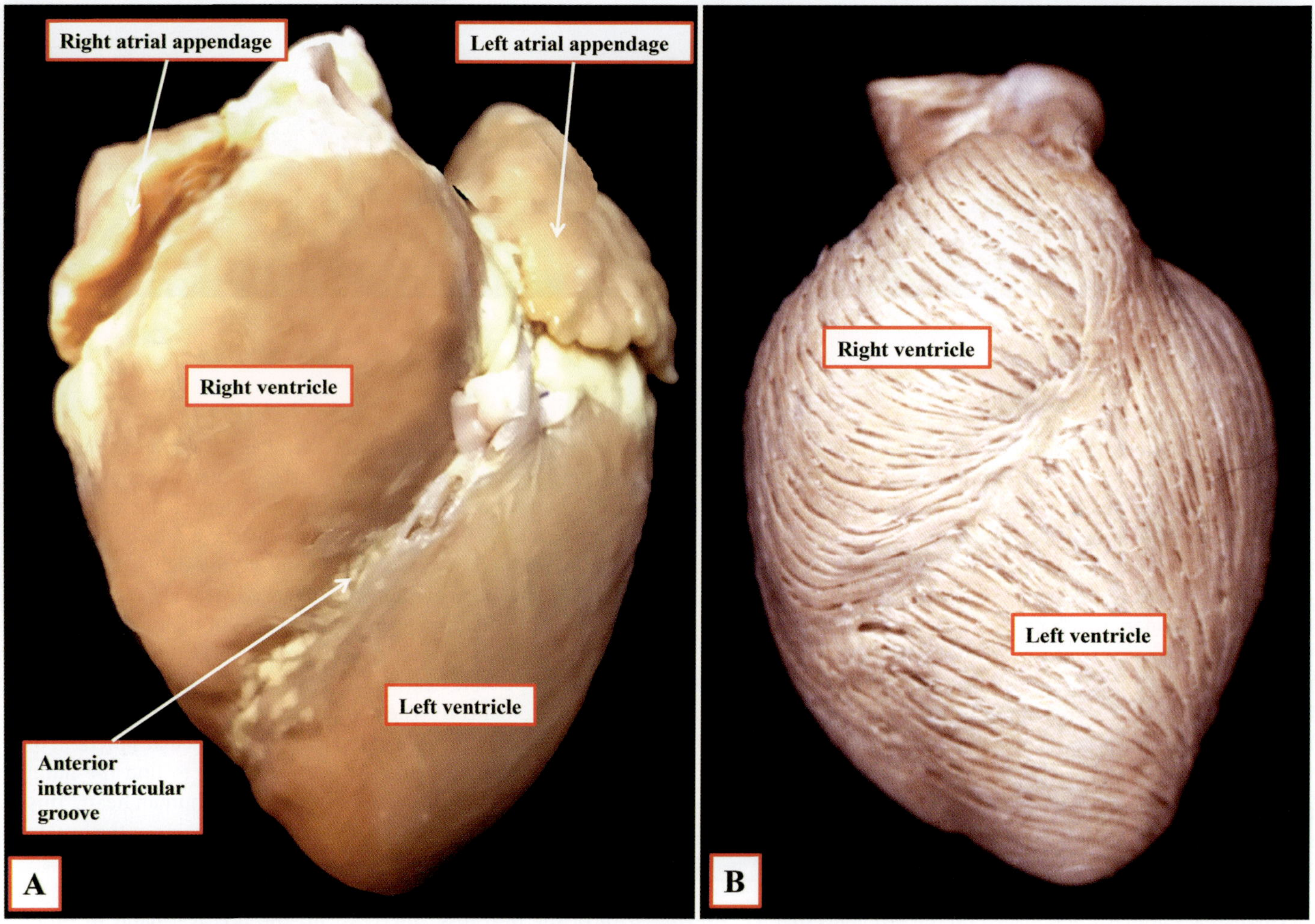

Figure 14.1. Panel A shows the arrangement of the porcine heart as seen when removed from the body and placed in approximately attitudinal arrangement for the pig. The atrial chambers sit above the ventricles in Valentine fashion, with the left ventricle forming the entirety of the apex of the ventricular cone. Panel B shows the "grain" that reflects the alignment of the chains of individual cardiomyocytes that make up the three-dimensional mesh within the ventricular walls of the rabbit heart. The arrangement is reminiscent of the features as observed in the human heart (see Chapter 9), except that the left ventricle forms the entirety of the apex of the ventricular cone, and the chambers themselves produce the Valentine arrangement within the body.

significant, since there is also a marked difference in the angulation of the aortic root relative to the left atrioventricular junction. This reflects the lack of an infero-septal recess in these hearts (Figure 14.7).[4] Along with the absence of a significant membranous part of the septum, this difference has significant consequences for the arrangement of the atrioventricular conduction axis. When taking note of all these subtle differences, the closest similarities with the arrangement in the human heart are found in the mouse.[5]

The Anatomy of the Murine Heart

The mouse is the most widely used experimental animal and is of particular value in that it can readily be genetically manipulated. It is an added bonus, therefore, that the heart of the mouse shares much more in common with the human heart than do the hearts of the other experimentally used species. As was the case with the non-primate species already discussed, the relationships of the cardiac components reflect the gait of the animal. As in the other species, therefore, the caval veins enter the morphologically right atrium at more or less right angles. In keeping with the other species, the left superior caval vein remains patent in postnatal life, opening to the right atrium through the relatively enlarged orifice of the coronary sinus (Figure 14.8 panel A). An unusual feature of the murine heart is the persistence of the venous valves into postnatal life. The inferior caval vein enters the right atrium directly adjacent to the oval fossa, but the structure of the atrial septum is very much in keeping with the arrangement seen in man. The pulmonary veins open through a solitary opening adjacent to the atrioventricular junction, but, as already emphasized, each atrium possesses a part of the initial developmental body, along with an appendage, a venous component, and a vestibule (Figure 14.9).

The septal components separate the atrial cavities. The ventricles are directly comparable with the arrangements seen in the human heart, with each chamber possessing an inlet, an apical component, and an outlet (Figures 14.8 panel B, 14.10). When comparing the two chambers directly, it is possible to appreciate the coarseness of the apical trabeculations of the right versus the left ventricle. The direct septal attachment of the leaflets of the tricuspid valve to the septal surface of the ventricle, along with the presence of the free-standing infundibular sleeve, also serve to distinguish the right ventricle from its morphologically left partner. The membranous septum, although

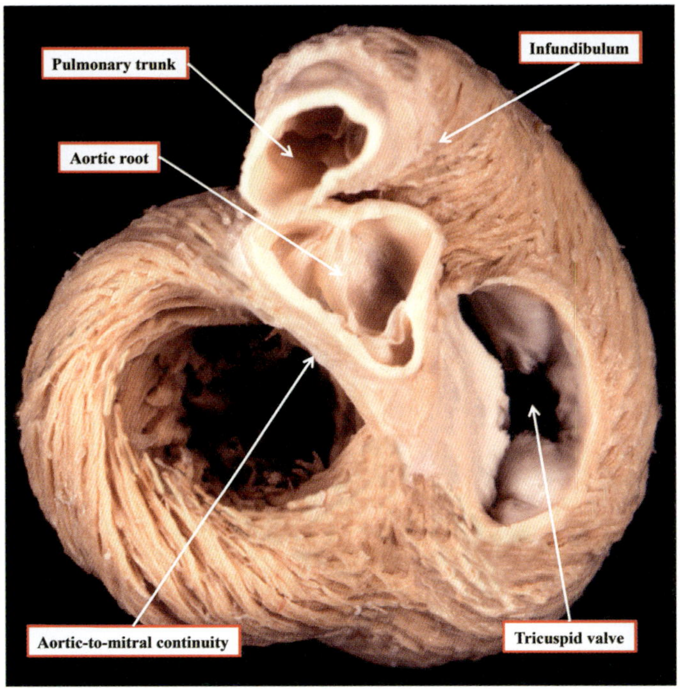

Figure 14.2. The image shows the base of the ventricular cone of the porcine heart, having removed the entirety of the atrial chambers, along with the leaflets of the mitral valve. The intrapericardial aorta has been cut back to the level of the sinutubular junction, and the pulmonary trunk sectioned proximal to its bifurcation. The arterial roots are positioned more directly in front of each other when compared to the human heart. The aortic root is not wedged as deeply between the aortic leaflet of the mitral valve and the septum when compared to the human arrangement. As will be described, this has significant consequences for the disposition of the atrioventricular conduction axis.

not as extensive as in man, is more obvious in the mouse than in the other non-primate species. The feature that makes the murine heart most similar to the human heart, however, is the presence of a well-formed infero-septal recess of the left ventricular outflow tract (Figure 14.10 panel B). The roof of the recess, as in the human heart, is formed by an area of fibrous continuity between the leaflets of the tricuspid and mitral valves, with the fibrous shelf providing the support for the antero-inferior buttress of the atrial septum.

Differences in the Arrangement of the Atrioventricular Conduction Axis

The similarity between the overall anatomy also means that the disposition of the conduction tissues is more comparable in the ***murine heart*** to the human arrangement than in the other non-primate species. The sinus node is formed at the lateral junction of the superior caval vein with the right atrium, with the parallel alignment of the working cardiomyocytes providing the substrate for preferential conduction into the left atrium (Figure 14.11 panel A). The compact atrioventricular node is similarly formed by contributions from both atrial vestibules (Figure 14.11 panel A), with the contributions from the antero-inferior buttress of the atrial septum completing the inputs to the compact node. Again, as with the human heart, it is likely that the vestibular inputs make up the slow pathways into the node, with the last septal connection functioning as the fast pathway (Figure 14.11 panel B).

The axis becomes the non-branching bundle as it is insulated from the atrial septal myocardium by the tongue of fibrous tissue that unites the leaflets of the tricuspid and mitral valves (Figure 14.12 panel A). The axis then branches astride the crest of the muscular

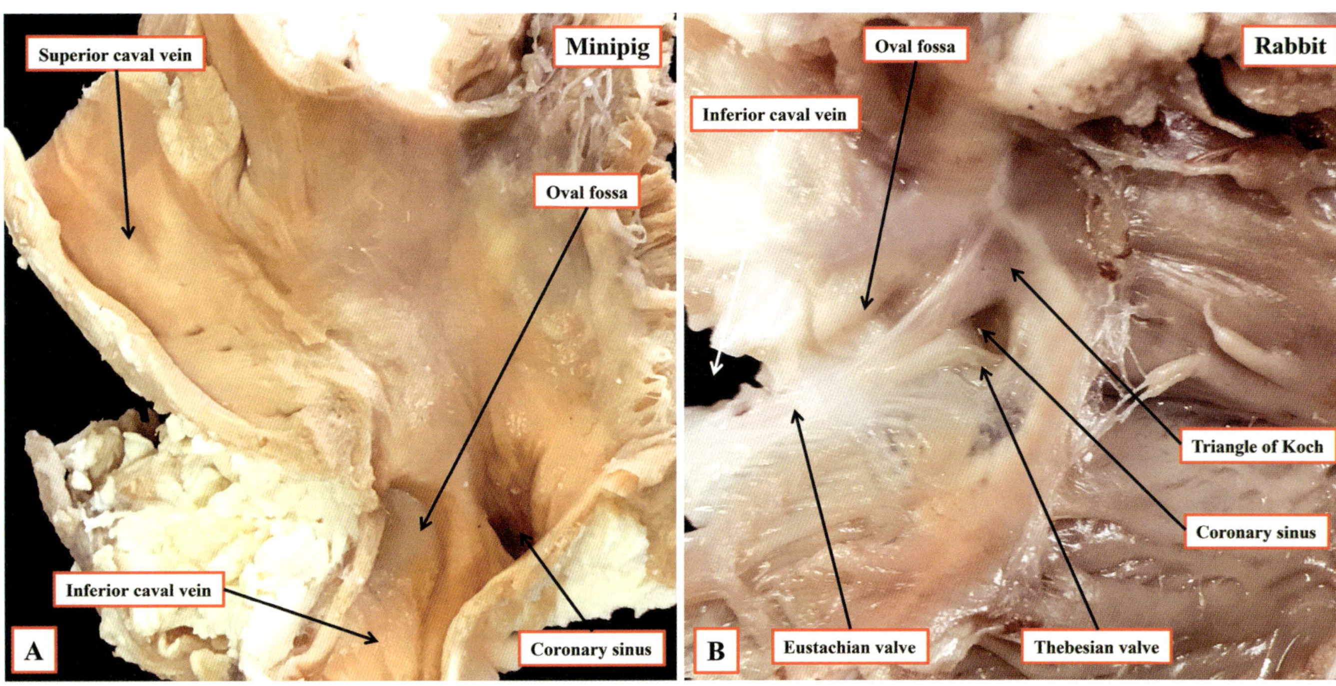

Figure 14.3. The images show the opened cavities of the right atrium in the minipig (panel A) and the rabbit (panel B). As can be seen in panel A, the long axes of the superior and inferior caval veins are almost at right angles to each other, rather than being cranial and caudal as in the human heart. Both panels show how the inferior caval vein opens to the right atrial cavity directly adjacent to the oval fossa. As shown in panel B, the Eustachian valve inserts into the myocardial fold between the opening of the coronary sinus and the oval fossa as the tendon of Todaro, demarcating an obvious triangle of Koch. In both species, the left superior caval vein persists as a confluent channel that opens to the right atrium through the mouth of the coronary sinus.

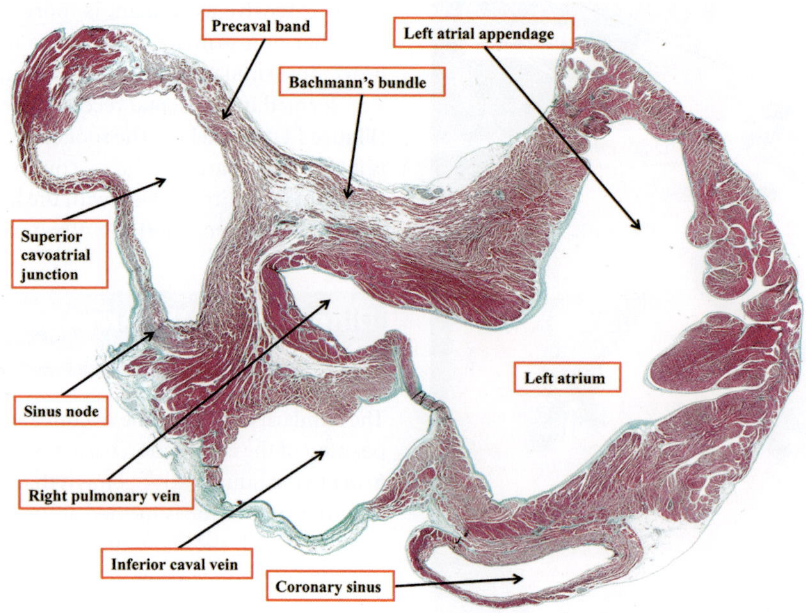

Figure 14.4. The image shows a section through the short axis of the atrial chambers of an adult pig, viewed from the apex looking towards the base and with the right side seen to the left hand. The section is stained using the trichrome technique. As in the human heart, it is possible to distinguish the site of the sinus node from the remainder of the atrial walls, which are made up of aggregated working atrial cardiomyocytes. The aggregation of the individual cardiomyocytes in parallel fashion favour preferential conduction in the precaval band and Bachmann's bundle. Unlike the situation in the human heart, however, the margins of the oval fossa do not contribute directly to Bachmann's bundle. Note the persistent left superior caval vein, with its cavity forming the coronary sinus.

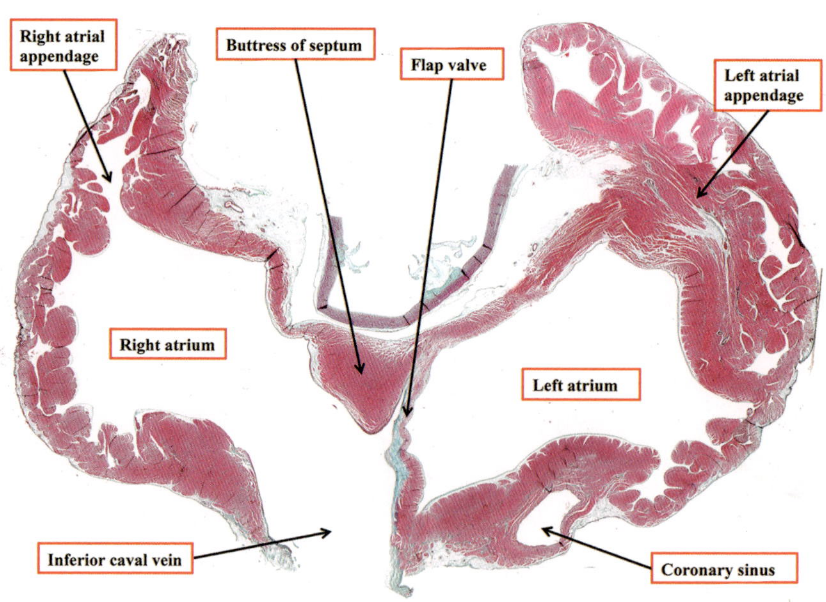

Figure 14.5. The image shows a short axis section taken from another minipig heart in a comparable plane to the section used to produce Figure 14.4, although the oval fossa is directly adjacent to the junction of the right atrium with the inferior caval vein. As in the human heart, the septum is made up predominantly of the flap valve which is anchored to the atrioventricular junctions by the antero-inferior buttress, although that relationship is not shown in this section.

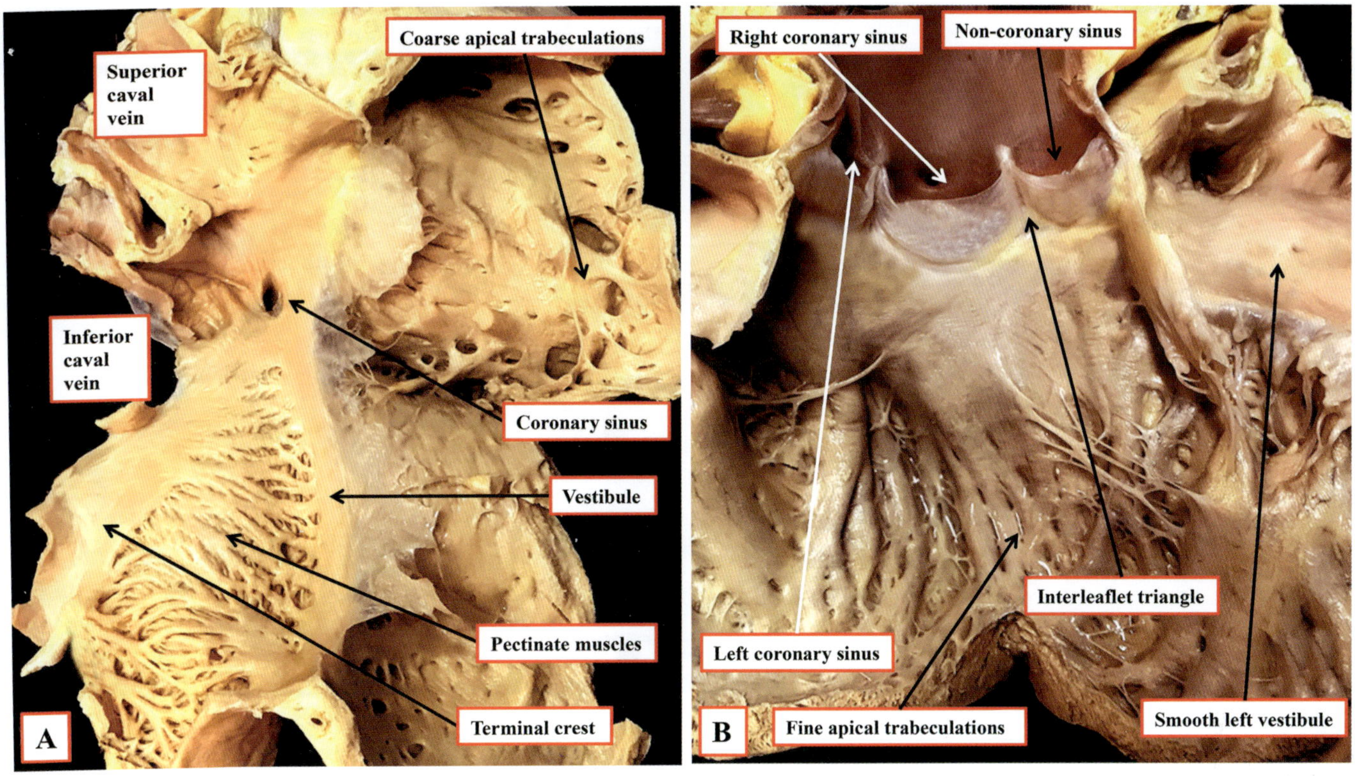

Figure 14.6. The images show the features of the right atrioventricular junction (panel A) and the left atrioventricular and ventriculo-arterial junctions (panel B) of the canine heart. The extent of the pectinate muscles relative to the vestibules of the atrioventricular junctions serves to distinguish between the morphologically right (panel A) and morphologically left (panel B) atrial appendages. The apical trabeculations of the morphologically right ventricle (panel A) are coarser than those of the morphologically left ventricle (panel B). Over and above these features, however, the ventricles can be distinguished because, on the right side, the septal leaflet of the tricuspid valve has direct attachments to the muscular septum, which is additionally trabeculated (panel A). These features are arranged as found in the human heart, with the exception that, in the canine heart, the non-coronary leaflet of the aortic valve is attached directly to the ventricular septum. In consequence, as in the porcine heart (see Figure 14.7), there is no formation of the infero-septal recess as seen in the human heart. In addition, there is no formation of an extensive membranous septum, with the space between the right and non-coronary leaflets filled by the interleaflet triangle.

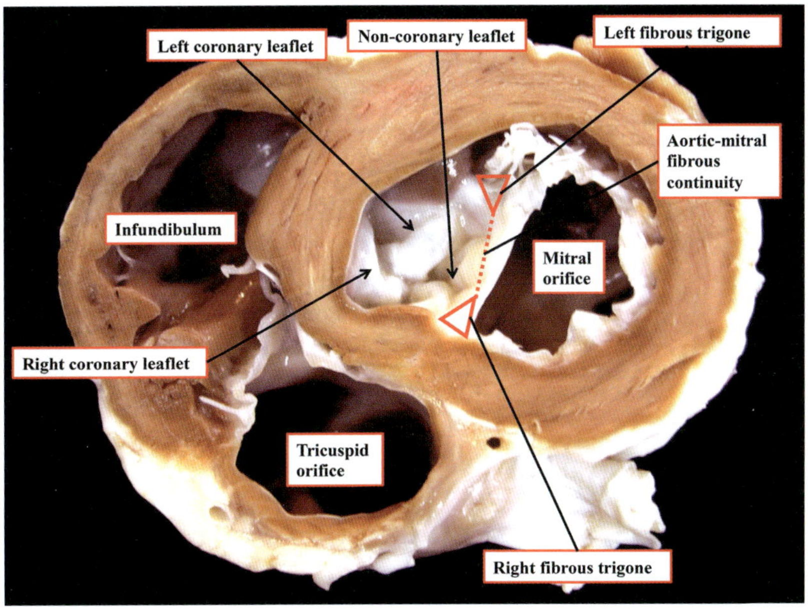

Figure 14.7. The image shows a short axis of the ventricular mass of the porcine heart viewed from the apex looking towards the base. Unlike in the human heart, where an infero-septal recess of the left ventricular outflow tract interposes between the aortic leaflet of the mitral valve and the surface of the ventricular septum, in the porcine heart, and also in the canine heart, the right fibrous trigone is attached directly to the septal surface, along with half of the hinge line of the non-coronary leaflet of the aortic valve. This has significant consequences for the arrangement of the atrioventricular conduction axis in these species.

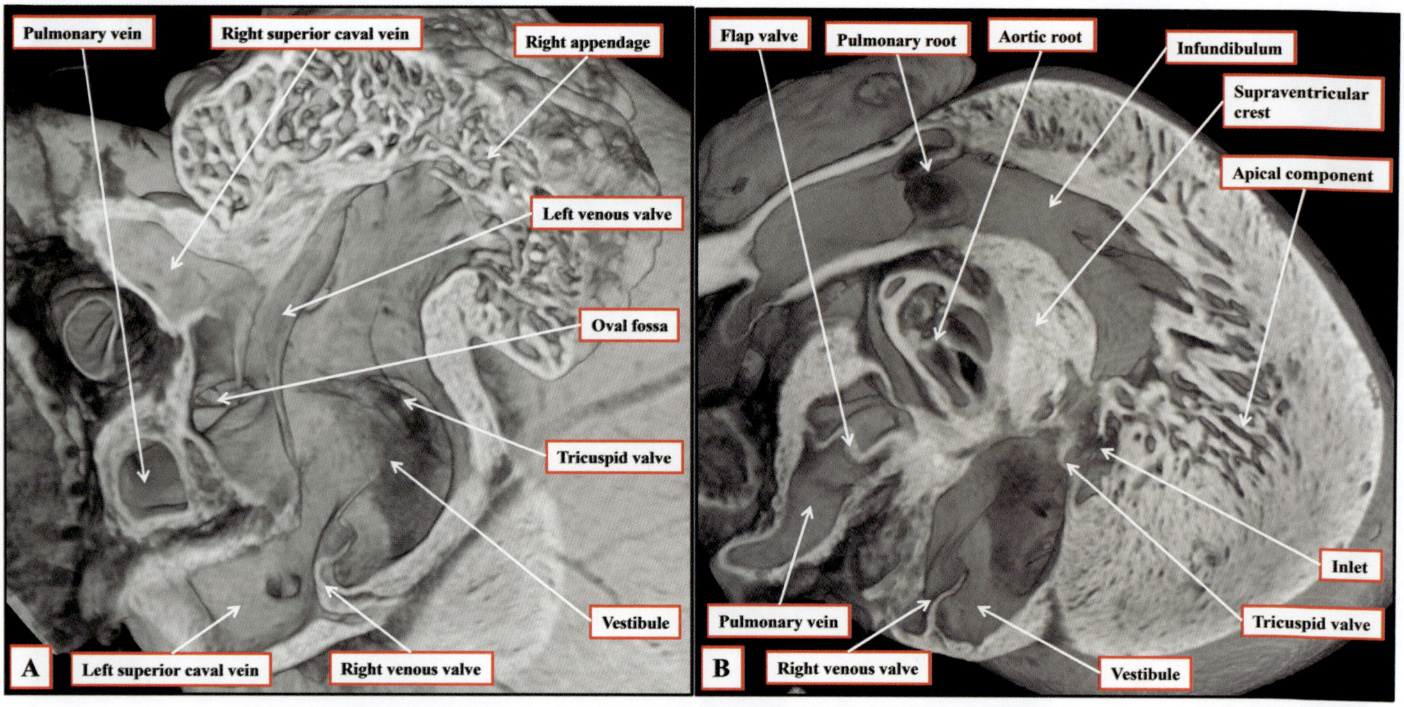

Figure 14.8. The images show the features of the right-sided chambers of the murine heart as revealed by taking sections from datasets prepared using episcopic microscopy. Panel A shows the right superior and left superior caval veins opening to the right atrium, with the left caval vein opening through a relatively enlarged coronary sinus, which is guarded by an extensive right venous valve. The section has cut across the inferior caval vein, which opens directly adjacent to the oval fossa. Note the solitary orifice of the pulmonary veins at their entrance to the left atrium. Panel B shows the typical features of the right ventricle, with its inlet, apical, and outlet components. The outlet component is a free-standing infundibular sleeve.

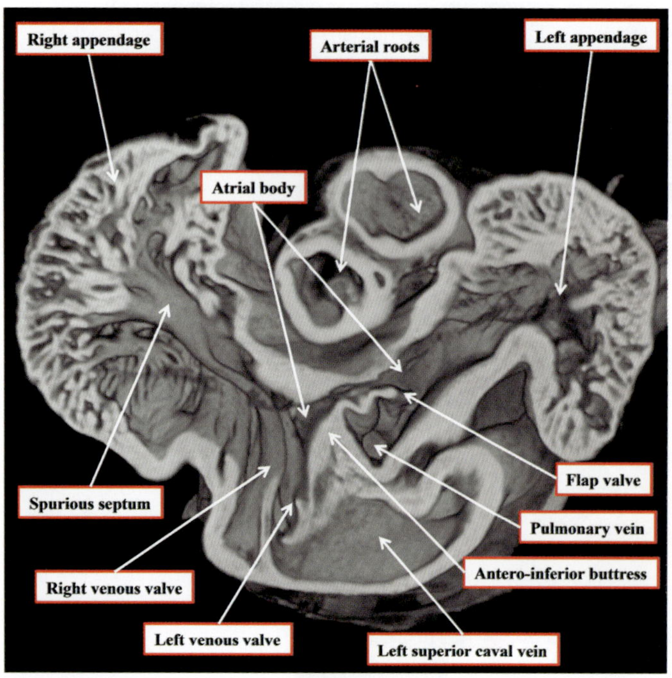

Figure 14.9. The image shows the short axis of the atrial chambers from the same episcopic dataset as shown in Figure 14.8. The right and left appendages can be distinguished on the basis of the extent of the pectinate muscles. Note the retention of both right and left venous valves in the right atrium and the solitary opening of the pulmonary vein in the morphologically left atrium. As in the human heart, each atrium possesses part of the body, along with a venous component, an appendage, and a vestibule. The chambers are separated by the atrial septum.

ventricular septum, sandwiched between the muscular and membranous parts of the septum (Figure 14.12 panel B).[6] The right bundle branch is more extensive in the mouse than the human heart, but the presence of extensive superior septal pathways is very reminiscent of the human arrangement. This is the more important in the murine heart, since there is evidence that the pathways underscore basal-to-apical excitation of the ventricular myocardium, rather than the base-to-apex pattern that is the anticipated sequence.[7–9]

The murine heart then becomes an even better copy of the human heart from the stance of investigating the conduction tissues, since histological sections show the presence of a well-formed retro-aortic node (Figure 14.13), the presence of the node having been confirmed in the mouse by its immunocytochemical identification.[10] Taken together, therefore, the similarities in anatomical and histological make-up between the murine and human hearts provide additional evidence for the continued use of the animal as a test bed for clinical studies.

Although the murine heart, as now shown above, serves as an excellent model for not only the anatomy of the human heart, but also the arrangement of the conduction tissues, the same cannot be said for the other animal species that have previously been used as models. It was the ***rabbit heart***, for example, that was used in the experiments that showed the presence of so-called atrionodal (AN), nodal (N), and nodal-His (NH) cardiomyocytes within the atrioventricular node.[11] In a subsequent correlative study, it proved possible to identify the location of cells with these electrophysiological characteristics.[12] At the time, the multilayered area identified histologically was described as the atrioventricular node. It is now clear that this area, when using the definition proposed by Tawara,[13]

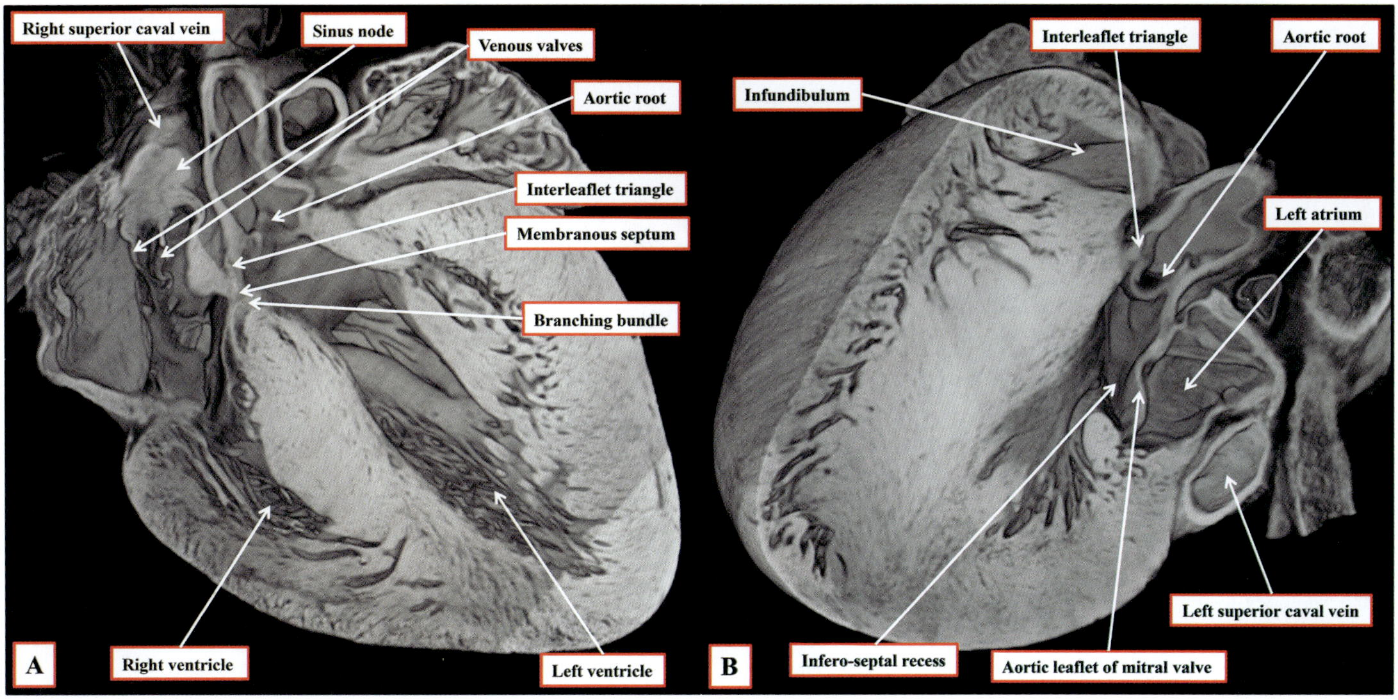

Figure 14.10. The images, again taken from the same episcopic dataset used to prepared Figures 14.8 and 14.9, show the features of the ventricular chambers. Panel A shows a four-chamber section incorporating the aortic root. The apical trabeculations are coarser in the right than the left ventricle, but an additional distinguishing feature is the attachments of the leaflets of the tricuspid valve to the septum. Panel B shows that, as in the human heart, there is an infero-septal recess of the subaortic outflow tract that interposes between the aortic leaflet of the mitral valve and the inferior part of the muscular ventricular septum. Note the persistently patent left superior caval vein in the left atrioventricular groove.

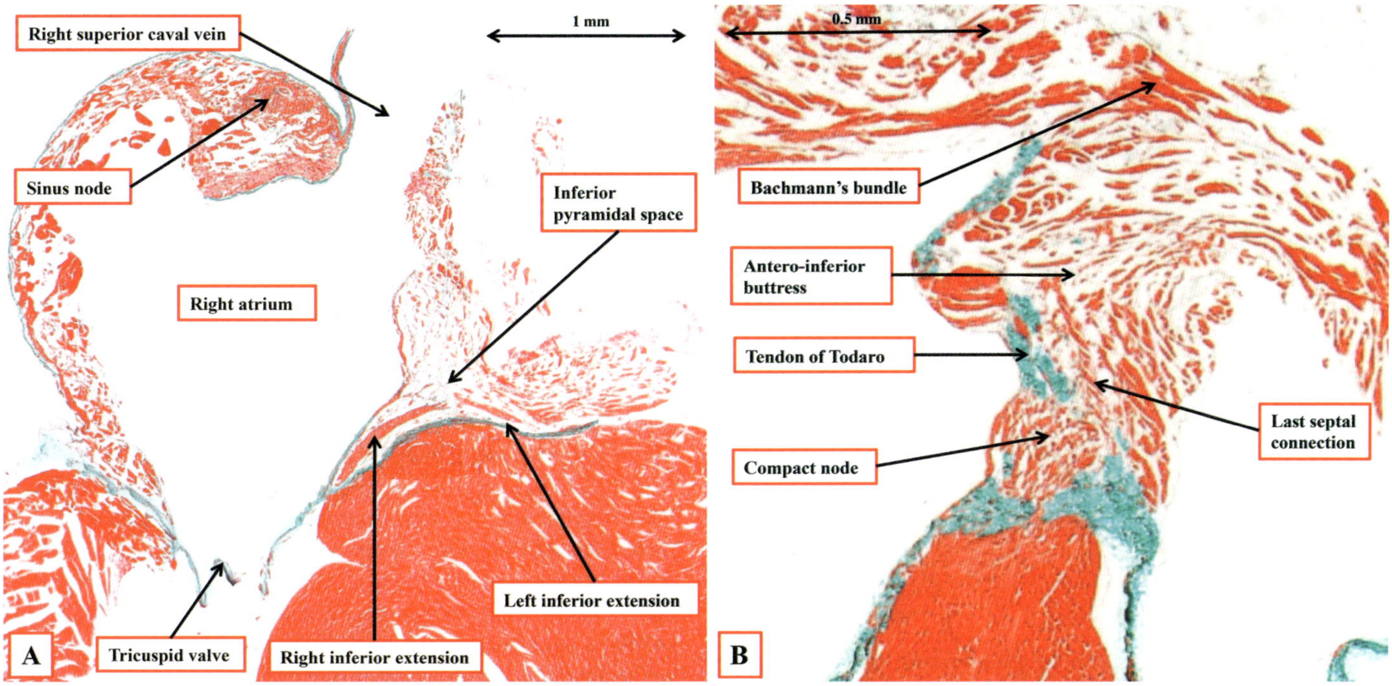

Figure 14.11. The images show serial sections, in four-chamber orientation, from a mouse heart. The sections are stained using the trichrome technique. Panel A shows the location of the sinus node and the inferior extensions of the atrioventricular node in the atrial vestibules. Panel B shows the parallel alignment of the working atrial cardiomyocytes in Bachmann's bundle, along with the last septal input to the atrioventricular node. As in the human heart, the vestibular inputs represent the slow nodal pathway, with the last septal connection providing the fast pathway.

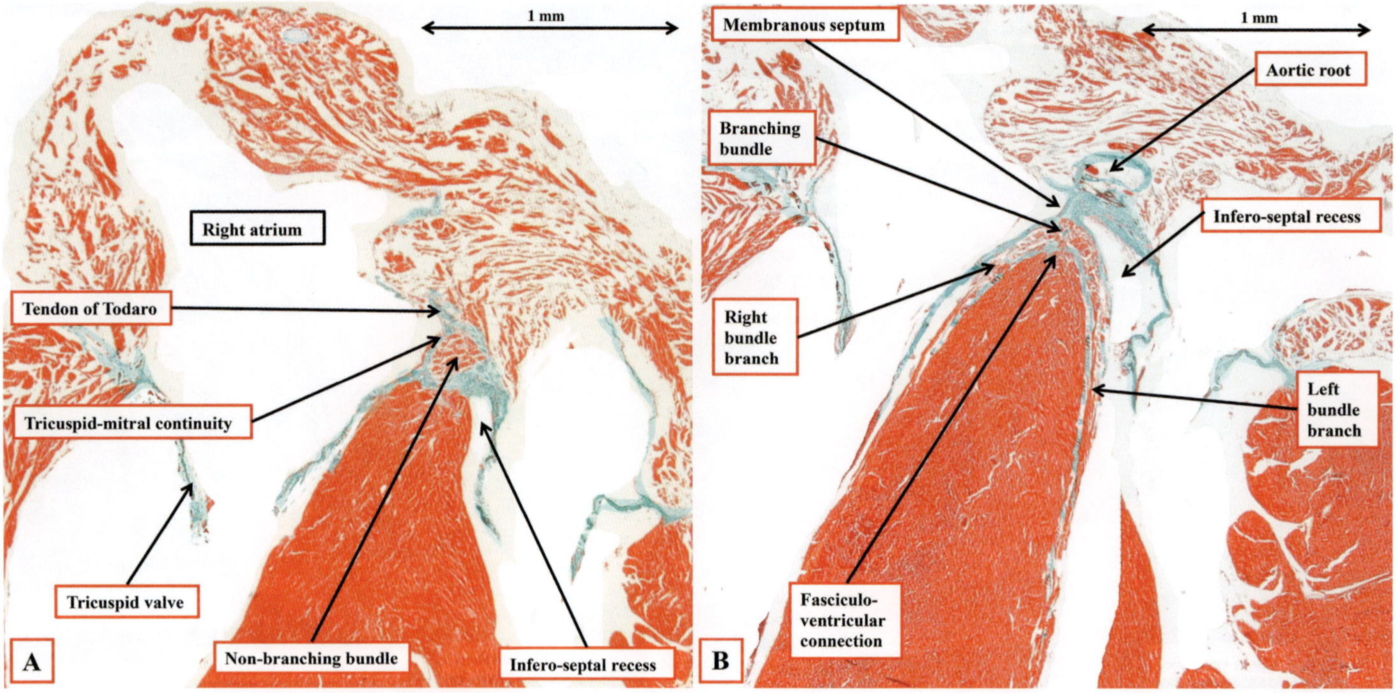

Figure 14.12. The images show further serial sections from the dataset used to illustrate Figure 14.10. The sections continue towards the outlet component of the heart and are again shown in four-chamber orientation. Panel A shows the non-branching atrioventricular bundle, with panel B showing the bundle branching on the crest of the muscular ventricular septum, wedged between the muscular and membranous parts of the septum. Note the extensive fasciculo-ventricular pathway. The right bundle branch is more extensive than in the human heart, but otherwise the arrangement is very similar to the pattern found in man.

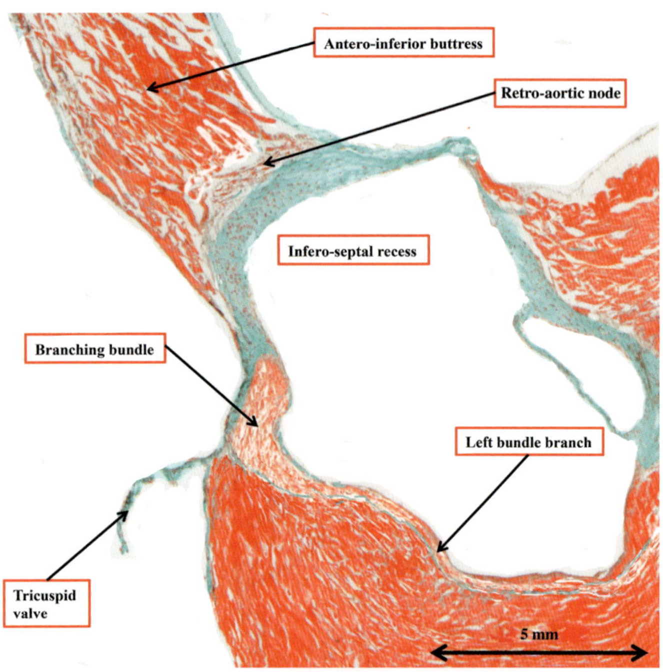

Figure 14.13. The section is from a different dataset from a murine heart, but is again stained using the trichrome technique. It shows the buttress of the atrial septum supported by the area of fibrous continuity between the tricuspid and mitral valves that forms the roof of the infero-septal recess. Note the presence of the retro-aortic node at the base of the buttress. The node is directly related to the non-coronary sinus of the aortic root.

is part of the non-branching atrioventricular bundle (Figure 14.14 panel C). It is questionable, therefore, whether the initial identification of the cell types in the rabbit heart should be used to provide a model for understanding nodal activation in the human heart.

There are then further problems when comparisons are made between the arrangement of the conduction axis in the human heart with either the porcine or canine models. In the ***porcine heart***, for example, the arrangement of the atrioventricular node is comparable with the arrangement found in the mouse and rabbit, with the contributions from the atrial vestibules merging with the inputs from the buttress of the atrial septum to form the compact atrioventricular node (Figure 14.15). The transition to form the non-branching bundle, however, is fundamentally different. This reflects the fact that, as in the ***canine heart*** (Figure 14.6), the aortic root is not wedged between the mitral valvar orifice and the septum, with lack of formation of an infero-septal recess (Figure 14.7).

In the absence of a well-formed membranous septum, the non-branching bundle skirts the aortic root on its right side (Figure 14.16). Since the anatomical arrangement reflects that found in the canine heart, it is no surprise that the arrangement of the conduction axis is directly comparable in the canine and porcine hearts (Figures 14.15, 14.16, 14.17).

The arrangement as found in the canine heart was well shown by Tawara in his initial monograph, with the difference from the human heart obvious from his illustraions.[13] The relationship of the conduction axis relative to the aortic root is then similar in the ox heart to the arrangement seen in the canine and porcine hearts.[14] Unlike all the other non-primate species discussed

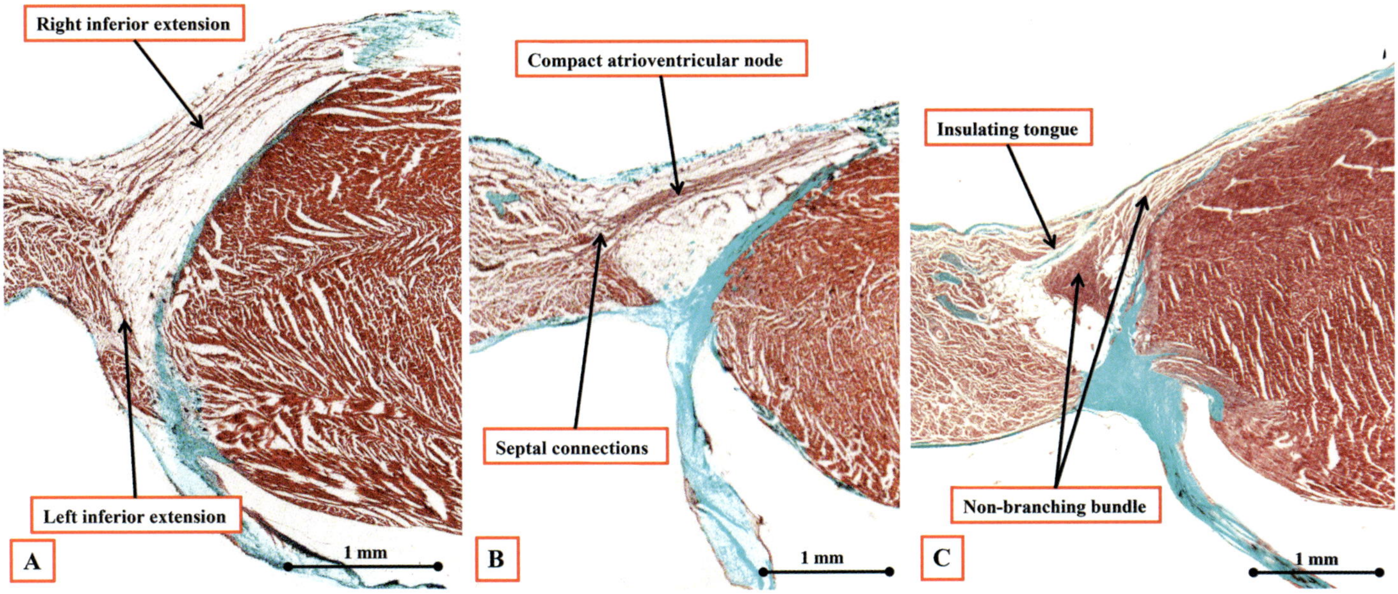

Figure 14.14. The images are serial sections, going from inferior to superior from panels A through C, from a dataset prepared using a rabbit heart. Panels A and B show that, as in the human and murine hearts, the compact node is formed by inputs from the atrial vestibules, along with septal inputs. The multi-layered area, however, in which it is possible to find AN, N, and NH cells, is part of the non-branching bundle, with this part of the axis insulated by a fibrous tongue from the adjacent atrial septal cardiomyocytes.

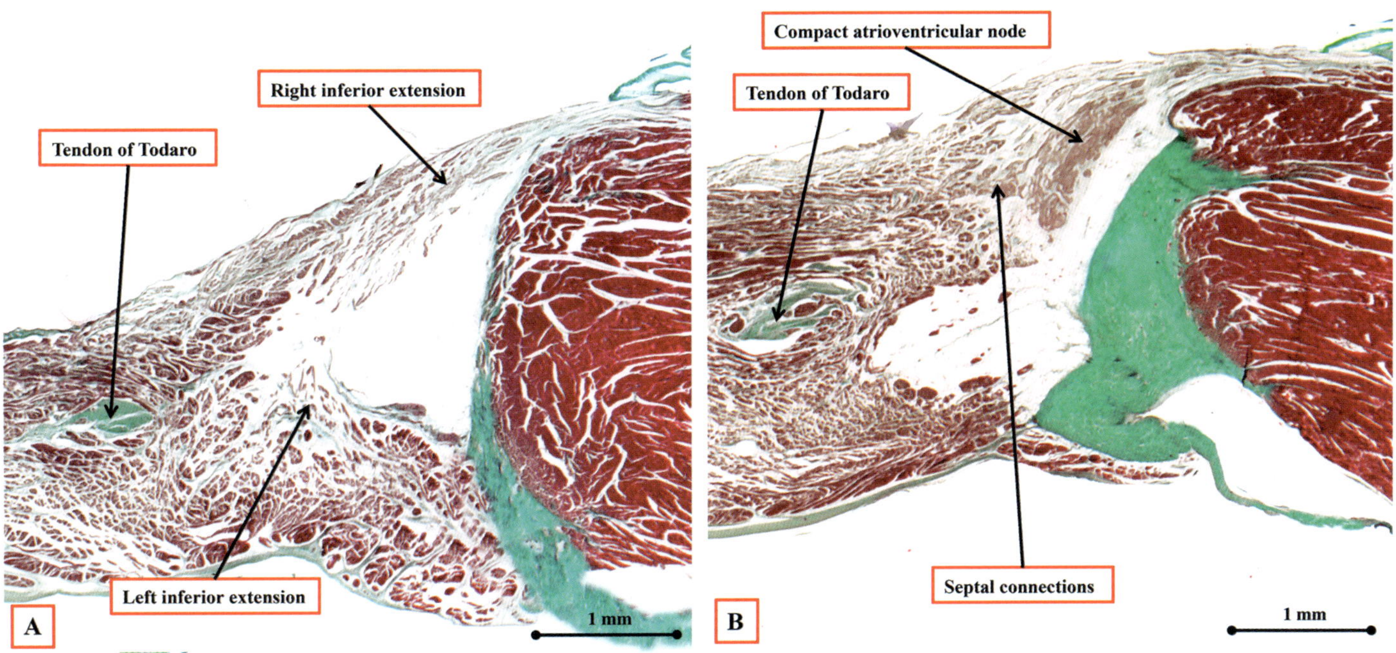

Figure 14.15. The images, shown in comparable orientation for those of the murine heart used to produce Figure 14.13, are taken from a dataset prepared using the porcine heart. As in the human, murine, and rabbit hearts, the vestibular inputs (panel A) join with the contributions from the septum to produce the compact atrioventricular node (panel B).

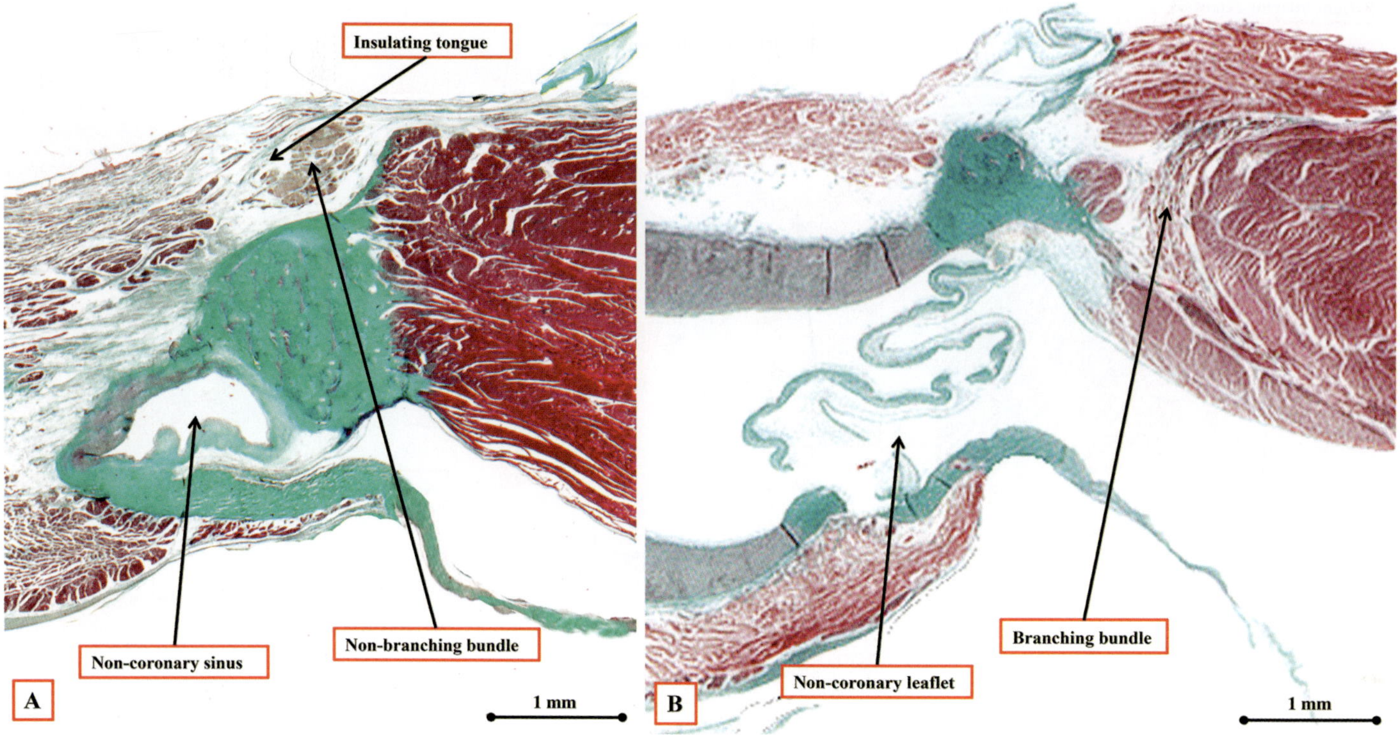

Figure 14.16. The images show further serial sections from the dataset prepared from the porcine heart used to produce Figure 14.15. Although the formation of the atrioventricular node was directly comparable with the arrangements found in man, mouse, and rabbit, the disposition of the ventricular component of the axis is fundamentally different. As shown in panel A, the non-branching bundle skirts on the right side of the aortic root and then branches directly on the crest of the muscular ventricular septum in intramyocardial fashion (panel B).

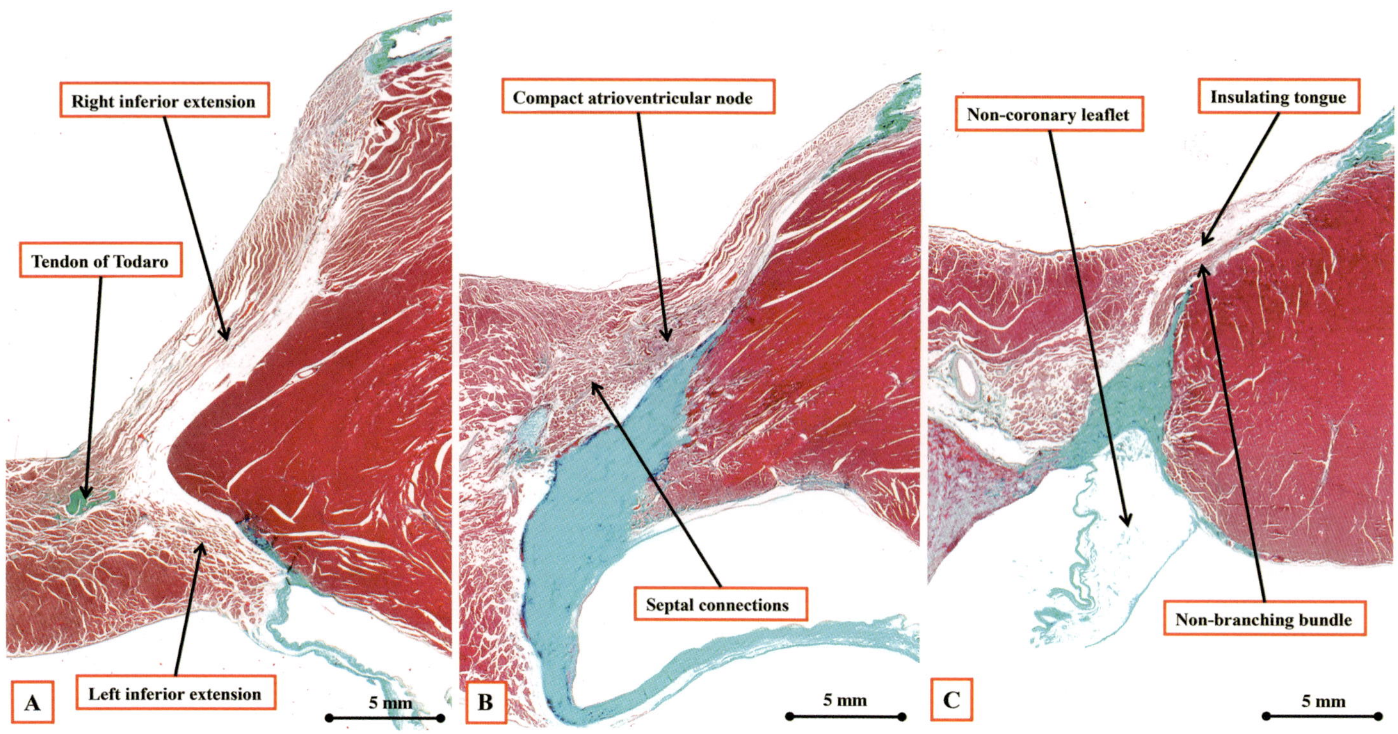

Figure 14.17. The images are taken from a histological dataset prepared using a canine heart, with the sections shown in comparable orientation for those illustrated in Figures 14.14 to 14.16. The canine node is formed in comparable fashion to that seen in all the other species, but as in the porcine heart, because of the absence of an infero-septal recess, the non-branching bundle skirts the aortic root on its right side.

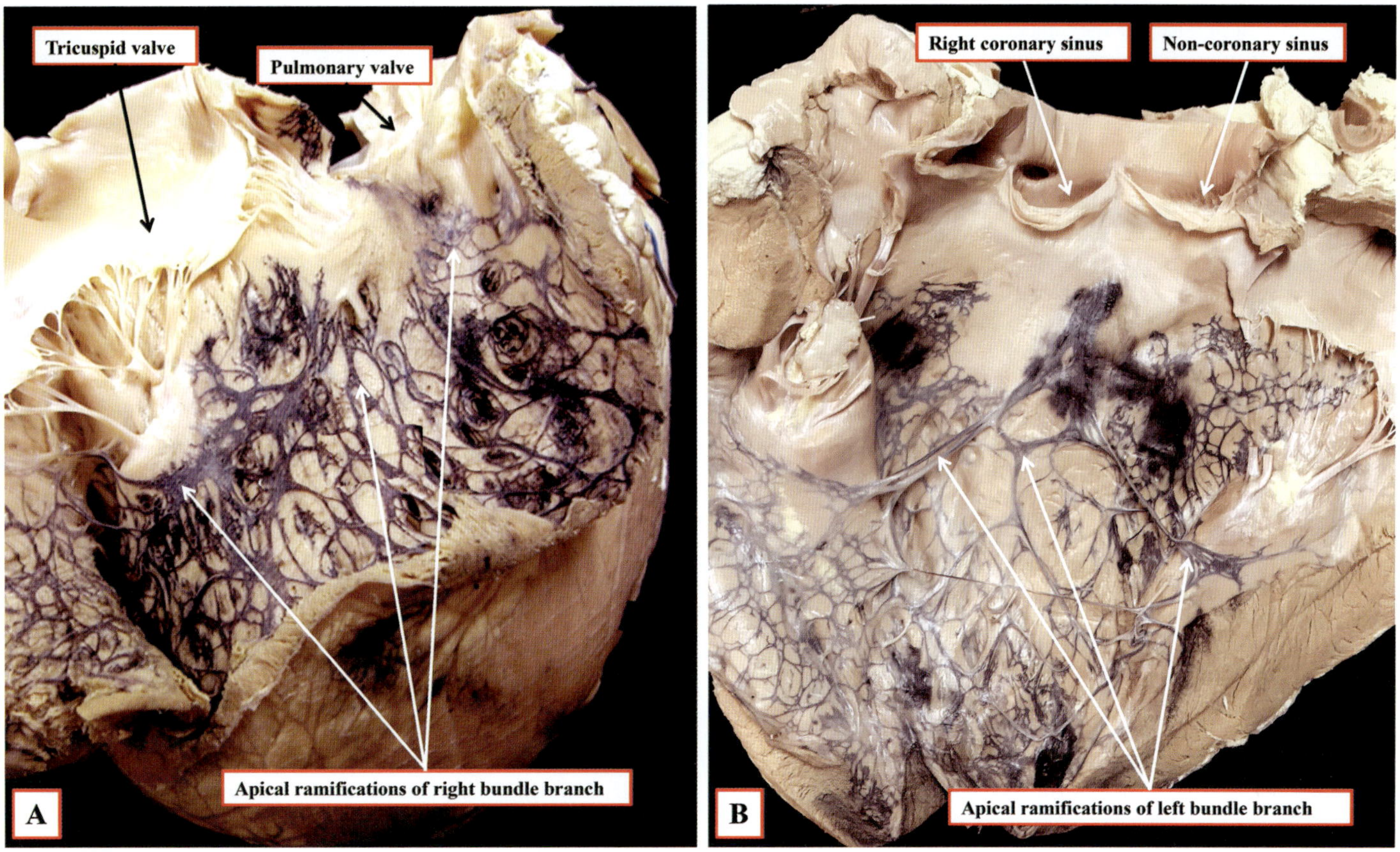

Figure 14.18. The images show the right (panel A) and the left (panel B) ventricles of the bovine heart. The sheaths enclosing the ramifications of the bundle branches have been injected with Indian ink, showing their extent. In each ventricle they form an interconnecting network, with the branches spreading throughout the apical component on the right side and extending into the proximal part of the infundibulum. In the left ventricle, the ramifications extend towards the papillary muscles of the mitral valve, but with an interconnecting septal network.

thus far, however, but similar to the ovine heart, which served to provide the answer to the problems confronted by Tawara,[15] the cardiomyocytes making up the ramifications of the ventricular bundle branches are true "Purkinje cells". This is not the case for the non-ungulate species, where the specialized cardiomyocytes are no larger than the working ventricular cardiomyocytes. An additional feature of the ungulate hearts, however, is the presence of dense sheaths that enclose the ramifications of the bundle branches. The fibrous tissue insulating the bundle branches from the septum in the human heart is far less dense. It is the robust nature of the sheaths as found in the ungulate hearts that makes it possible to demonstrate the extent of the ramification by injecting Indian ink proximally into the sheaths (Figure 14.18). Over and above the differences in anatomy, in order properly to comprehend both normal excitation and arrhythmias it is necessary to take note of ***conduction velocities***. Comparative data between human and animal hearts as derived from published reports are shown in Table 14.1.

In conclusion, there are many similarities in the disposition of the conduction tissues in the various species used for clinical experimentation. But there are also fundamental differences that do not allow projection of data from animal studies to the human heart. The same goes for the arrangement of the aortic root and its relationship to the left ventricle, and the specific interrelationships of the prominent working cardiomyocytes aggregated together within the atrial walls. It behoves those undertaking clinical investigations to be aware of the various similarities and differences.

Table 14.1. Conduction velocities in cardiac tissues (m/sec)

Cardiac tissue	Human	Animal
Atrium	0.53–0.83[16,17]	0.49–0.80[18]
AV nodal area	0.04[17]	0.08–0.16[19,20]
Non-branching bundle	1.3–1.7[21]	1.2–1.3[22]
Bundle branches	2[23]	2.5[24]
Ventricle	0.3–0.4[23]	0.4–0.9[18,24,25]

REFERENCES

1. Crick SJ, Sheppard MN, Ho SY, Gebstein L, Anderson RH. Anatomy of the pig heart: comparisons with normal human cardiac structure. *J Anat*. 1998;**193** (Pt 1):105–119. doi: 10.1046/j.1469-7580.1998.19310105.x
2. Rowlatt U. Comparative anatomy of the heart of mammals. *Zool J Linn Soc*. 1990;**98**:73–110. doi: 10.1111/j.1096-3642.1990.tb01220.x
3. Macias Y, de Almeida MC, Tretter JT, Anderson RH, Spicer DE, Mohun TJ, Sanchez-Quintana D, Farre J, Back Sternick

E. Miniseries 1—Part II: The comparative anatomy of the atrioventricular conduction axis. *Europace*. 2022;**24**:443–454. doi: 10.1093/europace/euab291

4. de Almeida MC, Macias Y, Tretter JT, Sanchez-Quintana D, Cabrera JA, Spicer DE, Anderson RH. Similarities and differences in the arrangement of the atrioventricular conduction axis in the canine compared to the human heart. *Heart Rhythm*. 2021;**18**:1990–1998. doi: 10.1016/j.hrthm.2021.07.065
5. Wessels A, Sedmera D. Developmental anatomy of the heart: a tale of mice and man. *Physiol Genomics*. 2003;**15**:165–176. doi: 10.1152/physiolgenomics.00033.2003
6. Sanchez-Quintana D, Macias Y, Nevado-Medina J, Spicer DE, Anderson RH. The atrioventricular conduction axis in man and mouse. *J Cardiovasc Dev Dis*. 2024;**11**:340. doi: 10.3390/jcdd11110340
7. van Rijen HV, van Veen TA, van Kempen MJ, Wilms-Schopman FJ, Potse M, Krueger O, Willecke K, Opthof T, Jongsma HJ, de Bakker JM. Impaired conduction in the bundle branches of mouse hearts lacking the gap junction protein connexin 40. *Circulation*. 2001;**103**:1591–1598. doi: 10.1161/01.cir.103.11.1591
8. van Veen TA, Hubens LE, de Bakker JM, van Rijen HV. Differences in the pattern of ventricular activation in small rodents determined by morphological organization of the cardiac ventricular conduction system. *Chin J Physiol*. 2010;**53**:52–61. doi: 10.4077/cjp.2010.amk015
9. van Veen TA, van Rijen HV, van Kempen MJ, Miquerol L, Opthof T, Gros D, Vos MA, Jongsma HJ, de Bakker JM. Discontinuous conduction in mouse bundle branches is caused by bundle-branch architecture. *Circulation*. 2005;**112**:2235–2244. doi: 10.1161/CIRCULATIONAHA.105.547893
10. Yanni J, Boyett MR, Anderson RH, Dobrzynski H. The extent of the specialized atrioventricular ring tissues. *Heart Rhythm*. 2009;**6**:672–680. doi: 10.1016/j.hrthm.2009.01.021
11. de Carvalho A, de Almeida D. Spread of activity through the atrioventricular node. *Circ Res*. 1960;**8**:801–809. doi: 10.1161/01.res.8.4.801
12. Anderson RH, Janse MJ, van Capelle FJ, Billette J, Becker AE, Durrer D. A combined morphological and electrophysiological study of the atrioventricular node of the rabbit heart. *Circ Res*. 1974;**35**:909–922. doi: 10.1161/01.res.35.6.909
13. Tawara S. *The Conduction System of the Mammalian Heart. An Anatomico-Histological Study of the Atrioventricular Bundle and the Purkinje Fibers*. London: Imperial College Press; 2000.
14. De Almeida MC, Sanchez-Quintana D, Davis N, Charles FR, Chikweto A, Sylvester W, Loukas M, Anderson RH. The ox atrioventricular conduction axis compared to human in relation to the original investigation of Sunao Tawara. *Clin Anat*. 2020;**33**:383–393. doi: 10.1002/ca.23524
15. De Almeida MC, Sanchez-Quintana D, Anderson RH. Sunao Tawara: further musings on his tribulations in providing the basis for the modern-day understanding of cardiac electrophysiology. *Anat Sci Int*. 2020;**95**:381–386. doi: 10.1007/s12565-020-00530-6
16. Zheng Y, Xia Y, Carlson J, Kongstad O, Yuan S. Atrial average conduction velocity in patients with and without paroxysmal atrial fibrillation. *Clin Physiol Funct Imaging*. 2017;**37**:596–601. doi: 10.1111/cpf.12342
17. Greener ID, Monfredi O, Inada S, Chandler NJ, Tellez JO, Atkinson A, Taube MA, Billeter R, Anderson RH, Efimov IR, et al. Molecular architecture of the human specialised atrioventricular conduction axis. *J Mol Cell Cardiol*. 2011;**50**:642–651. doi: 10.1016/j.yjmcc.2010.12.017
18. de Groot JR, Veenstra T, Verkerk AO, Wilders R, Smits JP, Wilms-Schopman FJ, Wiegerinck RF, Bourier J, Belterman CN, Coronel R, et al. Conduction slowing by the gap junctional uncoupler carbenoxolone. *Cardiovasc Res*. 2003;**60**:288–297. doi: 10.1016/j.cardiores.2003.07.004
19. Choi BR, Salama G. Optical mapping of atrioventricular node reveals a conduction barrier between atrial and nodal cells. *Am J Physiol*. 1998;**274**:H829–H845. doi: 10.1152/ajpheart.1998.274.3.H829
20. Efimov IR, Nikolski VP, Rothenberg F, Greener ID, Li J, Dobrzynski H, Boyett M. Structure–function relationship in the AV junction. *Anat Rec A Discov Mol Cell Evol Biol*. 2004;**280**:952–965. doi: 10.1002/ar.a.20108
21. Kupersmith J, Krongrad E, Waldo AL. Conduction intervals and conduction velocity in the human cardiac conduction system. Studies during open-heart surgery. *Circulation*. 1973;**47**:776–785. doi: 10.1161/01.cir.47.4.776
22. Alanis J, Lopez E, Pulido J. The H potential and the conduction velocity of the bundle of His. *J Physiol*. 1959;**147**:315–324. doi: 10.1113/jphysiol.1959.sp006245
23. Durrer D, van Dam RT, Freud GE, Janse MJ, Meijler FL, Arzbaecher RC. Total excitation of the isolated human heart. *Circulation*. 1970;**41**:899–912. doi: 10.1161/01.cir.41.6.899
24. Draper MH, Mya-Tu M. A comparison of the conduction velocity in cardiac tissues of various mammals. *Q J Exp Physiol Cogn Med Sci*. 1959;**44**:91–109. doi: 10.1113/expphysiol.1959.sp001379
25. Sano T, Takayama N, Shimamoto T. Directional difference of conduction velocity in the cardiac ventricular syncytium studied by microelectrodes. *Circ Res*. 1959;**7**:262–267. doi: 10.1161/01.res.7.2.262

Index

For the benefit of digital users, indexed terms that span two pages (e.g., 52–53) may, on occasion, appear on only one of those pages.